Dermatology and Diabetes

Emilia Noemí Cohen Sabban
Félix Miguel Puchulu • Kenneth Cusi
Editors

Dermatology and Diabetes

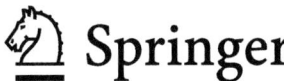 Springer

Editors
Emilia Noemí Cohen Sabban
Dermatology Department
Instituto de Investigaciones Médicas
A. Lanari, University of Buenos Aires (UBA)
Buenos Aires, Argentina

Félix Miguel Puchulu
Division of Diabetology
Department of Medicine
University of Buenos Aires
Buenos Aires, Argentina

Kenneth Cusi
Division of Endocrinology, Diabetes
and Metabolism
The University of Florida
Gainesville
Florida
USA

ISBN 978-3-030-10207-4   ISBN 978-3-319-72475-1   (eBook)
https://doi.org/10.1007/978-3-319-72475-1

Printed on acid-free paper

This Springer imprint is published by Springer Nature
The registered company is Springer International Publishing AG
The registered company address is: Gewerbestrasse 11, 6330 Cham, Switzerland

Preface

When we thought about this book on diabetes, our desire was to achieve something that would help the reader understand the disease from a wider point of view. Hence, this work, contributed by dermatologists and specialists in diabetes, not only reviews the dermatological manifestations of diabetes mellitus but also includes contributions from diabetologists, since we consider the disease in all its aspects in patients with diabetes. Thus, we approach the same issues from the perspective of both specialties, in the same way we face the daily task of taking care of our patients in a multidisciplinary team.

The book comprises a broad spectrum of skin conditions related to diabetes, its comorbidities, its most common complications—vasculopathy and neuropathy—as well as basic and necessary concepts regarding the epidemiology, classification, diagnosis, and treatment of the disease.

We hope that the effort invested in this work will be of great help to all those who, in one way or another, feel responsible for improving the quality of life of these patients.

Buenos Aires, Argentina   Emilia Noemí Cohen Sabban
Buenos Aires, Argentina   Félix M. Puchulu
Gainesville, FL, USA   Kenneth Cusi

Contents

Epidemiology of Diabetes

Mariano Javier Taverna

Introduction

Diabetes mellitus is a chronic, metabolic disease defined by increased concentrations of blood glucose which leads, over time, to progressive damage in most tissues and organs including heart, blood vessels, eyes, kidneys, skin, and nerves. The most common is type 2 diabetes, commonly in adults, which occurs as result of the combination of insulin resistance with pancreatic beta cell insufficiency, with 50% of patients requiring insulin treatment within 10 years [1]. Type 1 diabetes, more frequent in children and adolescents, is a chronic autoimmune disease in which autoreactive T lymphocytes and inflammation cause severe loss of beta cells [2]. The incidence of diabetes exhibits an alarming pandemic scenario, in large part due to the global obesity epidemic [3]. Diabetes causes premature death, severe disability and great economic burden. Therefore, there is a globally agreed target to stop the growing incidence of diabetes and obesity by 2025 [4].

Global Burden

The number of adults living with diabetes has approximately quadrupled since 1980 (108 millions) to 2014 (422 millions). The age-standardized prevalence of diabetes has nearly doubled since 1980, increasing from 4.7 to 8.5% in the adult population (Table 1.1) [3]. This is consequent to a rise in associated risk factors such as

M.J. Taverna, M.D., Ph.D.
Division of Diabetology, Clinical Hospital of the University of Buenos Aires, Buenos Aires, Argentina

National Research Council of Argentina (CONICET), Institute of Cardiological Investigations "Prof. Dr. Alberto C. Taquini" (ININCA), Buenos Aires, Argentina

School of Medicine, University of Salvador (USAL), Buenos Aires, Argentina
e-mail: taverna1@yahoo.fr

© Springer International Publishing AG 2018
E.N. Cohen Sabban et al. (eds.), *Dermatology and Diabetes*,
https://doi.org/10.1007/978-3-319-72475-1_1

Table 1.1 Global estimates of people with diabetes (adults 18+ years) in 1980 and 2014

World Health Organization region	Prevalence (%)		Number (millions)	
	1980	2014	1980	2014
African region	3.1	7.1	4	25
Region of the Americas	5	8.3	18	62
Eastern Mediterranean region	5.9	13.7	6	43
European region	5.3	7.3	33	64
Western Pacific region	4.4	8.4	29	131
South-East Asia region	4.1	8.6	17	96
Total	4.7	8.5	108	422

sedentary lifestyle, greater longevity, poor eating habits (high in salt, low in fiber, and rich in saturated fats and sugar) and, especially, overweight/obesity. Indeed, the obesity pandemic explains a large part of the global epidemic of diabetes (especially type 2 diabetes) [1, 3]. In 2014, global estimates showed that more than one in three adults aged over 18 years were overweight (body mass index, BMI 25–29.9 kg/m^2), and 10% were obese (BMI $\geq$30.0 kg/m^2). Both overweight and obesity were higher in women than men, lowest in the WHO South-East Asian region, and highest in the WHO region of the Americas. Moreover, the prevalence of overweight/obesity rises with country income level [3]. Physical inactivity is more common in women (27%) than men (20%) across all country income groups from all WHO regions, and is more common among adolescents (78% of boys, and 84% of girls), especially from high-income countries [5].

In the last decade, diabetes prevalence, in a pandemic scenario, has increased less faster in high-income nations than in low- and middle-income countries, including Africa and Asia, where most diabetic patients will probably be found by 2030. This rising incidence of diabetes in developing countries accompanies the trend of unhealthy lifestyle changes (low physical activity and Western pattern eating habits) and urbanization [3, 6]. The WHO Eastern Mediterranean region has showed the highest increases in diabetes prevalence, and nowadays exhibits the highest prevalence (13.7%) [3]. Of note, the risk of type 2 diabetes is strongly associated with lower socio-economic status [7].

Diabetes generated approximately 1.5 million deaths in 2012. In addition, suboptimal high blood glucose caused 2.2 million deaths, by increasing the risks of heart disease and other associated conditions such as kidney failure, stroke and tuberculosis. Forty-three percent of these 3.7 million deaths arise before the age of 70 years. The percentage of deaths secondary to hyperglycemia or diabetes that appear prior to age 70 is greater in low- and middle-income countries than in high-income countries. In 2012, diabetes was the eighth leading cause of death among both sexes and the fifth leading cause of death in women in 2012 [8].

Importantly, separate global estimates of diabetes prevalence for type 1 and type 2 do not exist. Approximately, 85% of people with diabetes, mostly adults and elderly people, are affected by type 2 diabetes. Unfortunately, in last decade, there is also a rising incidence of type 2 in children [9], especially in children of ethnic minority and from lower income families. Type 2 diabetes is frequently undiagnosed; therefore there are almost no data about its true incidence. Recently, it was reported that between 24 and 62% of diabetic patients from seven countries were undiagnosed and untreated [10]. A high proportion of undiagnosed diabetes can be found even among individuals from high-income countries [11]. Even though the prevalence of type 2 is frequently highest in wealthy subjects, this trend is changing in some middle-income countries. In addition, in high-income populations, type 2 diabetes is highest among individuals who are poor [12].

Type 1 diabetes occurs especially in children and adolescents [2, 3]. Most evidence about the incidence of type 1 diabetes has been obtained from population-based registries of new cases worldwide, such as the WHO DIAMOND project [13]. These registries reported large differences in the incidence of type 1 diabetes, ranging from under 0.5 to over 60 cases annually per 100,000 children (under 15 years). According to the WHO DIAMOND project, Scandinavia, Sardinia and Kuwait exhibit the highest incidence for type 1 diabetes, while is much less common in Asia and Latin American [13]. The worldwide epidemiology of type 1 diabetes shows a pandemic scenario with an annual increase of ~3%, especially in children from high income countries [14, 15].

Diabetic Complications

Chronic hyperglycemia, if not well controlled, may cause kidney failure, nerve damage, blindness, lower limb amputation, heart disease, stroke and several other long-term consequences that seriously affect the quality of life and induce premature death. There are no global estimates of diabetic complications. Where data are available—mostly from high-income countries—incidence and prevalence of chronic complications vary largely between countries [16–18].

End-Stage Renal Disease

Epidemiological data from 54 countries show that approximately 80% of cases of end-stage renal disease (ESRD) are secondary to diabetes and/or high blood pressure [7]. The percentage of ESRD due to diabetes alone ranges from 12 to 55%, and is ≤10 times higher in diabetic patients than non-diabetic individuals, especially in type 1 diabetes, elderly people, longer duration of diabetes, high blood pressure, obesity and low-income populations [19].

Loss of Vision

According to the WHO, prevalence of any retinopathy in persons with diabetes is 35% while vision-threatening retinopathy (proliferative retinopathy) is 7% [20, 21]. The proportion of diabetic retinopathy is higher among individuals with type 1 diabetes, longer duration of diabetes, high blood pressure, Caucasian populations, and among low-income populations [20, 21].

Lower Extremity Amputations

Diabetes strongly increases the risk of lower extremity non-traumatic amputation because of severe infected foot ulcers [18]. Amputation in diabetic patients is 10–20 times higher than in non-diabetic individuals. Its incidence ranges from 1.5 to 3.5 amputations per 1000 diabetic patients [18]. Amputation is higher in peripheral arterial occlusive disease, sensorimotor diabetic polyneuropathy, previous ulceration, elderly people, late complications of type 2 diabetes, male gender, long diabetes duration, and low-income populations [22].

Cardiovascular Events

Cardiovascular disease (CVD) is the leading cause of death in diabetes. Adults with diabetes (especially type 2 diabetes) have approximately three times higher incidence of cardiovascular events (myocardial infarction, stroke or CVD mortality) than non-diabetic adults [23]. The risk of cardiovascular disease rises continuously with increasing fasting plasma glucose concentrations [24, 25]. Two-thirds of deaths in diabetic patients are due to cardiovascular disease: 40% are from coronary artery disease, 15% from other types of heart disease, especially congestive heart failure, and ~10% from stroke [26]. Of note, a better management of diabetes and associated CVD risk factors has lead to a large reduction in thee incidence of cardiovascular events over the past 20 years, in particular in Scandinavia, United Kingdom and USA, in both type 1 and type 2 diabetes, albeit less reduction in non-diabetic people [27].

Economic Impact

Diabetes causes a great economic burden on the health care system that can be measured through direct medical costs, indirect costs associated with productivity loss, early mortality and the negative effect of diabetes on country's gross domestic product (GDP).

Direct medical costs secondary to diabetes include expenditures for preventing and especially treating diabetes and its complications, in particular outpatient and emergency care, inpatient hospital care, medications and medical supplies (self-monitoring consumables, injection devices etc.). Recently, it has been reported that the direct annual cost of diabetes to the world is more than US$ 827 billion [28, 29]. Moreover, total global health-care spending on diabetes more than tripled over the period 2003–2013 because of pandemic diabetes, according to the International Diabetes Federation [30].

It was reported that losses in GDP worldwide from 2011 to 2030, including both the indirect and direct costs of diabetes, will total US$ 1.7 trillion, including US$ 800 billion for low- and middle-income countries and US$ 900 billion for high-income populations [31].

Conclusions

Diabetes is a prominent cause of early death and disability. Chronic complications secondary to diabetes and associated CVD risk factors include, among others, heart disease, stroke, kidney failure, blindness, lower limb amputation, and nerve damage. In 2012, diabetes and associated conditions caused 3.7 million deaths. In 2014, 422 million people had diabetes (~85% type 2 diabetes), with a global prevalence of 8.5%. The global obesity epidemic explains, in large part, the current pandemic scenario of diabetes (especially type 2 diabetes). The growing epidemic of diabetes is higher in low- and middle-income countries than in developed populations.

Finally, diabetes is one of four priority noncommunicable diseases (NCDs) proposed by world leaders according to the 2011 Political Declaration on the Prevention and Control of NCDs. This declaration highlights that diabetes and its complications can be reduced and/or prevented with an appropriate strategy that include evidence-based, cost-effective, and population-level interventions [4].

References

1. Kahn SE, Cooper ME, Del Prato S. Pathophysiology and treatment of type 2 diabetes: perspectives on the past, present, and future. Lancet. 2014;383(9922):1068–83.
2. Pugliese A. Advances in the etiology and mechanisms of type 1 diabetes. Discov Med. 2014;18(98):141–50.
3. World Health Organization. Global report on diabetes, Geneva. 2016. Accessed 28 Aug 2017.
4. United Nations. Resolution 66/2. Political declaration of the high-level meeting of the general assembly on the prevention and control of noncommunicable diseases. In: Sixty-sixth session of the United Nations General Assembly. New York: United Nations; 2011.
5. World Health Organization. Global status report on noncommunicable diseases 2015. Geneva: World Health Organization; 2015.
6. Wild S, Roglic G, Green A, Sicree R, King H. Global prevalence of diabetes. Estimates for year 2000 and projections for 2030. Diabetes Care. 2004;27(5):1047–53.
7. Addo J, Agyemang C, de-Graft Aikins A, Beune E, Schulze MB, et al. Association between socioeconomic position and the prevalence of type 2 diabetes in Ghanaians in different geographic locations: the RODAM study. J Epidemiol Community Health. 2017;71(7):633–9.
8. WHO mortality database [online database]. Geneva: World Health Organization. http://apps.who.int/healthinfo/statistics/mortality/causeofdeath_query/. Accessed 28 Aug 2017.
9. Pulgaron ER, Delamater AM. Obesity and type 2 diabetes in children: epidemiology and treatment. Curr Diab Rep. 2014;14(8):508.
10. Gakidou E, Mallinger L, Abbott-Klafter J, Guerrero R, Villalpando S, et al. Management of diabetes and associated cardiovascular risk factors in seven countries: a comparison of data from national health examination surveys. Bull World Health Organ. 2011;89(3):172–83.
11. Beagley J, Guariguata L, Weil C, Motala AA. Global estimates of undiagnosed diabetes in adults. Diabetes Res Clin Pract. 2013;103(2):150–60.
12. World Health Organization. Diabetes: equity and social determinants. In: Blas E, Kuru A, editors. Equity, social determinants and public health programmes. Geneva: World Health Organization; 2010.
13. DIAMOND Project Group. Incidence and trends of childhood type 1 diabetes worldwide 1990-1999. Diabet Med. 2006;23(8):857–66.
14. Dabelea D. The accelerating epidemic of childhood diabetes. Lancet. 2009;373(9680):1990–2000.

15. Bendas A, Rothe U, Kiess W, Kapellen TM, Stange T, et al. Trends in incidence rates during 1999-2008 and prevalence in 2008 of childhood type 1 diabetes mellitus in Germany. Model-based national estimates. PLoS One. 2015;10(7):e0132716.
16. Gupta R, Misra A. Epidemiology of microvascular complications of diabetes in South Asians and comparison with other ethnicities. J Diabetes. 2016;8(4):470–82.
17. United States Renal Data System. International Comparisons. In United States Renal Data System. 2014 USRDS annual data report: epidemiology of kidney disease in the United States. Bethesda, MD: National Institutes of Health, National Institute of Diabetes and Digestive and Kidney Diseases; 2014. p. 188–210.
18. Moxey PW, Gogalniceanu P, Hinchliffe RJ, Loftus IM, Jones KJ, et al. Lower extremity amputations: a review of global variability in incidence. Diabet Med. 2011;28(10):1144–53.
19. Thomas MC, Cooper ME, Zimmet P. Changing epidemiology of type 2 diabetes mellitus and associated chronic kidney disease. Nat Rev Nephrol. 2016;12(2):73–81.
20. Ting DS, Cheung GC, Wong TY. Diabetic retinopathy: global prevalence, major risk factors, screening practices and public health challenges: a review. Clin Exp Ophthalmol. 2016;44(4):260–77.
21. Yau JW, Rogers SL, Kawasaki R, Lamoureux EL, Kowalski JW, et al. Global prevalence and major risk factors of diabetic retinopathy. Diabetes Care. 2012;35(3):556–64.
22. Volmer-Thole M, Lobmann R. Neuropthy and diabetic foot syndrome. Int J Mol Sci. 2016;17(6):E917.
23. Sarwar N, Gao P, Seshasai SR, Gobin R, Kaptoge S, Di Angelantonio E. Diabetes mellitus, fasting blood glucose concentration, and risk of vascular disease: a collaborative meta-analysis of 102 prospective studies. Lancet. 2010;375(9733):2215–22.
24. Danaei G, Lawes CM, Vander HS, Murray CJ, Ezzati M. Global and regional mortality from ischaemic heart disease and stroke attributable to higher-than-optimum blood glucose concentration: comparative risk assessment. Lancet. 2006;368(9548):1651–9.
25. Singh GM, Danaei G, Farzadfar F, Stevens GA, Woodward M, et al. The age-specific quantitative effects of metabolic risk factors on cardiovascular diseases and diabetes: a pooled analysis. PLoS One. 2013;8(7):e65174.
26. Low Wang CC, Hess CN, Hiatt WR, Goldfine AB. Atherosclerotic cardiovascular disease and heart failure in type 2 diabetes. Mechanisms, management, and clinical considerations. Circulation. 2016;133(24):2459–502.
27. Barengo NC, Katoh S, Moltchanov V, Tajima N, Tuomilehto J. The diabetes-cardiovascular risk paradox: results from a Finnish population-based prospective study. Eur Heart J. 2008;29(15):1889–95.
28. Seuring T, Archangelidi O, Suhrcke M. The economic costs of type 2 diabetes: a global systematic review. PharmacoEconomics. 2015;33(8):811–31.
29. NCD Risk Factor Collaboration (NCD-RisC). Worldwide trends in diabetes since 1980: a pooled analysis of 751 population-based studies with 4.4 million participants. Lancet. 2016;387(10027):1513–30.
30. International Diabetes Federation. IDF diabetes atlas. 6th ed. Brussels: International Diabetes Federation; 2013.
31. Bloom DE, Cafiero ET, Jané-Llopis E, Abrahams-Gessel S, Bloom LR, et al. The global economic burden of noncommunicable diseases (working paper series). Geneva: Harvard School of Public Health and World Economic Forum; 2011.

Definition, Diagnosis and Classification of Diabetes Mellitus

2

Félix Miguel Puchulu

Introduction

Diabetes Mellitus (DM) is a syndrome characterized by hyperglycemia and impaired metabolism of carbohydrates, proteins and fats, due to an absolute or relative deficiency of the secretion and/or insulin action.

Its prevalence is 7–10% approximately, of which 90% corresponds to type 2 diabetes and the rest is distributed among the different types of diabetes.

Diagnosis of DM

DM is defined by blood glucose levels. Patients with fasting plasma glucose (FPG) values $\geq$126 mg/dL (7.0 mmol/L) twice or 2 h plasma glucose $\geq$200 mg/dL (11.1 mmol/L) during an oral glucose tolerance test (OGTT) or glucose values $\geq$200 mg/dL (11.1 mmol/L) at any time of the day, will be considered diabetic.

Normal values are below 100 mg/dL fasting or under 140 mg/dL 2 h of testing glucose tolerance.

There are some people with glucose levels between 100 and 126 mg/dL on the fasting state, or $\geq$140 mg/dL but <200 mg/dL after 75 g of glucose (OGTT), they are considered non-diabetic but with alterations in carbohydrate metabolism. Both disorders are called prediabetes.

The first alteration is impaired fasting glucose (IFG), in which insulin resistance plays the most important role; the second disturbance is called impaired glucose

F.M. Puchulu, M.D.
Division of Diabetology, Department of Medicine,
University of Buenos Aires, Buenos Aires, Argentina
e-mail: fpuchulu@gmail.com

© Springer International Publishing AG 2018
E.N. Cohen Sabban et al. (eds.), *Dermatology and Diabetes*,
https://doi.org/10.1007/978-3-319-72475-1_2

7

Table 2.1 Oral Glucose Tolerance Test for the diagnostic of alterations on carbohydrate metabolism

Glycemia (min)	Normal (mg/dL)	IFG (mg/dL)	IGT (mg/dL)	Diabetes (mg/dL)
0	≤99	100–125	≤99	≥126
120	≤139	≤139	140–199	≥200
		Pre-diabetes		

OGTT oral glucose tolerance test, *IFG* impaired fasting glucose, *IGT* impaired glucose tolerance

tolerance (IGT), in which a disturbance in the normal secretion of insulin to the stimulus with glucose has the prevalence.

Both alterations can also be present in the same individual. The presence of IFG and IGT indicate a higher probability of evolving to T2DM. In the case of presenting one of the alterations, it has been seen that the IGT has a higher incidence of T2DM that the IFG (Table 2.1)

Current diagnostic criteria of the American Diabetes Association propose adding glycosylated hemoglobin A1c (HbA1c) within them. Values above 6.5% would define the presence of disease. In Argentina, due to the lack of standardization of the method for the determination of HbA1c, Argentine Diabetes Society (SAD) decided to exclude this criterion.

DM diagnostic criteria of the American Diabetes Association (ADA)

- FPG ≥ 126 mg/dL (7.0 mmol/L) Fasting is no caloric intake for at least 8 h*
- 2 h PG ≥ 200 mg/dL (11.1 mmol/L) during an OGTT (according to the technique described by WHO, using a glucose load of 75 g anhydrous dissolved in water)*
- A1c ≥ 6.5% (48 mmol/L) in laboratories with standardized methods*
- Classic symptoms of hyperglycemia or hyperglycemic crisis glucose and a random plasma glucose ≥200 mg/dL (11.1 mmol/L).

*In the absence of unequivocal hyperglycemia results should be confirmed by repeat testing.

Classification

The former classification of DM based on dependency insulin was modified with the intention of eliminating denominations as insulin dependent diabetes mellitus and non-insulin dependent diabetes mellitus (IDDM and NIDDM), taking into account the diversity of response to therapeutic. The current classification of DM is based on the etiology of the disease, considering than type 1 diabetes is the result of the destruction of pancreatic beta cells (autoimmune or unknown cause, etc.) and type 2 diabetes is related to the association of insulin resistance and insulin deficiency.

Etiologic Classification

1. Type 1 diabetes (due to β-cell destruction, usually leading to absolute insulin deficiency)
2. Type 2 diabetes (due to a progressive insulin secretory defect on the background of insulin resistance)
3. Gestational diabetes mellitus (GDM) (diabetes diagnosed in the second or third trimester of pregnancy that is not clearly overt diabetes)
4. Specific types of diabetes due to other causes, e.g., monogenic diabetes syndromes (such as neonatal diabetes and maturity-onset diabetes of the young [MODY]), diseases of the exocrine pancreas (such as cystic fibrosis), and drug- or chemical-induced diabetes (such as in the treatment of HIV/AIDS or after organ transplantation)

Type 1 Diabetes (T1DM)

T1DM is characterized by the sudden onset of severe symptoms associated with the absolute deficiency of insulin secretion, tendency to ketosis and dependence on exogenous insulin to sustain life. Represents around 10% of all cases of diabetes and is one of the most common chronic childhood conditions. T1DM is an autoimmune condition in which the immune system is activated to destroy the pancreatic cells which produce insulin. The cause of this auto-immune reaction is unknown. T1DM is not linked to modifiable lifestyle factors. There is no cure and it cannot be prevented yet.

The histopathology of T1DM is defined by a decreased β-cell mass in association with insulitis, a characteristic lymphocytic infiltrate limited to Langerhans islets and prominent in early stage of the disease in children.

It has similar characteristics with autoimmune inflammatory processes found in certain thyroid diseases (thyroiditis) and adrenal (adrenalitis). Insulitis is characterized by infiltration and resulting disruption of islets with destruction of beta cells by T lymphocytes of various types.

Pancreatic deficiency of insulin secretion is the main cause in this type of diabetes, is due to the specific loss of beta cells, with conservation within almost normal mass of alpha cells (glucagon), delta (somatostatin) and PP (pancreatic polypeptide). This can be demonstrated by measuring blood insulin (in patients who have not received the hormone exogenously, either fasting or basal, as to different stimuli for release (e.g., administration of glucose or glucagon). Also can measured values of C peptide, the residual product in the conversion of proinsulin to insulin, since they are not altered or masked by receiving replacement therapy.

T1DM usually occurs abruptly, with overt signs of hyperglycemia, and sometimes with significant deterioration of clinical status.

Hyperglycemia is the result of the destruction of 80–90% of the functioning beta cells mass.

Only the clinical manifestation is acute, there is a silent preclinical period and can be recognized by different immunological markers that reveal the underlying autoimmune process.

Most cases of T1DM are due to the autoimmune process and the destruction of beta islet cells in genetically susceptible individuals, autoimmune pathogenic process is called "type 1a" in the classification. It should be noted that not all T1DM 1 diabetes have the same clinical evolution.

Not all individuals with pathogenic autoimmune process of T1DM progress to clinical DM1 or they do it slowly, with a prior relatively long period without insulin dependence.

Antibodies have been detected years before the onset of hyperglycemia. Functional studies, such as intravenous glucose tolerance test, reveal a decrease in the first phase of insulin secretion months or weeks before the clinical onset of the disease or the presence of fasting hyperglycemia, according to the magnitude and extent of damage caused in the beta cells.

It must be considered a preclinical period in the natural history of the disease, which can be identified through different immunological and genetic markers.

Genetic Determinism

Autoimmune diabetes is a T-dependent specific organ disease, polygenic, mainly restricted by the human leukocyte antigen (HLA). **HLA-DR** is an MHC (mayor histocompatibility complex) class II cell surface receptor encoded by the HLA on chromosome 6 region 6p21.31. The complex of HLA-DR (**H**uman **L**eukocyte **A**ntigen—antigen **D R**elated) and its ligand, a peptide of nine amino acids in length or longer, constitutes a ligand for the T-cell receptor (TCR). HLA-DR molecules are upregulated in response to signaling.

While HLA genes are the most important genetic factors that determine predisposition or protection to T1DM, it is clear that predisposition is necessary, but is not enough.

It has been found other important genes that also confer susceptibility to T1DM: CCR5 (C-C motif chemokine receptor 5), CTLA4 (Cytotoxic T Lymphocyte Antigen 4), FOXP3 (forkhead box P3), HNF1A (HNF1 homeboxA), IL2RA (interleukin 2 receptor subunit alpha), IL6 (interleukin 6), INS (insulin gene), ITPR3 (inositol 1,4,5-trisphosphate receptor type 3), OAS1 (2′-5′-oligoadenylate synthetase 1), PTPN22 (protein tyrosine phosphatase, non-receptor type 22), SUMO4 (small ubiquitin-like modifier 4).

The VNTR region (variable number tandem repeat) which is adjacent to the 5′ end of the insulin gene is also related to T1DM predisposition.

It has also been found influence of the gene encoding the protein CTLA-4.

The HLA region is located in the short arm of chromosome 6. The association between HLA and T1DM was initially demonstrated by Nerup. Patients with T1DM have DR3 and/or DR4 by 94% compared with 60% in the healthy population.

People with positive HLA DR3 have a relative risk (RR) of 6.4 and diabetes carriers HLA DR4 3.7.

The presence of both markers increases the susceptibility to develop the disease, more than the sum of the relative risks (RR) of DR3 and DR4.

There are also markers that express a lower chance of developing diabetes. It has been found less frequently HLA DR2 in patients with T1DM, determining a RR for the disease of 0.26, so is considered as a protection factor.

HLA-DQB1 belongs to the HLA class II beta chain paralogs. This class II molecule is a heterodimer consisting of an alpha (DQA) and a beta chain (DQB), both anchored in the membrane. It plays a central role in the immune system by presenting peptides derived from extracellular proteins. Class II molecules are expressed in antigen-presenting cells (APC: B lymphocytes, dendritic cells, macrophages).

Different allelic variants of polymorphic gene DQB are circumscribed to the second exon of the gene and are encoding the amino terminal region of the antigen-presenting molecule.

Several alleles of HLA-DQB1 are associated with an increased risk of developing T1DM. The locus is the highest genetic risk for type 1 diabetes. Again, the DQB1*0201 and DQB1*0302 alleles, particularly the phenotype DQB1*0201/*0302 has a high risk of late onset type 1 diabetes. The risk is partially shared with the HLA-DR locus (DR3 and DR4 serotypes).

> **HLA**
> **Predisposition**: HLA DR3 (DQB1 0201) /DR4 (DQB1 0301).
> **Protection**: DR2 (DQB1 0602).

Autoimmunity

T1DM can be induced by a process of autoimmunity directed against the insulin-producing beta cells. This mechanism could be triggered by certain environmental factors in genetically determined individuals. The classic biomarkers that "predict" type 1 diabetes are serum autoantibodies against β-cell antigens, including insulin, GAD, IA-2, and zinc transporter 8. Autoantibodies to other antigens have been reported, but either occur infrequently or have been inadequately validated and are not used for prediction. The suspicion of an autoimmune process came from the striking association between T1DM and other endocrine autoimmune diseases, such as those affecting thyroid and adrenal, as the high percentage of specific antibodies present in the patient's serum. This event marks a discrete start of the disease process and is associated with a marked increase in the risk of the development of diabetes. The presence of two or more of the four autoantibodies can be considered asymptomatic disease, and usually progresses to hyperglycemia.

The first description of autoimmunity in diabetes was made in 1974 with the ICA (Islet Cell Antibodies). ICA are present in a 0.5–1.7% of the general population and 15–30% in T1DM, but at the time of onset of the disease, in patients less than 30 years, this percentage rises to 60–85%, descending to lower values after 2–3 years.

They are IgG class non-specific beta-cell autoantibodies, produced by activated T lymphocytes. They are determined by indirect immunofluorescence (IFI) and measured in JDFunits, values under 10 UJDF are considered negative. Currently this determination has been replaced by other antibodies described below.

The GADA (Glutamic Acid Decarboxylase Antibodies) of which there are two isoforms described, 65 kD (specific for diabetes) and 67 kD, are the most useful because of the ease of its determination. They can be measured by radiobinding assay (RBA).

GAD antigen is not beta cell specific, and participates in the formation of Gamma-Aminobutyric acid (GABA).

Islet antigen-2 (IA-2), previously known also as ICA-512, is a major target of islet cell autoantibodies.

They are present in 45–75% of the cases at the beginning of the disease. They are determined by RBA.

Insulin autoantibodies (IAA) are positive in 20–50% of patients with recent onset diabetes. They are positive previous the treatment with insulin. The use of insulin determines the presence of insulin antibodies (IA) to the exogenous insulin (IA instead of IAA) as they would be related of the exogenous antigen of the hormone injection. They are measured by RBA. They have inverse correlation with age, being more common at younger ages.

It has recently been discovered the antibodies against the Zinc transporter 8 islet (ZnT8A) that also predicts T1DM. ZnT8 is specifically expressed in the pancreatic β-cells and has been identified as a novel target autoantigen in patients with T1DM. Antibodies to ZnT8 have been detected in 60–80% of Caucasian and 33–58% of Asian population with T1DM.

IAAs are the first to appear, GADAs and IAAs are the most frequent islet autoantibodies in childhood, GADA is the hallmark of adult-onset type 1 diabetes, and IA-2 antigens are very specific for the development of diabetes. A study by Annette and coworkers showed that the age of onset of antibodies, and the association between them determined a greater predisposition to develop T1DM, and also that some antibodies are more specific to develop it. They showed that the subgroup of children with two islet autoantibodies, progression to diabetes within 10 years after seroconversion was increased in children with the combination of autoantibodies against insulin and IA2 than in children with autoantibodies against insulin and GAD65 and children with autoantibodies against GAD65 and IA2.The addition of zinc transporter 8 autoantibodies identified seven more children (6%) who progressed to diabetes but did not substantially alter the estimates of diabetes progression.

The sensitivity and predictive capacity increase with the association of markers. The association of GADA, IA- 2A and IAA determines a sensitivity of 90% and a positive predictive value close to 100% for the next 5 years (Fig. 2.1).

The appearance of autoantibodies does not follow a distinct pattern; the presence of multiple autoantibodies has the highest positive predictive value for T1DM.

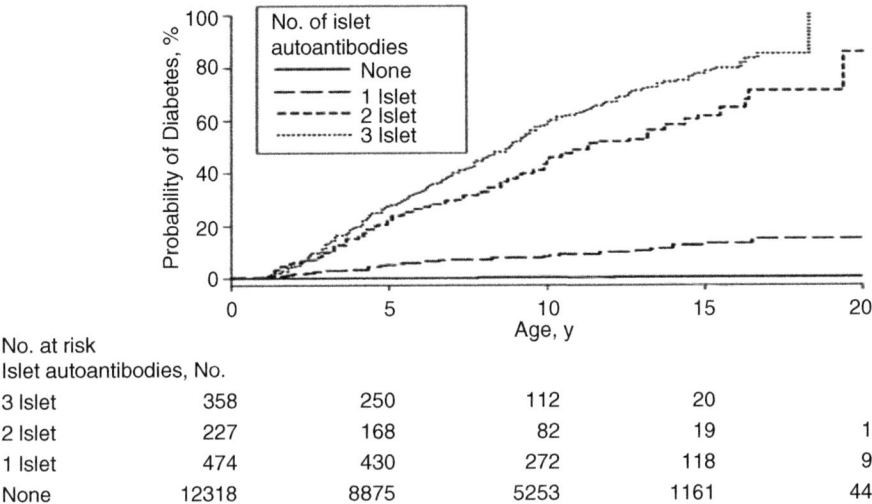

No. at risk Islet autoantibodies, No.					
3 Islet	358	250	112	20	
2 Islet	227	168	82	19	1
1 Islet	474	430	272	118	9
None	12318	8875	5253	1161	44

Fig. 2.1 Development of Diabetes in Children Stratified for Islet Autoantibody Outcome The numbers at risk represent the children receiving follow-up at age 0, 5, 10, 15, and 20 years. Positive predictive value (PPV) for the development of T1DM in a risk group (Ziegler et al.)

Environmental Factors

Given the evidence of the genetic predisposition for diabetes and autoimmune origin, is still in search those factors that act as trigger determining the process of aggression to the pancreas to generate diabetes.

The mechanism of action involved in environmental factors is not known precisely, but it is postulated that they may act in two different ways: by direct toxicity against beta cell; and by triggering the autoimmune mechanism against beta cell.

Age is an important factor, being less common to develop T1DM in the first 9 months of life, probably related to the protection provided by the maternal antibodies to the newborn. There is an increase incidence at 5–6-year-old, a peak at 12–14-year-old and a slight decrease between 20 and 35 years comes later. There are also geographical variations, with significant differences between different areas; (e.g., in Finland the incidence is 29.5/100,000 people per year while in Hokkaido, Japan, is 1.6/100,000 per year). Migrant studies indicate that the incidence of T1DM has increased in population groups who have moved from a low incidence region to a high incidence area, also emphasizing the influence of environmental conditions.

There have been described factors as chemical agents and specific drugs (alloxan, streptozotocin, pentamidine and a rodenticide vacor).

A large number of epidemiological studies were conducted to determine the influence of viral infections in the development of T1DM in humans, accepting its association mainly with four viruses: mumps, coxsackie, rubella and cytomegalovirus, which would act as a trigger for immune process.

Currently, although genetic and immunological markers are involved, the use of immunosuppressants in the preclinical period is not approved, since its safety and effectiveness are not demonstrated, and that might be unnecessary in patients who undergo to an spontaneous remission without developing the disease.

Type 2 Diabetes Mellitus (T2DM)

T2DM is a chronic metabolic condition characterized by insulin resistance (that is, the body's inability to effectively use insulin) and insufficient pancreatic insulin production, resulting in high blood glucose levels (hyperglycaemia). When insulin resistance is present, the β-cell maintains normal glucose tolerance by increasing insulin output. It is only when the β-cell is incapable of releasing sufficient insulin in the presence of insulin resistance that glucose levels rise. T2DM is commonly associated with obesity, physical inactivity, hypertension, disturbed blood lipid levels and a prothrombotic state, and therefore is recognized to have an increased cardiovascular risk. It is associated with long-term microvascular and macrovascular complications, along with poor quality of life and life expectancy reduced.

T2DM has a polygenic origin of variable expression, where environmental factors play an important role in its determinism.

The variable expression of genes implies that the presence of the predisposition not invariably determines an evolution towards the disease, and that their presence only involves the risk of developing T2DM. This risk is enhanced with some environmental factors as unhealthful food, refined carbohydrates, barriers to physical activity and stress.

T2DM accounts for 90–95% of all diabetes types. This form encompasses individuals who have insulin resistance and usually relative (rather than absolute) insulin deficiency. Insulin resistance alone is insufficient to develop diabetes, so it requires the alteration in insulin secretion. The IR has two determining factors, the genetic, and the environmental, which is influenced by diet, sedentary lifestyle, overweight, medication, etc. It is more common in adults; its onset is insidious by the lack of symptoms, being common to ignore the presence of the disease.

> **T2DM= Insulin Resistance + β-cell dysfunction**

Other Specific Types

Among the other specific types of diabetes, it is important to identify the monogenic types of diabetes.

It is worth noting the MODY diabetes (Maturity Onset Diabetes of the Young), which is characterized by diabetes that appears early in life, but behaves like type 2 diabetes and not as Type 1, and are characterized by impaired insulin

Table 2.2 Genetic classification and clinical phenotypes of the MODY subtypes (Attiya K. et al.)

Type	Gene name	Locus	Gene function	Primary defect
MODY 1	Hepatocyte nuclear factor 4α (HNF4A)	20q	Transcription factor (nuclear factor)	Pancreas
MODY 2	Glucokinase (GCK)	7p15-p13	Hexokinase IV	Pancreas/liver
MODY 3	Hepatocyte nuclear factor 1α (HNF1A)	12q24.2	Transcription factor (homeodomain)	Pancreas/kidney
MODY 4	Insulin promoter factor-1 (IPF-1)	13q12.1	Transcription factor (homeodomain)	Pancreas
MODY 5	Hepatocyte nuclear factor 1 β (HNF1B)	17q12	Transcription factor (homeodomain)	Kidney/pancreas
MODY 6	Neurogenic differentiation 1 (NEUROD1)	2q	Transcription factor(bHLH)	Pancreas
MODY 7	Kruppel-like factor 11 (KLF11)	2p25	Transforming growth factor-beta-inducible-early growth response 2.	Pancreas
MODY 8	Bile salt dependent lipase (CELL)	9q34.3	The endocrine cells of pancreas synthesize insulin and are involved in the pathogenesis of diabetes mellitus and exocrine cells are involved in the pathogenesis of pancreatic malabsorption	Pancreas
MODY 9	Paired domain gene 4 (PAX4)	7q32	Transcription factor (paired domain gene 4)	Pancreas
MODY 10	Insulin (INS)	11p15.5.	Beta cells of the islets of Langerhans	NF-kappa-B
MODY 11	Tyrosine kinase, B-lymphocyte specific	8p23-p22	Tyrosine kinase (B lymphocytes)	MIN6 beta cells

secretion with minimal or no defects in insulin action. They are inherited in an autosomal dominant pattern, MODY is caused by a mutation in a single gene. If a parent has this gene mutation, their offspring has a 50% chance of inheriting it from them.

It commonly appears before 25 years of age, usually occurs in three or more generations of the same family. It is monogenic type, with dominant inheritance,

They have been described 11 types of maturity onset diabetes of the young whose recognition is difficult to perform, but is important to consider the presence of this type of DM because their treatment and prognosis differ from the T1DM (Table 2.2).

The diagnosis of monogenic diabetes should be considered in children with the following findings:

- Diabetes diagnosed within the first 6 months of life
- Strong family history of diabetes but without typical features of type 2 diabetes (non-obese, low-risk ethnic group)
- Mild fasting hyperglycemia (100–150 mg/dL [5.5–8.5 mmol/L]), especially if young and non-obese
- Diabetes with negative autoantibodies and without signs of obesity or insulin resistance

Gestational Diabetes (GD) GD has been defined as any degree of glucose intolerance with onset or first recognition during pregnancy regardless of whether the condition may have predated the pregnancy or persisted after the pregnancy. It has 7% prevalence with a range from 1 to 14%, depending on the population studied and the diagnostic criteria used. For the diagnosis of GD an oral glucose tolerance test is performed between weeks 24 and 28 of pregnancy; if negative and there are risk factors for, is repeated between 31 and 33 weeks. It is made with 75 g of anhydrous glucose dissolved in 375 mL of water, to be ingested in 5 min (Table 2.3).

The diagnostic criteria are different according to different medical societies that are considered.

Classical risk factors for developing gestational diabetes are:

- Policystic Ovary Syndrome
- A previous diagnosis of gestational diabetes or prediabetes, impaired glucose tolerance, or impaired fasting glycemia.
- A family history revealing a first-degree relative with T2DM
- Maternal age—a woman's risk factor increases as she gets older (especially for women over 35 years of age).
- Ethnicity (those with higher risk factors include African-Americans, Afro-Caribbeans, Native Americans, Hispanics, Pacific Islanders, and people originating from South Asia).
- Being overweight, obese or severely obese increases the risk by a factor 2.1, 3.6 and 8.6, respectively.
- A previous pregnancy which resulted in a child with a macrosomia [high birth weight: >90th centile or >4000 g (8 lbs 12.8 oz)].
- Previous poor obstetric history.

Table 2.3 Oral glucose tolerance test for the diagnostic of Gestational Diabetes

Time (min)	ADA (75 g OGTT) (2 h) (mg/dL)	Carpenter (100 g OGTT) (3 h) (mg/dL)
0	≥92	≥95
60	≥180	≥180
120	≥153	≥155
180	–	≥140

- Other genetic risk factors: There are at least ten genes where certain polymorphism are associated with an increased risk of gestational diabetes, most notably TCF7L2.

LADA: In the classification of the ADA the place of this type of diabetes is not defined. It is known as LADA for its acronym in English Autoimmune Latent Diabetes of the Adult. It is characterized, as indicated by its name, its autoimmune origin that occurs in adults, but with a less abrupt onset and may not require the use of insulin than 6 months periods. It is important to consider this possibility in adult individuals (over 35 years) and who are not overweight. GADA determination is indicated in this group of patients, being important to understand the type of diabetes present because they tend to insulin dependence and must be distinguished from T2DM with failure to oral agents. Other antibodies that may be useful for diagnosis include IA-2A and ZnT8-A. The determination of IAA is not recommended (less frequent in adults).

Considerations

Diabetes is the generic name of a syndrome that is defined by a blood glucose value, however it can be concluded that there are different causes of this condition so should be identified the type of diabetes in a newly diagnosed diabetic patient, to understand the nature of the disease, since this knowledge will make a difference in the treatment, prognosis and complications.

Bibliography

1. Vaccaro O, et al. Risk of diabetes in the new diagnostic category of impaired fasting glucose: a prospective analysis. Diabetes Care. 1999;22:1490–3.
2. International Expert Committee. International Expert Committee report on the role of the A1C assay in the diagnosis of diabetes. Diabetes Care. 2009;32:1327–34.
3. American Diabetes Association. Diagnosis and classification of diabetes mellitus. Diabetes Care. 2017;40(Supplement 1):s11–24.
4. National Institute for Health and Care Excellence. NICE guidance 2017, Type 2 diabetes in adults: management [NG28].
5. National Center for Biotechnology Information, U.S. National Library of Medicine Policies and Guidelines. Gene ID: 3119. HLA-DQB1 major histocompatibility complex, class II, DQ beta 1 [Homo sapiens (human)], updated on 23 July 2017.
6. Bonifacio E. Predicting Type 1 diabetes using biomarkers. Diabetes Care. 2015;38(6):989–96.
7. Ziegler AG, Rewers M, Simell O, Simell T, Lempainen J, Steck A, Winkler C, Ilonen J, Veijola R, Knip M, Bonifacio E, Eisenbarth GS. Seroconversion to multiple islet autoantibodies and risk of progression to diabetes in children. JAMA. 2013;309(23):2473–9.
8. In't Veld P. Insulitis in human type 1 diabetes. The quest for an elusive lesion. Islets. 2011;3(4):131–8. https://doi.org/10.4161/isl.3.4.15728.
9. Mehers KL, Gillespie KM. The genetic basis for type 1 diabetes. Br Med Bull. 2008;88(1):115–29. https://doi.org/10.1093/bmb/ldn045.
10. Pihoker C, Lernmark Å, et al. Autoantibodies in diabetes. Diabetes. 2005;54(suppl 2):S52–61.

11. Skyler J. Insulin therapy in type 1 diabetes mellitus. In: De Fronzo R, editor. Current therapy of diabetes mellitus. St. Louis, MO: Mosby; 1998. p. 36–49.
12. Poskus E, Ermácora M. Los avances en Diabetes Mellitus impulsados por los inmunobiológicos recombinantes. En Bioquímica y Patología Clínica. 1998;62(1):18–31.
13. Frechtel G, Poskus E. Diabetes autoinmune de inicio en edad infanto-juvenil y adulta. Bases racionales para el diagnóstico y tratamiento. Separata; Lugar: Buenos Aires; 2005.
14. Caputo M, Cerrone GE, López AP, González C, Mazza C, Cédola N, Puchulu FM, Targovnik HM, Frechtel GD. Genotipificación del gen HLA DQB1 en diabetes autoinmune del adulto (LADA). Medicina. 2005;65:235–40.
15. Poskus E. Autoinmunidad, marcadores inmunológicos en diabetes mellitus. En Diabetes mellitus. Tercera Edición. Ruiz M. Editorial; 2004. p. 20–55.
16. Valdez SN, Iacono RF, Villalba A, Cardoso Landaburu A, Ermácora M, Poskus E. A radioligando-binding assay for detecting antibodies specific for proinsulin and insulin using 355-proinsulin. J Immunol Methods. 2003;279:173–81.
17. De Grijse J, Asanghanwa M, Nouthe B, et al. Belgian diabetes registry. Predictive power of screening for antibodies against insulinoma-associated protein 2 beta (IA-2beta) and zinc transporter-8 to selectfirst-degree relatives of type 1 diabetic patients with risk of rapid progression to clinical onset of the disease: implications for prevention trials. Diabetologia. 2010;53:517–24.
18. Wenzlau JM, Moua O, Sarkar SA, Yu L, Rewers M, Eisenbarth GS, et al. SlC30A8 is a major target of humoral autoimmunity in type 1 diabetes and a predictive marker in prediabetes. Ann N Y Acad Sci. 2008;1150:256–9.
19. Yang L, Luo S, Huang G, Peng J, Li X, Yan X, et al. The diagnostic value of zinc transporter 8 autoantibody (ZnT8A) for type 1 diabetes in Chinese. Diabetes Metab Res Rev. 2010;26:579–84.
20. Kawasaki E. ZnT8 and type 1 diabetes. Endocr J. 2012;59(7):531–7. Epub 2012 Mar 8.
21. Verge GF, et al. Prediction of type 1 diabetes mellitus in first-degree relatives using a combination of insulin, GAD and ICA512/IA-2 autoantibodies. Diabetes. 1996;45:926–33.
22. Reaven GM. Insulin resistance-how important is it to treat? Exp Clin Endocrinol Diabetes. 2000;108(Suppl 2):S274–80.
23. Recomendaciones para gestantes con diabetes. Conclusiones del Consenso reunido por convocatoria del Comité de Diabetes y Embarazo de la SAD. Octubre 2008.
24. Ross G. Gestational diabetes. Aust Fam Physician. 2006;35(6):392–6.
25. American Diabetes Association. Standards of medical care in diabetes. Diabetes Care. 2016;39(suppl 1):S1–S106.
26. Attiya K, Sahar F. Maturity-onset diabetes of the young (MODY) genes: literature review. Clin Pract. 2012;1(1):4–11.
27. Kahn S, Cooper M, Del Prato S. Pathophysiology and treatment of type 2 diabetes: perspectives on the past, present and future. Lancet. 2014;383(9922):1068–83.

Basic Concepts in Insulin Resistance and Diabetes Treatment

3

Fernando Bril and Kenneth Cusi

Introduction

Type 2 diabetes mellitus (T2DM) should be understood as the final common pathway that results from an imbalance between increased insulin resistance (i.e., decreased insulin action) and relative insulinopenia (i.e., impaired insulin secretion) [1].

There is consensus that for most patients with T2DM the earliest defect observed is insulin resistance. For many patients this is genetically determined, but a common acquired factor that worsens insulin resistance is obesity [2]. However, the relative contribution of acquired versus genetic factors is unclear and varies from patient to patient. At early stages, the pancreas is able to compensate for insulin resistance by increasing insulin secretion so that glucose tolerance is preserved. Thus, a state of normal glucose tolerance is maintained at the expense of hyperinsulinemia. Over time, and by mechanisms that are still incompletely understood, pancreatic β-cells fail to maintain this high rate of insulin secretion, and impaired glucose tolerance and overt T2DM develop [3].

In the current chapter, the mechanisms leading to insulin resistance and the spectrum of therapeutic approaches for patients with T2DM will be described.

F. Bril, M.D.
Division of Endocrinology, Diabetes and Metabolism, University of Florida, Gainesville, FL, USA

K. Cusi, M.D., F.A.C.P., F.A.C.E. (✉)
Division of Endocrinology, Diabetes and Metabolism, University of Florida, Gainesville, FL, USA

Division of Endocrinology, Diabetes and Metabolism, Malcom Randall VAMC, Gainesville, FL, USA
e-mail: Kenneth.Cusi@medicine.ufl.edu

© Springer International Publishing AG 2018
E.N. Cohen Sabban et al. (eds.), *Dermatology and Diabetes*,
https://doi.org/10.1007/978-3-319-72475-1_3

Causes of Insulin Resistance: Acquired vs. Genetic

The interplay between acquired and genetic defects in the development and promotion of insulin resistance is complex and incompletely understood [4–6]. Moreover, the relative contribution of each of these factors varies from case to case, and ranges from monogenic insulin resistance syndromes to fully-acquired cases in the setting of obesity.

Monogenic syndromes of insulin resistance are rare, but they have been consistently reported in the literature in the last few decades [6]. Over 15 different culprit genes have been identified including insulin receptor, peroxisome proliferator-activated receptor-γ (PPAR-γ), pericentrin, perilipin, protein kinase B (Akt2), etc. Of note, most single-gene causes of insulin resistance do not affect insulin signaling pathways, but adipose tissue function, inducing insulin resistance only as a consequence of the dysfunctional adipose tissue. Other responsible genes identified are involved in DNA repair, but their link to severe insulin resistance has not been fully elucidated [6]. These genetic syndromes range from infantile fatal disease to mild insulin resistance in later life, and have been reviewed in depth elsewhere [7, 8].

As for the acquired defects, obesity has received significant attention, as it is commonly associated with insulin resistance [4, 5]. However, teasing out the contribution of genetic factors from that directly attributed to obesity has been difficult. Moreover, the severity of obesity does not always correlate with the severity of insulin resistance, implying that there are other mechanisms that regulate the degree of obesity-related insulin resistance. Accumulating evidence suggests that the initiating event of insulin resistance may not be the presence of obesity itself, but the presence of dysfunctional adipose tissue [4, 5]. This concept helps to explain why non-obese individuals with a family history of T2DM (i.e., with a genetic background) are insulin resistant long before the development of obesity [9]. Based on the same principles, the development of obesity (even in the absence of a genetic background) results in adipose tissue insulin resistance due to a distinctive fat distribution (favoring visceral accumulation, in contrast of subcutaneous adipose tissue), but most importantly, due to the development of ectopic accumulation of fat in insulin sensitive tissues, such as the liver and skeletal muscle [4, 5]. Other common causes of insulin resistance include some medications and are described in Table 3.1 [8, 10].

Physiology of Insulin Resistance

Adipose Tissue

As mentioned above, adipose tissue is likely the tissue where insulin resistance begins [5]. By molecular mechanisms that are beyond the scope of this article and that have been reviewed elsewhere [5, 11, 12], adipose tissue can become insulin resistant in the setting of obesity and/or genetic predisposition. As a

Table 3.1 Causes of insulin resistance

Genetic causes of insulin resistance
Mutations in insulin receptor or insulin pathway 1. INSR [insulin receptor]—autosomal recessive (e.g., Donohue and Rabson Mendenhall syndromes) 2. INSR [insulin receptor]—autosomal dominant (e.g., type A IR and HAIR-AN syndromes) 3. IRS-1 4. Akt/PKB (e.g., Lipodystrophy with familial diabetes) 5. Insulin receptor kinase inhibitor (PC-1)
Mutations directly affecting adipose tissue function 1. Genetic lipodystrophy (generalized or partial) (e.g., PPAR-γ, perilipin1, etc.) 2. Genetically determined obesity (e.g., Alstrom syndrome)
Mutations affecting DNA repair 1. WRN gene (adult progeria or Werner syndrome) 2. BLM gene (DNA helicase) (Bloom syndrome) 3. ATM gene (ataxia-telangiectasia)
Acquired causes of insulin resistance
Obesity ± sedentary life
Increased plasma FFA (i.e., "lipotoxicity")
Hyperglycemia
Subclinical/clinical inflammation
Pregnancy
Medications 1. Highly active antiretroviral treatment (e.g., protease inhibitors) 2. Glucocorticoids 3. Nicotinic acid 4. Atypical antipsychotics (e.g., olanzapine)

consequence of this, hormone-sensitive lipase fails to be inhibited by insulin, which results in increased rates of lipolysis. This, in turn, results in an oversecretion of free fatty acids (FFA) into the circulation, where they can reach other organs promoting lipotoxicity [5]. The term "lipotoxicity" was originally introduced by Unger [13] to describe the harmful effects of increased FFA levels on β-cell function. However, since its original use, the term lipotoxicity has attained a much broader meaning, and it is now applied to any deleterious effects of FFAs on tissues that would not normally be destined to store large amounts of lipids, such as the liver [14, 15].

In addition to FFA oversecretion, insulin-resistant adipose tissue is also characterized by a pro-inflammatory phenotype [5, 12]. Adipocytokines, such as tumor necrosis factor (TNF)-α and interleukin (IL)-6 are secreted by dysfunctional adipocytes and may contribute to insulin resistance in an autocrine, paracrine, and endocrine fashion. This consolidates a "closed loop" in which insulin resistance promotes inflammation, and inflammation reinforces insulin resistance. Reduced levels of beneficial molecules, such as adiponectin, have also been described in obesity and insulin-resistant states [16]. Moreover, there exists a closed cross-talk between adipocytes and macrophages in the adipose tissue, further expanding the systemic impact of adipose tissue-derived inflammation [11, 12].

Liver

The liver receives FFAs from three different sources: adipose tissue lipolysis, diet, and *de novo* lipogenesis [14, 17]. Of these, adipose tissue lipolysis is the most important one, contributing with approximately ~60% of all FFAs in normal conditions. In the setting of adipose tissue insulin resistance (increased lipolysis, as described above), the flux of FFA to the liver increases. When FFA supply surpasses the metabolic needs of the organ, the liver begins to accumulate them as triglycerides, which results in hepatic steatosis [18]. In addition, increased hepatic FFA oxidation leads to an incomplete oxidation, with the generation of lipid intermediates (e.g., ceramides and diacylglycerols) and reactive oxygen species (ROS) that promote hepatic insulin resistance and inflammation [18].

Hepatic insulin resistance translates into increased rates of hepatic glucose production (HGP) and of very low density lipoprotein (VLDL) secretion, as insulin is unable to suppress them as under normal conditions [19, 20]. In turn, increased HGP promotes a compensatory hyperinsulinemia in order to maintain normal plasma glucose levels. However, such hyperinsulinemia turns to be deleterious as it increases the rate of intracellular *de novo* lipogenesis (DNL), further contributing to hepatocyte triglyceride accumulation.

Nonalcoholic fatty liver disease, defined as an intracellular triglyceride accumulation greater than 5.5% in the absence of any secondary cause of steatosis (e.g., alcohol, drugs, viral hepatitis, autoimmune hepatitis, etc.), is increasingly common in patients with obesity and/or T2DM [17, 21–23]. It is closely linked to insulin resistance, and in some patients, it can progress to its more severe form known as nonalcoholic steatohepatitis (NASH), characterized by the presence of hepatic steatosis combined with inflammation, necrosis, and/or fibrosis [21, 22]. In the absence of treatment, this liver condition may progress to cirrhosis and hepatocellular carcinoma [21, 22].

Skeletal Muscle

In the setting of this "lipotoxic" environment promoted by insulin resistance, skeletal muscle insulin resistance also develops, resulting in impaired insulin-stimulated muscle glucose uptake. Several factors contribute to the development of insulin resistance in this tissue. For instance, increased plasma FFA levels promote intramyocellular steatosis and impaired insulin signaling. This is observed among healthy lean individuals, in a dose-dependent manner, when plasma FFA are experimentally increased during an intravenous lipid infusion [24]. This also occurs within 24–48 h after plasma FFA are just slightly increased experimentally to achieve plasma FFA levels typically observed in obesity [25, 26]. However, intramyocellular triglyceride accumulation *per se* appears not to play a role in the development of insulin resistance. Human studies report that athletes paradoxically have a high triglyceride content despite their normal (or above normal) insulin sensitivity [27]. Thus, the current hypothesis is that insulin resistance-related steatosis is characterized by accumulation of toxic lipid metabolites and pro-inflammatory lipid intermediates that impair insulin signaling and are responsible for insulin resistance [27].

Chronic hyperinsulinemia, secondary to increased hepatic glucose production, can also promote insulin resistance by downregulating the number of insulin receptors and their downstream signaling steps. An approximately 2 to 3-fold increase in plasma insulin levels causes skeletal muscle insulin resistance after a 72-hour insulin infusion in otherwise insulin-sensitive individuals [28]. The combination of elevated FFA and hyperinsulinemia is the perfect storm for skeletal muscle insulin resistance, which in turn contributes to glucose intolerance.

Pancreatic ß-Cells

In order to keep plasma glucose levels in the normal range in the setting of insulin resistance, a compensatory hyperinsulinemia is required, which results in a demanding burden to the pancreatic ß-cells [29]. While ß-cells can keep up with the workload, glucose tolerance remains within the normal range. However, when this compensation fails, hyperglycemia develops. However, subtle defects in ß-cell function can be detected long before the development of frank hyperglycemia [29]. The underlying mechanisms responsible for this relentless decline in ß-cell function over time are incompletely understood. However, basic and clinical evidence suggests that hyperglycemia (i.e., glucotoxicity) and chronic elevated plasma FFAs (i.e., lipotoxicity) play key roles in this progression [30–32].

In the setting of obesity and insulin resistance, ß-cells are forced to manage the FFA oversupply. In ideal conditions, this chronic increase of plasma FFA should enhance basal and glucose-stimulated insulin secretion. However, in predisposed patients (e.g., family history of T2DM) increased plasma FFA produces the opposite effect, inducing insulin secretion impairment and favoring the progression to T2DM [31]. These patients appear to have a genetically-determined reduced ß-cell adaptation to excess FFA supply. Once hyperglycemia develops, this generates a positive feedback, where hyperglycemia impairs ß-cell function, further perpetuating the increased plasma glucose levels [30].

Management of T2DM

The management of T2DM requires a multidisciplinary approach, focused on lifestyle modifications, as well as diabetes self-management education and support [33]. At center stage of this approach are nutrition therapy, physical activity, and smoking cessation counseling [33]. Health care providers should focus on how to optimize lifestyle in every patient with T2DM, as modest weight reductions have been shown to improve glycemic control and reduce the need for glucose-lowering medications [34]. Relatively modest reductions of body weight (of approximately 5%) are frequently enough to observe beneficial effects in glycemic control, although weight loss ≥7% are optimal and associated with further benefits on blood pressure, lipids, and NASH [33, 35].

While hypocaloric diets (~500–750 kcal/day energy deficit) should be strongly encouraged in patients with T2DM in order to achieve the desired weight reduction, diet composition appears to be of lesser importance [33]. A variety of different diets have proven to be effective, as long as total calorie intake targets are kept in mind. Therefore, diets should be individualized to patients' preferences and needs. Foods higher in fiber and lower in glycemic load and added sugars should be emphasized (whole grains, vegetables, fruits, legumes, low-fat dairy, nuts, and seeds). Regarding physical activity, the American Diabetes Association recommends for most adults with T2DM at least 150 min of moderate-to-vigorous intensity aerobic physical activity per week. In addition, adults with T2DM should engage in 2–3 sessions/week of resistance exercise on nonconsecutive days [33].

Nevertheless, reaching sufficient weight loss, and especially sustaining such reduction over time is challenging. Even in intensive intervention groups during well-controlled clinical trials (i.e., Look AHEAD) weight loss was only 4.7% after 8 years of follow-up [34]. Weight loss medications (e.g., orlistat, lorcaserin, phentermine/topiramate ER, naltrexone/bupropion, liraglutide 3 mg) can be used as adjunctive therapy in patients with BMI ≥ 27 kg/m². In addition, metabolic surgery should be considered in patients with a BMI ≥ 40 kg/m² or ≥35 kg/m² if hyperglycemia is not adequately controlled despite optimal therapy [33]. Several review articles have addressed the benefits and risks of metabolic surgery in the management of T2DM [36, 37].

Due to the limitations of lifestyle modification to achieve hemoglobin A1c targets (<7% for most adults, but potentially <6.5% or <8% for selected individuals based on risk of hypoglycemia, life expectancy, comorbidities, etc.), pharmacologic treatment should be considered early-on in patients with T2DM [33]. In recent years, we have witnessed an exponential increment in our pharmacological options, with several new drug groups with distinctive mechanisms of action.

Briefly, glucose-lowering agents can be divided based on their mechanisms of action in the following groups: (a) drugs that mainly improve insulin resistance; (b) drugs that mainly improve insulin secretion; (c) drugs with an incretin-mimetic effect; and finally, (d) drugs that are glucose-lowering agents by inducing glycosuria. In this section, we will describe the mechanisms of action, best indications, side effects, and special considerations of each pharmacological agent.

Insulin Sensitizers

Metformin

Metformin is a biguanide that has been available worldwide for the prevention and treatment of T2DM for over 50 years. Its exact mechanism of action remains incompletely understood, although it is clear that it decreases hepatic gluconeogenesis and improves insulin sensitivity at the level of the liver, and to a lesser extent, skeletal muscle [38]. There are several proposed molecular mechanisms for this drug:

inhibition of mitochondrial complex I, leading to a reduction in ATP synthesis with the consequent increase in AMP and AMP kinase activation; delayed glucose absorption in the gastrointestinal tract, inhibition of glucagon signaling and gluconeogenic enzymes, glucagon-like peptide (GLP)-1 secretion, and others [38]. Nevertheless, it is debatable whether these actions occur at physiological concentrations or not. A recent study suggested that at the regular doses used in humans, metformin inhibited mitochondrial glycerophosphate dehydrogenase in rats, resulting in a reduction in the contribution of both glycerol and lactate to hepatic gluconeogenesis [39].

Given its proven efficacy, overall safety, and cardiovascular benefits, metformin has consolidated over time as the first line of therapy for patients with T2DM and is used at doses that range from 500 to 2000 mg daily [33]. It can be safely used in patients with an eGFR $\geq$30 mL/min/1.73 m^2, but patients should be advised to stop the medication in cases of nausea, vomiting, dehydration, or before a contrast-enhanced computed tomography study. Metformin has also been associated with vitamin B12 deficiency, and therefore, periodic testing of vitamin B12 levels is now recommended [33]. It is usually well tolerated, although a minority may suffer metformin-associated gastrointestinal side effects. Most patients usually develop tolerance to these side effects and slow titration should be always recommended to help to avoid them. Only ~5% of patients are unable to tolerate metformin due to GI side effects. Other side effects, such as lactic acidosis and skin rashes are extremely rare [33].

Thiazolidinediones (TZDs)

Currently, only two available drugs are included in this group: pioglitazone and rosiglitazone. While they both share the same main mechanism of action (i.e., peroxisome proliferator-activated receptor [PPAR]-γ agonism), they have important distinctive effects on lipid metabolism, as well as in the liver and cardiovascular system in humans [5, 17, 40, 41]. By activating PPAR-γ, these molecules improve insulin sensitivity mainly at the level of the adipose tissue, which leads to a reduction in adipocyte triglyceride breakdown (lipolysis) and in plasma FFA levels [42]. This, in turn, results in a reduction of lipotoxicity in other tissues, with the consequent improvements in skeletal muscle and liver insulin sensitivity [43].

In 2007 it was claimed that rosiglitazone could potentially be associated with myocardial infarction and increased cardiovascular disease [44]. However, while the fear among primary care physicians remains, the FDA actually removed that black box warning some years ago, after finding that there was no evidence for that association. Moreover, several studies have shown that pioglitazone actually reduces the progression of cardiovascular disease and cardiovascular events in patients with and without T2DM [45–48].

Of particular interest, pioglitazone has consistently shown to improve hepatic steatosis and NASH in patients with and without T2DM [43, 49]. This is important as ~70% of patients with T2DM are believed to have nonalcoholic fatty liver disease, of whom ~50% may have the more severe form with inflammation and necrosis (i.e., NASH) [23]. In patients with T2DM and NASH, current guidelines suggest that pioglitazone should be strongly considered early-on after metformin [21, 22]. This has also been embraced by the American Diabetes Association 2018 guidelines for patients with T2DM and NASH. Unlike pioglitazone, rosiglitazone did not show any significant liver histological benefit in patients with NASH [50], suggesting that pioglitazone may have additional mechanisms of action to improve liver histology other than the currently known classical PPAR-γ pathways.

Thiazolidinediones' benefits (glycemic control, resolution of NASH, reduction of cardiovascular disease, and improvement of polycystic ovarian syndrome) should be weighed against the potential risks of this group of drugs. Fluid retention and peripheral edema may occur in ~7–10% of patients on TZDs, and this percentage increases when combined with insulin [42]. Several mechanisms are likely to contribute to this side effect, being enhanced renal water and sodium reabsorption probably the most important one. Thiazolidinediones can also increase heart failure symptoms in patients with pre-existing disease, and therefore, are contraindicated in patients with known heart failure. They also produce weight gain (in the range of 1–5 kg with chronic use), mild anemia, and a slight increase in bone fractures probably due to a reduction in bone mineral density. In 2011, pioglitazone was associated with bladder cancer [51]. Since then, several studies have tried to replicate those results in retrospective and prospective studies with varying results [52–54]. A recent meta-analysis has reported that out of the 23 epidemiological studies published to date, 18 showed no association between bladder cancer and pioglitazone, while those that have reported an association were not confirmed in the same population in subsequent analysis, or either had a significant detection bias or patients on the TZD had significantly more risk factors for bladder cancer than the comparison group [55].

Insulin, Insulin Analogues, and Insulin Secretagogues

Insulin and Insulin Analogs

It is beyond the scope of this review to describe the pharmacodynamic and pharmacokinetic properties of the different insulin preparations, the most appropriate insulin regimen for patients with T2DM, as well as the practical issues to starting or adjusting insulin dosing. We refer the reader to dedicated articles where they have been reviewed in-depth [56, 57].

Insulin analogs can be classified based on their distinctive half-lives: (a) rapid-acting analogs (e.g., aspart, lispro, glulisine, and inhaled insulin); (b) short-acting insulin (e.g., regular); (c) intermediate-acting insulin (e.g., human NPH); (d) long-acting analogs (e.g., glargine, detemir, and degludec); (e) concentrated insulins (e.g., glargine U-300, degludec U-200, NPH U-500) and (f) premixed insulin products (e.g., NPH/regular 70/30, 70/30 aspart mix, 75/25 lispro mix, 50/50 lispro mix). For most patients with T2DM, basal insulin alone is the most convenient initial insulin regimen, beginning with 10–20 IU daily or 0.1–0.3 IU/kg daily. However, many of these patients will require mealtime bolus insulin dosing with disease progression [33]. Rapid-acting analogs are preferred for bolus dosing due to their faster onset of action.

The most common side effect of insulin is hypoglycemia, and special care should be paid to try to avoid them as much as possible, to reduce the risk of cognitive decline and other important deleterious outcomes. Another common side effect of insulin therapy are weight gain and peripheral edema. Less frequent side effects include: self-limited blurred vision (usually at the beginning of therapy, it is likely the result of a disbalance in the osmotic equilibrium between the lens and ocular fluids) or electrolyte disturbances most commonly observed during treatment of an acute decompensation as in diabetic ketoacidosis (e.g., hypokalemia, hypomagnesemia, and/or hypophosphatemia). Dermatologic reactions to insulin can result in lipohypertrophy (as insulin is lipogenic) or lipoatrophy (probably immunologically mediated). The frequency of lipoatrophy has significantly reduced since the introduction of biosynthetic human insulin, and can also be reduced by alternating the injection site. Less than 1% of patients may present with hypersensitivity at injection sites, with inflammation and/or subcutaneous nodules [33].

Sulfonylureas

The main mechanism of sulfonylureas is to increase insulin secretion by binding to the sulfonylurea receptor (SUR1). They act by inhibiting the ATP-dependent K^+ channel on pancreatic ß-cells [58]. As a consequence of this, ß-cells become depolarized, which produces an influx of calcium into the cytosol and insulin exocytosis. Of note, sulfonylureas induce insulin secretion independently of glucose levels, and they can therefore increase the risk of hypoglycemia [58].

They should be taken 30 min before meals and the typical starting dose should be low and up-titrated every 2 weeks if glycemic control has not been reached [33]. They should be given once or twice per day as they have a prolonged biological effect that lasts longer than their plasma half-life due to receptor interaction and active metabolites. Shorter-duration sulfonylureas, such as glipizide, are preferred due to lower risk of hypoglycemia [33].

While they are usually well tolerated, they still have significant side effects that should be considered. As mentioned above, the most common side effect is hypoglycemia and these episodes can be even more frequent and serious in the elderly, undernourished, in the setting of alcohol abuse, or after exercise or a missed meal. They also produce significant weight gain. Other less common side effects include skin reactions such as erythema multiforme, exfoliative dermatitis, and photosensitivity. Abnormal liver function tests have also been observed. The most important deleterious aspect is their potential for increasing the risk of acute myocardial infarction, stroke, or death, compared with metformin or other agents [58–60].

The only advantage of this class of oral agents is their low cost. However, their risk of causing hypoglycemia is high, which combined with their potential to increase cardiovascular disease, makes them the least desirable option for the management of patients with T2DM.

Meglitinides

Meglitinides (repaglinide and nateglinide) have a similar mechanism of action as sulfonylureas, but they use a different pancreatic ß-cell receptor. They are also structurally different, and therefore they can be used despite sulfonylurea allergy. They have a rapid onset of action and short half-life. Like sulfonylureas, they should be administered with meals. Side effects include weight gain and hypoglycemia. Repaglinide is mainly metabolized in the liver, therefore it can be used safely in patients with chronic kidney disease [61]. However, the fact that they must be given with each meal (making adherence challenging), and that other agents may be more effective to lower postprandial glucose levels, has largely relegated this class of agents to an infrequent use.

Incretin-Mimetics

Glucagon-Like Peptide (GLP)-1 Receptor Agonists (GLP-1RAs)

The incretin effect is responsible for 50–70% of total insulin secretion after oral glucose administration, but it is absent if intravenous glucose is administered. One of such incretin hormones is GLP-1, which has a short half-life because it is quickly inactivated by dipeptidyl peptidase (DDP)-4. In addition to increasing insulin secretion in a glucose-dependent manner, GLP-1RAs also suppress elevated glucagon levels, delay gastric emptying, suppress appetite, and induce weight loss [33]. Beyond their beneficial effects in glycemic controls, some members of this class, such as liraglutide [62] and semaglutide [63], have shown to reduce cardiovascular events, cardiovascular mortality, and even overall mortality. Similar results have not been reported with other GLP-1 agonists, such as lixisenatide [64] or long-acting once weekly exenatide [65], and therefore it remains unclear whether differences are attributable to the different populations studied or really unique properties of some GLP-1RAs in the class.

Glucagon-like peptide-1 agonists have become widely used in patients with T2DM and their metabolic effects have been quite consistent across studies. They are administered by subcutaneous injections and can be classified based on their half-lives in short-acting (exenatide twice daily [BID], lixisenatide once daily [QD]) or long-acting (liraglutide QD, albiglutide once weekly [QW], dulaglutide QW, semaglutide QW, and exenatide long-acting release QW) [33]. Among their side effects, nausea, vomiting, and diarrhea are probably the most common ones, but patients usually develop tolerance to them with chronic use. However, they are contraindicated in patients with gastroparesis. The risk of hypoglycemia is low as insulin secretion is stimulated only if the plasma glucose levels are elevated [62]. These medications have been found to slightly increase heart rate, most likely as a reflex secondary to blood pressure reduction [33]. Injection site reactions, such as rash, erythema, or pruritus are frequent with these drugs. Patients may develop antibodies against the GLP-1 agonists, but the clinical significance of such antibodies is unclear (although more injection site reactions are observed in patients with positive antibodies). In most cases, they appear not to affect efficacy of the drugs [33]. There has been some concern regarding the association of this group of drugs with pancreatitis, pancreatic cancer, and medullar thyroid carcinoma. However, studies have shown conflicting results regarding these associations, and therefore more research is needed before final conclusions can be drawn. A recent meta-analysis that included 113 randomized controlled trials did not find an increased incidence of pancreatitis or of pancreatic cancer with GLP1-RA therapy versus comparator arms, but there was a small but significant greater risk of cholelithiasis (OR [95% CI] 1.30 [1.01–1.68], P = 0.041) [66]. Of note, there have also been reports of GLP-1RAs resulting in significant improvements in patients with psoriasis [67]. While this awaits further confirmation in larger studies, a potential explanation for this effect comes from studies showing an overexpression of GLP-1 receptors in psoriatic plaques likely due to infiltration with immune cells [68].

Dipeptidyl Peptidase (DDP)-4 Inhibitors

In the United States, this class of drugs includes saxagliptin, sitagliptin, linagliptin, and alogliptin. They inhibit DPP-4, the enzyme responsible for the degradation of GLP-1 (among other peptides), potentiating endogenous GLP-1 action on pancreatic β-cells. However, they are likely to have a broader spectrum of effects that are just now being better understood, as reviewed elsewhere [69]. While they share the incretin effect with GLP-1 agonists, they have several important differences with that drug group.

This class of oral medications leads to a modest improvement in hemoglobin A1c (~0.7% compared to decreases between 1.0 and 1.5% with other classes of oral agents or GLP-1RA) [33]. As DPP-4 is an enzyme expressed on most cell types and deactivates many different bioactive peptides in addition to GLP-1, its inhibition probably affects plasma glucose by different mechanisms [69]. They only show a modest effect on plasma GLP-1 levels when compared to GLP-1RAs. Unlike GLP-1RAs, they do not produce significant weight loss, and although they have proven to be safe from a cardiovascular standpoint, they have not shown any cardiovascular improvement like some GLP-1RAs [70, 71]. Moreover, in a large randomized controlled trial with saxagliptin, there was a small but significant increase in hospitalizations for heart failure [71]. This has not been found with other members of this class and it remains unclear if it is a real effect or not, as some observational studies have failed to observe such effect on heart failure with saxagliptin [33, 69].

This group of drugs have been usually very well tolerated and they have a low risk of hypoglycemia. They are popular among clinicians given their good safety profile, relative low-cost and that they all have been combined in a tablet formulation with metformin to improve patient adherence. The most commonly reported side effects are headache, nasopharyngitis, and upper respiratory tract infection [33]. While acute pancreatitis has been reported with these drugs, and there is some concern for pancreatic cancer, it is still unknown whether there is a causal relationship [33, 69, 72]. There have been several reports of skin lesions with these drugs, including hypersensitivity reactions, angioedema, and blistering skin conditions (e.g., Stevens–Johnson syndrome). Of note, use of a DPP-4 inhibitor in combination with an ACE inhibitor may further increase the risk of angioedema due to prolongation of bradykinin and substance P half-lives [33]. Linagliptin is the only member of the group that is primarily eliminated via the enterohepatic system, and therefore, it does not require dose adjustment for chronic kidney disease as the other drugs of the group.

Sodium-Glucose Cotransporter (SGLT)-2 Inhibitors

This group of drugs is composed of canagliflozin, dapagliflozin, and empagliflozin [33]. Their mechanism of action is inhibition of SGLT-2 transporters in the renal proximal tubule, promoting urinary glucose excretion. Their glucose-lowering effect therefore depends on the filtered glucose load (i.e., baseline hyperglycemia) [33].

In addition to their glucose-lowering effects, these drugs have shown to have a number of other beneficial metabolic effects. Both empagliflozin and canagliflozin have shown to reduce the composite primary outcome of death from cardiovascular causes, nonfatal myocardial infarction, or nonfatal stroke in large randomized controlled trials [73, 74]. Moreover, they both significantly decreased heart failure hospitalization compared to placebo. While empagliflozin [73], but not canagliflozin [74], significantly reduced overall cardiovascular mortality, both had similar mean reductions despite different confident intervals [73, 74]. Additional benefits of these drugs are to reduce blood pressure, delay the progression of microvascular disease, and produce modest weight loss. These benefits occur despite a small increase in plasma LDL-C [73, 74].

As these drugs produce an osmotic diuresis, it is important to pay attention to the volume status of patients when starting these drugs and during follow-up [33]. They have been associated with orthostatic hypotension, dehydration, and/or acute kidney injury. This is even more frequent in elderly patients or those concomitantly taking diuretics, ACE inhibitors or angiotensin receptor blockers (ARB) [75]. Potential hyperkalemia has also been observed. Because of this, use in elderly populations should be done with care [33]. Patients taking these medications are at increased risk of urinary tract infections (especially in women), acute balanitis or balanoposthitis, and vulvovaginal candida infections [75]. Among other less frequent, but potentially more serious adverse events, there may be an increase risk of bone fractures, especially in patients taking canagliflozin [75]. While the mechanism remains elusive, it is suspected that increased falls (due to volume depletion) may play an important role in this increase. However, reduced bone mineral density has also been reported [76]. Euglycemic diabetes ketoacidosis has also been reported in patients with T2DM on SGLT-2 inhibitors. This occurs mainly in patients with type 1 diabetes mellitus or T2DM concomitantly using insulin, after decreasing insulin doses due to better control when a SGLT-2 inhibitor is added or after prolonged fasting [77]. Canagliflozin has also been associated with increased amputation risk [74]. Patients on canagliflozin with a previous amputation, peripheral vascular disease, and/or neuropathy were at highest risk for amputation. At the current time, it is unclear whether other members of this drug class can also lead to amputations. Dapagliflozin has been associated with bladder cancer, but it is unknown whether this is a causal association [78].

Conclusions

Hyperglycemia in T2DM develops as pancreatic β-cells fail to meet the demands of chronic insulin resistance and acquired insults, such as obesity, in genetically predisposed subjects. As more drugs become available for the treatment of T2DM, health care providers are more frequently faced with the burden of making decisions regarding the most appropriate medication for each patient. Due to its safety profile, efficacy, low cost, cardiovascular benefits and long-term clinical experience, metformin has consolidated as the first-line therapy for T2DM. The question remains what the best second line of therapy is. The results from recent large randomized controlled trials of diabetes medications showing cardiovascular risk reduction will make some GLP-1RAs (liraglutide, semaglutide) and SGLT2 inhibitors (empagliflozin, canagliflozin) second-line therapy for patients with T2DM and proven cardiovascular disease. In patients with T2DM and NASH, pioglitazone will become the agent of choice given its benefit in this population. Ultimately, physicians must individualize care to the unique medical and social situation of each patient. However, optimizing therapy is a challenge when we do not routinely measure insulin resistance or insulin secretion in our patients when we choose treatment. Doctors would probably benefit from understanding in each patient what is their predominant metabolic defect leading to hyperglycemia. Unfortunately, we basically choose treatment based on their cost, safety profile, and physicians'/patients' personal preferences. A more targeted treatment approach will likely be beneficial in the future. The choices mentioned above based on liver or cardiovascular disease are a beginning. Clearly, more work is needed to better tailor treatment in the future.

References

1. DeFronzo RA, Ferrannini E, Groop L, Henry RR, Herman WH, Holst JJ, et al. Type 2 diabetes mellitus. Nat Rev Dis Primers. 2015;1:15019.
2. Cusi K. The epidemic of type 2 diabetes mellitus: its links to obesity, insulin resistance, and lipotoxicity. In: Regensteiner JG, Reusch JEB, Stewart KJ, Veves A, editors. Diabetes and exercise. 1st ed. New York: Humana Press; 2009. p. 3–54.
3. Cusi K. The role of adipose tissue and lipotoxicity in the pathogenesis of type 2 diabetes. Curr Diab Rep. 2010;10:306–15.
4. Caprio S, Perry R, Kursawe R. Adolescent obesity and insulin resistance: roles of ectopic fat accumulation and adipose inflammation. Gastroenterology. 2017;152:1638–46.
5. Cusi K. Role of obesity and lipotoxicity in the development of nonalcoholic steatohepatitis: pathophysiology and clinical implications. Gastroenterology. 2012;142:711–25. e716
6. Parker VE, Semple RK. Genetics in endocrinology: genetic forms of severe insulin resistance: what endocrinologists should know. Eur J Endocrinol. 2013;169:R71–80.
7. Semple RK, Savage DB, Cochran EK, Gorden P, O'Rahilly S. Genetic syndromes of severe insulin resistance. Endocr Rev. 2011;32:498–514.
8. Semple RK. EJE PRIZE 2015: how does insulin resistance arise, and how does it cause disease? Human genetic lessons. Eur J Endocrinol. 2016;174:R209–23.
9. Cusi K. Lessons learned from studying families genetically predisposed to type 2 diabetes mellitus. Curr Diab Rep. 2009;9:200–7.
10. Repaske DR. Medication-induced diabetes mellitus. Pediatr Diabetes. 2016;17:392–7.
11. Asghar A, Sheikh N. Role of immune cells in obesity induced low grade inflammation and insulin resistance. Cell Immunol. 2017;315:18–26.
12. Sell H, Habich C, Eckel J. Adaptive immunity in obesity and insulin resistance. Nat Rev Endocrinol. 2012;8:709–16.
13. Unger RH. Lipotoxicity in the pathogenesis of obesity-dependent NIDDM. Genetic and clinical implications. Diabetes. 1995;44:863–70.
14. Bril F, Lomonaco R, Cusi K. The challenge of managing dyslipidemia in patients with nonalcoholic fatty liver disease. Clin Lipidol. 2012;7:471–81.

15. Lomonaco R, Ortiz-Lopez C, Orsak B, Webb A, Hardies J, Darland C, et al. Effect of adipose tissue insulin resistance on metabolic parameters and liver histology in obese patients with nonalcoholic fatty liver disease. Hepatology. 2012;55:1389–97.
16. Unger RH, Scherer PE, Holland WL. Dichotomous roles of leptin and adiponectin as enforcers against lipotoxicity during feast and famine. Mol Biol Cell. 2013;24:3011–5.
17. Bril F, Cusi K. Nonalcoholic fatty liver disease: the new complication of type 2 diabetes mellitus. Endocrinol Metab Clin N Am. 2016;45:765–81.
18. Sunny NE, Bril F, Cusi K. Mitochondrial adaptation in nonalcoholic fatty liver disease: novel mechanisms and treatment strategies. Trends Endocrinol Metab. 2017;28:250–60.
19. Bril F, Barb D, Portillo-Sanchez P, Biernacki D, Lomonaco R, Suman A, et al. Metabolic and histological implications of intrahepatic triglyceride content in nonalcoholic fatty liver disease. Hepatology. 2017;65:1132–44.
20. Bril F, Sninsky JJ, Baca AM, Superko HR, Portillo Sanchez P, Biernacki D, et al. Hepatic steatosis and insulin resistance, but not steatohepatitis, promote atherogenic dyslipidemia in NAFLD. J Clin Endocrinol Metab. 2016;101:644–52.
21. Chalasani N, Younossi Z, Lavine JE, Charlton M, Cusi K, Rinella M, et al. The diagnosis and management of nonalcoholic fatty liver disease: practice guidance from the American Association for the Study of Liver Diseases. Hepatology. 2017. https://doi.org/10.1002/hep.29367.
22. European Association for the Study of the Liver (EASL), European Association for the Study of Diabetes (EASD), European Association for the Study of Obesity (EASO). EASL-EASD-EASO clinical practice guidelines for the management of non-alcoholic fatty liver disease. Diabetologia. 2016;59:1121–40.
23. Bril F, Cusi K. Management of nonalcoholic fatty liver disease in patients with type 2 diabetes: a call to action. Diabetes Care. 2017;40:419–30.
24. Belfort R, Mandarino L, Kashyap S, Wirfel K, Pratipanawatr T, Berria R, et al. Dose-response effect of elevated plasma free fatty acid on insulin signaling. Diabetes. 2005;54:1640–8.
25. Kashyap SR, Belfort R, Berria R, Suraamornkul S, Pratipranawatr T, Finlayson J, et al. Discordant effects of a chronic physiological increase in plasma FFA on insulin signaling in healthy subjects with or without a family history of type 2 diabetes. Am J Physiol Endocrinol Metab. 2004;287:E537–46.
26. Kashyap S, Belfort R, Cersosimo E, Lee S, Cusi K. Chronic low-dose lipid infusion in healthy subjects induces markers of endothelial activation independent of its metabolic effects. J Cardiometab Syndr. 2008;3:141–6.
27. Amati F, Dube JJ, Alvarez-Carnero E, Edreira MM, Chomentowski P, Coen PM, et al. Skeletal muscle triglycerides, diacylglycerols, and ceramides in insulin resistance: another paradox in endurance-trained athletes? Diabetes. 2011;60:2588–97.
28. Iozzo P, Pratipanawatr T, Pijl H, Vogt C, Kumar V, Pipek R, et al. Physiological hyperinsulinemia impairs insulin-stimulated glycogen synthase activity and glycogen synthesis. Am J Physiol Endocrinol Metab. 2001;280:E712–9.
29. Abdul-Ghani MA, Tripathy D, DeFronzo RA. Contributions of beta-cell dysfunction and insulin resistance to the pathogenesis of impaired glucose tolerance and impaired fasting glucose. Diabetes Care. 2006;29:1130–9.
30. Del Prato S, Leonetti F, Simonson DC, Sheehan P, Matsuda M, DeFronzo RA. Effect of sustained physiologic hyperinsulinaemia and hyperglycaemia on insulin secretion and insulin sensitivity in man. Diabetologia. 1994;37:1025–35.
31. Kashyap S, Belfort R, Gastaldelli A, Pratipanawatr T, Berria R, Pratipanawatr W, et al. A sustained increase in plasma free fatty acids impairs insulin secretion in nondiabetic subjects genetically predisposed to develop type 2 diabetes. Diabetes. 2003;52:2461–74.
32. Solomon TP, Knudsen SH, Karstoft K, Winding K, Holst JJ, Pedersen BK. Examining the effects of hyperglycemia on pancreatic endocrine function in humans: evidence for in vivo glucotoxicity. J Clin Endocrinol Metab. 2012;97:4682–91.
33. American Diabetes Association. Standards of medical care in diabetes-2017: summary of revisions. Diabetes Care. 2017;40:S4–5.

34. Look AHEAD Research Group, Wing RR, Bolin P, Brancati FL, Bray GA, Clark JM, et al. Cardiovascular effects of intensive lifestyle intervention in type 2 diabetes. N Engl J Med. 2013;369:145–54.
35. Vilar-Gomez E, Martinez-Perez Y, Calzadilla-Bertot L, Torres-Gonzalez A, Gra-Oramas B, Gonzalez-Fabian L, et al. Weight loss through lifestyle modification significantly reduces features of nonalcoholic steatohepatitis. Gastroenterology. 2015;149:367–78.
36. Keidar A. Bariatric surgery for type 2 diabetes reversal: the risks. Diabetes Care. 2011;34(Suppl 2):S361–266.
37. Adams TD, Davidson LE, Litwin SE, Kim J, Kolotkin RL, Nanjee MN, Gutierrez JM, Frogley SJ, Ibele AR, Brinton EA, Hopkins PN, McKinlay R, Simper SC, Hunt SC. Weight and metabolic outcomes 12 years after gastric bypass. N Engl J Med. 2017;377:1143–55.
38. Rena G, hardie DG, Pearson ER. The mechanisms of action of metformin. Diabetologia. 2017;60:1577–85.
39. Madiraju AK, Erion DM, Rahimi Y, Zhang XM, Braddock DT, Albright RA, et al. Metformin suppresses gluconeogenesis by inhibiting mitochondrial glycerophosphate dehydrogenase. Nature. 2014;510:542–6.
40. Goldberg RB, Kendall DM, Deeg MA, Buse JB, Zagar AJ, Pinaire JA, et al. A comparison of lipid and glycemic effects of pioglitazone and rosiglitazone in patients with type 2 diabetes and dyslipidemia. Diabetes Care. 2005;28:1547–54.
41. Soccio RE, Chen ER, Lazar MA. Thiazolidinediones and the promise of insulin sensitization in type 2 diabetes. Cell Metab. 2014;20:573–91.
42. Yau H, Rivera K, Lomonaco R, Cusi K. The future of thiazolidinedione therapy in the management of type 2 diabetes mellitus. Curr Diab Rep. 2013;13:329–41.
43. Cusi K, Orsak B, Bril F, Lomonaco R, Hecht J, Ortiz-Lopez C, et al. Long-term pioglitazone treatment for patients with nonalcoholic steatohepatitis and prediabetes or type 2 diabetes mellitus: a randomized trial. Ann Intern Med. 2016;165:305–15.
44. Nissen SE, Wolski K. Effect of rosiglitazone on the risk of myocardial infarction and death from cardiovascular causes. N Engl J Med. 2007;356:2457–71.
45. Mazzone T, Meyer PM, Feinstein SB, Davidson MH, Kondos GT, D'Agostino RB Sr, et al. Effect of pioglitazone compared with glimepiride on carotid intima-media thickness in type 2 diabetes: a randomized trial. JAMA. 2006;296:2572–81.
46. Nissen SE, Nicholls SJ, Wolski K, Nesto R, Kupfer S, Perez A, et al. Comparison of pioglitazone vs glimepiride on progression of coronary atherosclerosis in patients with type 2 diabetes: the PERISCOPE randomized controlled trial. JAMA. 2008;299:1561–73.
47. Dormandy JA, Charbonnel B, Eckland DJ, Erdmann E, Massi-Benedetti M, Moules IK, et al. Secondary prevention of macrovascular events in patients with type 2 diabetes in the PROactive study (PROspective pioglitAzone clinical trial in macroVascular events): a randomised controlled trial. Lancet. 2005;366:1279–89.
48. Kernan WN, Viscoli CM, Furie KL, Young LH, Inzucchi SE, Gorman M, et al. Pioglitazone after ischemic stroke or transient ischemic attack. N Engl J Med. 2016;374:1321–31.
49. Belfort R, Harrison SA, Brown K, Darland C, Finch J, Hardies J, et al. A placebo-controlled trial of pioglitazone in subjects with nonalcoholic steatohepatitis. N Engl J Med. 2006;355:2297–307.
50. Ratziu V, Giral P, Jacqueminet S, Charlotte F, Hartemann-Heurtier A, Serfaty L, et al. Rosiglitazone for nonalcoholic steatohepatitis: one-year results of the randomized placebo-controlled fatty liver improvement with rosiglitazone therapy (FLIRT) trial. Gastroenterology. 2008;135:100–10.
51. Lewis JD, Ferrara A, Peng T, Hedderson M, Bilker WB, Quesenberry CP Jr, et al. Risk of bladder cancer among diabetic patients treated with pioglitazone: interim report of a longitudinal cohort study. Diabetes Care. 2011;34:916–22.
52. Lewis JD, Habel LA, Quesenberry CP, Strom BL, Peng T, Hedderson MM, et al. Pioglitazone use and risk of bladder cancer and other common cancers in persons with diabetes. JAMA. 2015;314:265–77.

53. Tuccori M, Filion KB, Yin H, Yu OH, Platt RW, Azoulay L. Pioglitazone use and risk of bladder cancer: population based cohort study. BMJ. 2016;352:i1541.
54. Korhonen P, Heintjes EM, Williams R, Hoti F, Christopher S, Majak M, et al. Pioglitazone use and risk of bladder cancer in patients with type 2 diabetes: retrospective cohort study using datasets from four European countries. BMJ. 2016;354:i3903.
55. Levin D, Bell S, Sund R, Hartikainen SA, Tuomilehto J, Pukkala E, et al. Pioglitazone and bladder cancer risk: a multipopulation pooled, cumulative exposure analysis. Diabetologia. 2015;58:493–504.
56. Lasserson DS, Glasziou P, Perera R, Holman RR, Farmer AJ. Optimal insulin regimens in type 2 diabetes mellitus: systematic review and meta-analyses. Diabetologia. 2009;52:1990–2000.
57. Fonseca VA, Haggar MA. Achieving glycaemic targets with basal insulin in T2DM by individualizing treatment. Nat Rev Endocrinol. 2014;10:276–81.
58. Roumie CL, Hung AM, Greevy RA, et al. Comparative effectiveness of sulfonylurea and metformin monotherapy on cardiovascular events in type 2 diabetes mellitus: a cohort study. Ann Intern Med. 2012;157:601–10.
59. Pladevall M, Riera-Guardia N, Margulis AV, Varas-Lorenzo C, Calingaert B, Perez-Gutthann S. Cardiovascular risk associated with the use of glitazones, metformin and sufonylureas: meta-analysis of published observational studies. BMC Cardiovasc Disord. 2016;16:14.
60. Azoulay L, Suissa S. Sulfonylureas and the risks of cardiovascular events and death: a methodological meta-regression analysis of the observational studies. Diabetes Care. 2017;40:706–14.
61. Guardado-Mendoza R, Prioletta A, Jimenez-Ceja LM, Sosale A, Folli F. The role of nateglinide and repaglinide, derivatives of meglitinide, in the treatment of type 2 diabetes mellitus. Arch Med Sci. 2013;9:936–43.
62. Marso SP, Daniels GH, Brown-Frandsen K, Kristensen P, Mann JF, Nauck MA, et al. Liraglutide and cardiovascular outcomes in type 2 diabetes. N Engl J Med. 2016;375:311–22.
63. Marso SP, Bain SC, Consoli A, Eliaschewitz FG, Jodar E, Leiter LA, et al. Semaglutide and cardiovascular outcomes in patients with type 2 diabetes. N Engl J Med. 2016;375:1834–44.
64. Pfeffer MA, Claggett B, Diaz R, Dickstein K, Gerstein HC, Kober LV, et al. Lixisenatide in patients with type 2 diabetes and acute coronary syndrome. N Engl J Med. 2015;373:2247–57.
65. Holman RR, Bethel MA, Mentz RJ, Thompson VP, Lokhnygina Y, Buse JB, Chan JC, Choi J, Gustavson SM, Iqbal N, Maggioni AP, Marso SP, Öhman P, Pagidipati NJ, Poulter N, Ramachandran A, Zinman B, Hernandez AF, EXSCEL Study Group. Effects of once-weekly exenatide on cardiovascular outcomes in type 2 diabetes. N Engl J Med. 2017;377:1228–39.
66. Monami M, Nreu B, Scatena A, Cresci B, Andreozzi F, Sesti G, Mannucci E. Safety issues with glucagon-like peptide-1 receptor agonists (pancreatitis, pancreatic cancer and cholelithiasis): data from randomized controlled trials. Diabetes Obes Metab. 2017;19:1233–41.
67. Drucker DJ, Rosen CF. Glucagon-like peptide-1 (GLP-1) receptor agonists, obesity and psoriasis: diabetes meets dermatology. Diabetologia. 2011;54:2741–4.
68. Faurschou A, Pedersen J, Gyldenlove M, Poulsen SS, Holst JJ, Thyssen JP, et al. Increased expression of glucagon-like peptide-1 receptors in psoriasis plaques. Exp Dermatol. 2013;22:150–2.
69. Andersen ES, Deacon CF, Holst JJ. Do we know the true mechanism of action of the DPP-4 inhibitors? Diabetes Obes Metab. 2017. https://doi.org/10.1111/dom.13018. [Epub ahead of print].
70. Green JB, Bethel MA, Armstrong PW, Buse JB, Engel SS, Garg J, et al. Effect of sitagliptin on cardiovascular outcomes in type 2 diabetes. N Engl J Med. 2015;373:232–42.
71. Scirica BM, Bhatt DL, Braunwald E, Steg PG, Davidson J, Hirshberg B, et al. Saxagliptin and cardiovascular outcomes in patients with type 2 diabetes mellitus. N Engl J Med. 2013;369:1317–26.
72. Gokhale M, Buse JB, Gray CL, Pate V, Marquis MA, Sturmer T. Dipeptidyl-peptidase-4 inhibitors and pancreatic cancer: a cohort study. Diabetes Obes Metab. 2014;16:1247–56.
73. Zinman B, Wanner C, Lachin JM, Fitchett D, Bluhmki E, Hantel S, et al. Empagliflozin, cardiovascular outcomes, and mortality in type 2 diabetes. N Engl J Med. 2015;373:2117–28.

74. Neal B, Perkovic V, Mahaffey KW, de Zeeuw D, Fulcher G, Erondu N, et al. Canagliflozin and cardiovascular and renal events in type 2 diabetes. N Engl J Med. 2017;377:644–57.
75. DeFronzo RA, Norton L, Abdul-Ghani M. Renal, metabolic and cardiovascular considerations of SGLT2 inhibition. Nat Rev Nephrol. 2017;13:11–26.
76. Bilezikian JP, Watts NB, Usiskin K, Polidori D, Fung A, Sullivan D, et al. Evaluation of bone mineral density and bone biomarkers in patients with type 2 diabetes treated with canagliflozin. J Clin Endocrinol Metab. 2016;101:44–51.
77. Peters AL, Buschur EO, Buse JB, Cohan P, Diner JC, Hirsch IB. Euglycemic diabetic ketoacidosis: a potential complication of treatment with sodium-glucose cotransporter 2 inhibition. Diabetes Care. 2015;38:1687–93.
78. Jabbour S, Seufert J, Scheen A, Bailey CJ, Karup C, Langkilde AM. Dapagliflozin in patients with type 2 diabetes mellitus: a pooled analysis of safety data from phase 2b/3 clinical trials. Diabetes Obes Metab. 2017. https://doi.org/10.1111/dom.13124.

Introduction to Cutaneous Manifestations of Diabetes Mellitus

Emilia Noemí Cohen Sabban

Diabetes mellitus (DM) is a chronic endocrinopathy affecting almost every organ and system; and the skin, the largest organ in the body, is not an exception.

It affects individuals regardless of ethnicity, age or socio-economic level, and the number of patients drastically increased and tends to continue to increase globally.

The term "diabetes" comes from the Greek language and means "to go through" making reference to the quick passing of fluids the patient drinks due to increased thirst, from intake to urination. Physicians used to taste urine, therefore, the term "mellitus," which comes from the Latin and refers to the sweet or honey-like flavor glucose gives [1].

DM is caused by a deficiency or improper use (resistance) of insulin (I). The pancreas produces insulin which is necessary for glucose to be transported from the bloodstream into cells, thus providing energy.

I deficit is accompanied by chronic hyperglycemia, responsible for glucose following other non-insulin dependent metabolic pathways in order to reduce sugar concentration on the skin, through the polyols pathway, sugar autoxidation, non-enzymatic glycation (NEG)—[2]. But in turn, they create an unbalance between the antioxidant capacity, which is diminished, and a higher free radical (FR) production, which results in "oxidative stress" with the subsequent vascular inflammation and prothrombotic state, thus playing an essential role in the development of DM complications [3].

Unfortunately, this mechanism reinforces itself, since under hyperglycemia or oxidative stress conditions, as in the case of DM, NEG is accelerated and more AGEs products are generated. There is sufficient evidence showing that the interaction

E.N. Cohen Sabban, M.D.
Dermatology Department, Instituto de Investigaciones Médicas A. Lanari,
University of Buenos Aires (UBA), Buenos Aires, Argentina
e-mail: emicohensabban@gmail.com

between AGEs and their AGE receptor (RAGE) causes oxidative stress, thus closing a vicious circle. More recently, it was also proven that the AGE-RAGE axis is in turn interrelated to the renin-angiotensin system and that both are involved in vascular damage, one of the most significant complications of diabetes [4, 5].

Therefore, all these biochemical alterations (hyperglycemia, insulin deficiency, NEG increase) are responsible for DM complications (microangiopathy, neuropathy, alteration of the immune response, etc.) and they are closely linked to its cutaneous manifestations [6, 7].

Insulin, a multifunctional hormone involved in regulating many cellular processes, is essential for normal proliferation, differentiation and cutaneous metabolism at skin level. It acts on the epidermal cells, specially, on keratinocytes and on the dermal cells, such as fibroblasts. These cells express the insulin receptor (IR), which is activated through its binding to I. Since the I-IR binding accelerates cellular processes, it is logical that higher activity levels are found in proliferating or differentiating epithelia; while IR activation is minimal in keratinocytes which are already fully differentiated.

Hyperglycemia and the alteration of I signaling pathways with a lower IR expression are directly involved in the development of chronic complications of DM because they lower the use of glucose by keratinocytes, as well as differentiation and proliferation [8].

Since DM is a disease that progresses with chronic hyperglycemia due to an I deficiency, the skin will be directly affected in multiple cellular processes, such as poor wound healing [9, 10].

Many theories have been formulated in order to explain how hyperglycemia may generate neural and vascular disorders which are typical of this disease. They may be divided into those emphasizing the direct toxic effect of hyperglycemia and its derivatives on tissue (such as oxidants, hyperosmolarity or glycosylated products), among which the skin is no an exception, and those assigning pathophysiological relevance to a continued alteration of cellular signaling pathways (such as changes in phospholipids or kinases) induced by glucose metabolism products [11].

Diabetes mellitus (DM) expresses itself on the skin through a wide range of signs and symptoms, some of which remain unexplained despite extensive research work [12]. But it has been proven that the impact of DM on the skin stems from the acute metabolic disorder, dermatosis being a sign of increased blood glucose, as in the case of candidiasis, and more frequently, from chronic complications of a prolonged diabetes, such as ulcers [13].

It is estimated that 30% of diabetic patients present cutaneous manifestations during the course of their disease. If we add lesions due to frequent complications, such as vasculopathy and neuropathy, this percentage would increase to ALMOST 100%. Sometimes, cutaneous disease is the first sign of undiagnosed DM. But more frequently, cutaneous changes are observed in patients with diagnosed but poorly managed DM, in that case, their identification by the dermatologist, together with proper metabolic control, may help prevent some of these dermatoses as well as more serious complications. Most of them are related to the long-term effects of

Table 4.1 DM cutaneous manifestations classification [17, 18]

Group 1	Cutaneous markers of DM	30%
Group 2	Cutaneous infections	
Group 3	Dermatoses most frequently related to DM	
Group 4	Cutaneous alterations caused by DM treatment	
Group 5	Vasculopathy-related cutaneous manifestations	almost 100%
Group 6	Neuropathy-related cutaneous manifestations	

DM on skin collagen and microcirculation. In fact, some cutaneous disorders may be a warning to suspect microvascular complications such as diabetic dermopathy or bullous diabeticorum [14]. It is worth highlighting that skin may also be affected by the adverse effects of glucose-lowering drugs.

Cutaneous infections are more frequent in patients diagnosed with T2DM, while autoimmune alterations are more common in Type 1 diabetic patients [15].

There is a correlation between the duration of the disease and the onset of cutaneous lesions, being long-standing diabetics the ones that present the most devastating cutaneous lesions; although they may also appear in the short term [16].

There are different classifications for cutaneous manifestation of DM, below we include one that divides them into six groups (Table 4.1).

In the following chapters, we will refer to each group and their cutaneous manifestations.

References

1. Real Academia Española. Diccionario de la lengua española. Madrid: RAE; 2001.
2. Cohen Sabban E. La glicosilación no enzimática: una vía común en la diabetes y el envejecimiento. Med Cutan Ibero Lat Am. 2011;39:243–6.
3. Yamagishi S. Advanced glycation end products and receptor-oxidative stress system in diabetic vascular complications. Ther Apher Dial. 2009;13:534–9.
4. Yamagishi S. Role of advanced glycation end products (AGEs) and receptor for AGEs (RAGE) in vascular damage in diabetes. Exp Gerontol. 2011;46:217–24.
5. Yamagishi SI, Maeda S, Matsui T, Ueda S, Fukami K, Okuda S. Role of advanced glycation end products (AGEs) and oxidative stress in vascular complications in diabetes. Biochim Biophys Acta. 2012;1820:663–71.
6. Huntley AC. Cutaneous manifestations of diabetes mellitus. Diabetes Metab Rev. 1993;9:161–76.
7. Ahmed K, Muhammad Z, Qayum I. Prevalence of cutaneous manifestations of diabetes mellitus. J Ayub Med Coll Abbottabad. 2009;21:76–9.
8. Spravchikov N, Sizyakov G, Gartsbein M, Accili D, Tennenbaum T, Wertheimer E. Glucose effects on skin keratinocytes: implications for diabetes skin complications. Diabetes. 2001;50:1627–35.
9. Wertheimer E. Diabetic skin complications: a need for reorganizing the categories of diabetes-associated complications. Isr Med Assoc J. 2004;6:287–9.
10. Wertheimer E, Trebicz M, Eldar T, Gartsbein M, Nofeh-Moses S, Tennenbaum T. Differential roles of insulin receptor and insulin-like growth factor-1 receptor in differentiation of murine skin keratinocytes. J Invest Dermatol. 2000;115:24–9.
11. Sheetz MJ, King GL. Molecular understanding of hyperglycemia's adverse effects for diabetic complications. JAMA. 2002;288(20):2579–88.

12. Chatterjee N, Chattopadhyay C, Sengupta N, Das C, Sarma N, Pal SK. An observational study of cutaneous manifestations in diabetes mellitus in a tertiary care Hospital of Eastern India. Indian J Endocrinol Metab. 2014;18(2):217–20.
13. Goyal A, Raina S, Kaushal SS, Mahajan V, Sharma NL. Pattern of cutaneous manifestations in diabetes mellitus. Indian J Dermatol. 2010;55(1):39–41.
14. Horton WB, Boler PL, Subauste AR. Diabetes mellitus and the skin: recognition and management of cutaneous manifestations. South Med J. 2016;109(10):636–46.
15. Van Hattem S, Bootsma AH, Thio HB. Skin manifestations of diabetes. Cleve Clin J Med. 2008;75(11):772–87.
16. Ahmed I, Goldstein B. Diabetes mellitus. Clin Dermatol. 2006;24:237–46.
17. Cabo HA. Diabetes y piel [tesis doctoral]. Facultad de Medicina, UBA; 1983.
18. American Diabetes Association. Standards of Medical Care in Diabetes-2009. Diabetes Care. 2009;32:13–61.

Cutaneous Barrier, Innate Immunity and Diabetes

5

Patricia Troielli and Lucrecia Juarez

Cutaneous Barrier

CB is defined as a dynamic, functional and morphological structure made up of cells and non-cellular components of the skin which provides an effective isolation of the individual from his environment. It prevents infections, maintains body temperature and electrolyte balance, avoids water loss and limits the damage of oxidative stress and effects of ultraviolet radiation (Table 5.1).

The complex lipid structure that makes up the CB is regulated to keep homeostasis in the skin.

A disturbance of the epidermal barrier function induces a rapid response from the keratinocytes that involves upregulation of the inflammatory signal cytokines, adhesion molecules and growth factors. This leads to epidermal hyperplasia and an increase in lipid synthesis in order to restore normal function.

Several diseases a variety of drugs and therapeutic options may delay repair or alter the healthy barrier's kinetics [1].

The physical barrier localized primarily in the stratum corneum (SC) is crucial in the activity of the epidermal permeability barrier. The viable epidermis and outer nucleated layers also contribute to this skin function. On other hand, the SC is more than just an inert brick wall. In the presence of physiologic stress, it can regulate the rate of corneocytes shedding or desquamation.

In the SC, the corneocytes produced from terminal keratinocyte differentiation build a platform of protein-enriched cells, the cornified envelope, formed through

P. Troielli, M.D. (✉)
School of Medicine, University of Buenos Aires, Buenos Aires, Argentina
e-mail: ptroielli@gmail.com

L. Juarez, M.D.
School of Medicine, University of Buenos Aires, Buenos Aires, Argentina

School of Medicine, University of La Plata, Buenos Aires, Argentina
e-mail: dralucreciajuarez@gmail.com

© Springer International Publishing AG 2018
E.N. Cohen Sabban et al. (eds.), *Dermatology and Diabetes*,
https://doi.org/10.1007/978-3-319-72475-1_5

Table 5.1 Cutaneous barrier functions

Barrier	Role	Effector
Permeability	Prevent excess water loss Protects from harmful chemicals, allergens and microbial pathogens Maintains body temperature	Components of skin structure
Antimicrobial	Protects against multiple pathogens (bacteria fungi and some viruses)	Acidic pH Sphingoid bases Innate immune (antimicrobial peptides)
Antioxidant	Protects skin from oxidative stress	Tocopherol Vitamin C-E Glutathione Ubiquinol Uric acid Small proline rich region proteins (SPRR) Superoxide dismutase
UV	Protects skin from UV DNA damage Protects skin from oxidative stress	Urocanic acid Structure components

specific precursor proteins crosslinking, including involucrin, loricrin, small proline-rich regions proteins (SPRR), transglutaminase, filagrin and corneodesmosomes, surrounded by an enriched neutral lipid, covalently binded into the extracellular space.

Fillagrin, the principal water ligand compound, is a component of the natural moisturizing factor (NMF) cross-linked to the cornified envelope and aggregates keratin filaments into macrofibrils.

The enriched neutral lipid-lamellar membranes localized in the extracellular spaces of the SC are synthesized in the keratinocytes as lamellar bodies (LB) during epidermal differentiation.

LB are secretory organelles 0.2 Å~ 0.3 μ with a predominant role in the maintenance of cutaneous permeability and other activities such as antimicrobial, chemical defense and movement of molecules and proteins from intra to extracellular space.

LB are first observed in the upper stratum spinosum layer of the epidermis, with increasing numbers found in the stratum granulosum layer. This organelles contain phospholipids, glucosylceramides, sphingomyelin, cholesterol and several enzymes. These precursor lipids are converted into non-polar lipid products by enzymes (Fig. 5.1).

Beta-glucocerebrosidase converts glucosylceramides into ceramides, phospholipases convert phospholipids into free fatty acids and glycerol acidic sphingomyelinase converts sphingomyelin into ceramides.

In addition, others enzymes, proteases such as chemotryptic enzymes (kallikreins) and cathepsins, are present in LBs. Enzyme inhibitors, such as the serine protease inhibitor, elafin, are packaged into LBs.

Moreover, antimicrobial peptides (AMP), such as human β-defensin 2 and the cathelicidin LL-37 are also present in LBs [2–5].

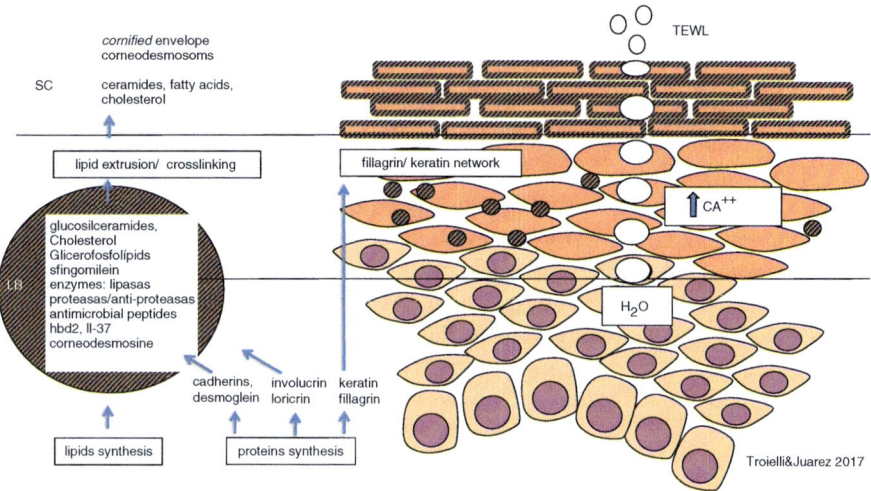

Fig. 5.1 Cutaneous barrier. *LB* lamellar bodies, *SC* stratum corneum, *TEWL* transepidermal water loss (reproduced from Cutaneous Manifestations of Diabetes. Cohen Sabban E.N. 2017)

The SC contains an abundance of cholesterol from the LB, and cholesterol sulfate, that is converted into cholesterol by the Cholesterol Sulfatase enzyme which plays an important role in regulating SC cohesion and desquamation.

Lipids, cholesterol, ceramides and fatty acids must be present in appropriate distribution in stratum granulosum cells in order to synthesize structurally normal LB. Altered metabolism, either in excess or a deficiency of a particular lipid can result in abnormal lamellar bilayer formation and affect normal skin function.

The extracellular processing of lipids leads to a balance of 50% ceramides, 25% cholesterol, and 15% free fatty acids with very little phospholipid.

Topically applied lipids may interfere with the skin barrier function and treatment with formulations containing physiological lipids such as cholesterol, ceramide 3, oleic acid and palmitic acid are suggested as strategy to recover dry skin and inflammatory disorders [2, 6–8].

Lipids required for LB formation are derived from de novo synthesis by keratinocytes and from extra-cutaneous sources not as yet completely identified.

Impaired nutritional status may alter the structural integrity of the skin, as well as a proper nutritional intake. The intake of Ca^{++} and vitamin C complements endogenous factors in regulating skin barrier function [9].

The pH of the skin surface and outer layers is acidic with a pH range from 5 to 5.5 leading to a defense environment against invading organisms and it is necessary for the activity of several enzymes in the SC.

The acidic PH stimulates sphingomyelinase and beta-glucocerebrosidase activity, allowing a normal regulation of ceramides level but also blocks other enzymes such as proteases that need an optimum PH 7 or higher to increase proteolytic activity and induce corneocyte desquamation.

The increase in serine protease activity with pH 7 or higher leads to the activation of protease activated receptor 2 (PAR-2) which can increase the differentiation of keratinocytes into corneocytes and inhibit LB secretion, with severe effect in the homeostasis of the skin.

The importance of preserving an acidic skin PH remains an under recognized topic.

Elderly patients have skin PH increased and ceramide deficit [10]. This is explained by high levels of alkaline enzymes activity, like alkaline ceramidases which are involved in barrier lipid degradation in aged human skin.

Changes in PH predispose to infections. Candidal intertrigo is more frequent in flexural areas with higher PH than in other skin sites.

Diabetics are prone to develop Candidal intertrigo and it has been reported that PH was significantly higher in the intertriginous zones of non-insulin dependent diabetics compared to healthy individuals [11, 12].

Permeability Barrier

Skin hydration level depends on four factors:

1. Presence of natural hygroscopic agents, the NMF within the corneocytes.
2. Presence of endogenous glycerol as a natural moisturizer and hyaluronic acid in the epidermis and dermis.
3. Ordered lamellar arrangement of intercellular lipids in the SC that form a barrier to transepidermal water loss (TEWL).
4. Presence of tight junctions within the stratum granulosum to further impede water loss.

Dry skin can be a symptom in a number of systemic diseases such as psoriasis, diabetes and renal transplantation. The mechanism of xerosis in these disorders is not yet fully understood.

Amino acids (AAs) play important roles in maintaining an optimal hydration state of SC as a component of the natural moisturizing factor (NMF).

These groups of small hydrophilic compounds account for 5–30% of the total dry weight of SC and are the main components to which water binds directly. Small amounts of bound water are associated with the hydrophilic polar groups of intercellular lipids such as sphingomyelin and corneocytes.

The upper SC works like a "sponge" where solutes, ions and antimicrobial peptides contained in the sweat, flow in-out and some are retained.

It has been suggested, that skin hydration depends of arginine, the major component of fillagrin-derived natural moisturizing factors, that is concentrated in the middle layer of the SC.

The low arginine levels in the upper SC are probably due to further metabolic modification, i.e., citrullination, or direct loss to the external environment [13].

Watabe et al., have demonstrated that also sweat contains several NMF, lactate, urea, sodium, and potassium. Lactate and potassium significantly affect the hydration state of SC and reduced sweat delivery to the SC may cause xerosis in several chronic diseases [14].

A case control study found no difference in SC hydration and transepidermal water loss between diabetics and controls [15].

On the other hand, studies suggest that patients with diabetes mellitus tend to show a normal hydration state with decreased sebaceous and sweat gland activity and impaired skin elasticity without impairment of the SC barrier function [16].

It has been proven that hydration state of SC and lipids on the diabetics skin surface decreases with glycemic index over 110 mg/dl.

A long-standing hyperglycemia condition impairs skin barrier by accelerating skin ageing process.

Insulin plays a decisive role in the skin homeostasis. Epidermis constitutes a glycolytic tissue. Keratinocytes insulin receptors make up the system of insulin uptake which regulates the glycemic level in epidermal cells inducing transitory states of hyperglycemia [17].

The properties of the SC in patients with diabetes mellitus have similarities to senile xerosis. Studies show that diabetic rats have normal levels of ceramides and aminoacids but show low levels of triglycerides in SC [18].

The epidermal barrier retains moisture, regulates water flux, and modifies the rate and magnitude of TEWL.

Nowadays, cutaneous barrier recovery and inflammation are instrumentally monitored as TEWL and skin blood flow using the Evaporimeter and Laser Doppler Flowmeter, respectively.

Pathological states of the skin may be detected by measuring the TEWL rate.

The barrier has the ability to detect homeostatic abnormalities at an early stage through mild TEWL increase. The alteration of the Ca^{+2} gradient, the loss of elevated Ca^{+2} in the granular layer is the signal that induces in a few minutes the physiological self-repair mechanism by releasing the lipid stored in the SC. This lipid movement increases the production of fillagrin and fillagrin degradation products like free aminoacids. These pyrrolidone carboxylic acid and urocanic acid with sugar ions form the NMF to restore hydration.

Dermatologic conditions or metabolic diseases with permeability barrier impairment diminish the capacity to adapt to different exogenous physical, infectious and chemical insults. The repair mechanisms are not able to keep up with the magnitude or velocity to restore normal function and without therapeutic intervention the progression of xerosis leads to dry skin with different signs and symptoms of inflammation and infection.

Antioxidant Barrier

Reactive oxygen species (ROS) contribute to the processes of skin ageing and impaired skin barrier function. ROS are particularly harmful in that they destabilize other molecules and promote chain reactions that damage biomolecules rapidly, such as telomere shortening and deterioration, mitochondrial damage, membrane degradation and oxidation of structural and enzymatic proteins [19, 20].

The CB disturbance decreased antioxidant capacity and alters its functions.

The quantity of ROS in the skin is higher than in any other organ and in many cases a clear correlation between ROS (from internal and external origen) and a proaging state can be found.

The skin is at the interface between the body and the environment and is therefore in constant contact with pollutants, xenobiotics, and UV irradiation. These exogenous factors represent the main contributor to ROS production in human skin, therefore being very specific for this organ. Additionally, alcohol intake, nutritional factors and physiological and mechanical stress are believed to contribute to this kind of ROS production. In addition, the skin is also one of the very few organs that are in direct contact with atmospheric oxygen which can contribute to ROS.

Enzymes that are ROS producing, on purpose or as a byproduct, include the mitochondrial electron transport chain, NADPH oxidases, xanthine oxidoreductase (XOR), several peroxisomal oxidases, enzymes of the cytochrome P450 family, cyclooxygenases, and lipoxygenases.

To deal with ROS production, there are specific antioxidant mechanisms in the skin present at an intra and extracellular level. Most of the antioxidants are at higher concentration in the epidermis than in the dermis. This correlates well with the fact that ROS load is higher in the epidermis than in the dermis. Vitamin C, vitamin E, glutathione, ubiquinol, and uric acid are detectable in the SC but their concentration increases steeply towards deeper cell-layers of the SC. These comparably low concentrations of non-enzymatic and lipophilic anti-oxidants in the outer layers of the SC are possible because the cornified envelope itself has anti-oxidative capabilities. These antioxidant capabilities of the cornified envelope rely on the small proline rich region proteins (SPRR).

The highest concentrations of enzymes and antioxidants are found in the stratum granulosum constantly declining towards the stratum basale. In this way, the suprabasal cells have lower ROS levels and are protected against UVB-induced apoptosis. The importance of the SC as an anti-oxidant/UV barrier is also stressed by the fact that UV can completely deplete the stratum corneum of antioxidants/vitamins. Therefore, only the remaining SC proteins (mainly SPRR2 subfamily) can exert their antioxidant properties and protect the epidermal cells.

The formation of structures known as advanced glycation end products (AGEs) can be significantly accelerated by oxidative stress. AGEs originate from the non-enzymatic glycation reaction between sugars and proteins, nucleic acids or lipids. AGEs are a heterogeneous group of molecules and can either be ingested through food consumption or formed inside the cell. Diabetic patients have higher concentrations of AGEs (see Chap. 15).

UV Barrier

Photon energy carried in UV (particularly UVB at 280–315 nm, and UVA at 315–400 nm) induces alterations that accumulate and promote the majority of the typical manifestations of skin ageing and cancer. UVB makes up only 5% of the UV radiation that reaches the earth's surface and has little penetrance but it displays great biological activity. UVA makes up the remaining 95% of incident light and is more penetrating, promoting photo aging. However, UVA carries less energy and therefore promotes carcinogenesis to a lower extent than UVB.

The main effects of acute and chronic exposure to UV radiation are DNA damage, inflammation and immunosuppression. These effects are direct as well as indirect due to ROS production [20].

It has recently been established that ultraviolet (UV) irradiation activates the inflammasome in human keratinocytes [21].

Skin Innate Immune System

The innate immune system employs cells of different tissues, organs and molecules to protect the body from a variety of pathogenic microbes and toxins present in the environment.

The skin innate immune system has numerous functions, including:

1. Action as antimicrobial barrier
2. Activation of the complement cascade
3. Recruitment of innate immune cells.

Controlling the extent of an immune response is thus a major challenge for maintaining skin integrity, which is of paramount importance for host survival [22, 23].

The skin innate immune system can detect and respond to the insults of microbes and danger signals from the environment and from inside the body.

The skin, can sense pathogens and mediate immune response by different types of cell receptors present in keratinocytes, macrophages, mast cells, fibroblasts and nerve-related cell types and in many specialized immune cells, including DCs, CD4$^+$ T helper (T_H) cells, $\gamma\delta$ T cells and natural killer T (NKT) cells.

The Pattern Recognition Receptors (PRRs) including membrane bound Toll Like Receptors (TLRs) and C-type lectin receptors (CLRs), detect Pathogen Associated Molecular Patterns (PAMPs) sensing byproduct microorganisms, such as lipopolysaccharides (LPS), lipopeptides, flagellin, bacterial DNA, double stranded viral RNA, *Candida sp.* wall, components β-Glucans mannans, phospholipomannans of fungus.

The intracellular PRRs are TLRs of the endosomal compartment and Nucleotide-binding Oligomerization Domain proteins (NOD- Like receptors NOD1 and NOD2) that sense Danger Associated Molecular Pattern (DAMPs).

DAMPS are derived from dying cells, small molecules from damaged cell nuclei, ATP, DNA, β Defensins, HMGB1, exogenous particles like asbestos, endogenous like crystals of uric acid, ultraviolet radiation.

NOD1 and NOD2 are intracellular PRRs that recognize bacterial molecules produced during the breakdown of peptidoglycan (PGN), N0D1 recognizes products of gram negative PGN and NOD 2 products of both gram negative and positive PGN.

The differential activation of these receptors results in various complex signaling pathways, NF-KB, MAPK, inflammasomes and leads to the release of regulatory factors and multiple cytokines (IL-1β, IL6, IL8, IL-18, and IL-33) and chemokines.

IL-33, a newly discovered member of the IL-1 family, has been identified as a potent inducer of Th2 type immunity. Emerging evidence implies that IL-33 may also act as an alarm to alert the immune system when released by epithelial barrier tissues during trauma or infection [24].

Wound healing is impaired in diabetic patients owing to overproduction of inflammatory cytokines, and IL-33 has been involved in modulation of uncontrolled inflammatory responses.

Even though the pathology of diabetic wound healing is not totally explained, recent scientific evidence shows that IL-33 supplement may promote induction of M2 macrophages in diabetic mice and accelerate wound closure.

Macrophages are implicated in all stages of wound healing stimulating angiogenesis, fibrosis and reepithelization. Their polarization state (M1 inflammatory type and M2 proliferative type) depends on the microenvironment present in the wound and is essential for tissue repair.

The functional/phenotypic switch Macrophage M1 to M2 does not readily occur in diabetic wounds and the macrophages remain predominantly in a pro-inflammatory M1-activation state and continue the chronic inflammation [25].

Manipulation of IL-33-mediated signal might be a potential therapeutic approach for diabetic skin wounds.

Keratinocytes participate in the innate immune response of the skin. They can sense danger and infections, toxins, irritants via expressing TLRs and inflammasome activation.

They produce lipids, chemokines, cytokines and peptides with antimicrobial activity, antimicrobial peptides (AMPs). Several AMPs are extruded from the LBs to the extracellular space in the SC [3].

The AMPs lead to pores in the microbial membrane with subsequent osmotic lysis and microbial cell death while cationic antimicrobial peptides associate with negatively charged bacterial membrane, many of which have chemotactic properties. There are others AMPs skin sources (Table 5.2).

Human β-defensins (HBD) are generally short and positively charged, and have hydrophobic or amphipathic domains in their folded structure. They are recognized as HBD 1, 2, 3, 4. HBD 3, 4 are predominantly expressed in the skin and have potent

Table 5.2 AMPs skin sources

AMPs	Sources
α defensins	Azurophilic granules of infiltrating neutrophils
β defensins	Keratinocytes and macrophages
Cathelicidin LL37	Keratinocytes, ductal epithelium, eccrine glands, mast cells
Granulysin	Infiltrating T cells
Psoriasin	Keratinocytes, follicular epithelium, sebocytes
Dermcidin	Eccrine glands
RNase	Keratinocytes

antimicrobial activity against gram-positive. Almost all of HBD have activity against gram-negative bacteria and HBD 2, 3, 4 against yeast and viruses.

Cathelicidins antimicrobial peptides (CAMPs) represent another AMPs family. Human cathelicidin hCAP-18 is constitutively expressed by neutrophils and squamous epithelium in response to inflammatory challenge; it is processed by proteinase 3 to generate the active peptide LL-37.

Recent studies demonstrated that ceramide metabolites, ceramide-1-phosphate and sphingosine-1-phosphate produced in human keratinocytes in response to subtoxic levels of endoplasmic reticulum (ER) stress stimulate production of these major epidermal innate immune elements, β defensins and cathelicidin antimicrobial peptides, via STAT1/3- or NF-κB-dependent mechanisms, respectively.

However, patients with T2DM have lower levels of CAMP (LL-37) and DEFB4 (HBD-2) gene expression in peripheral blood cells which probably makes them susceptible to infectious diseases. Furthermore, it has been reported that the expression of DEFB4 is lower in diabetic foot ulcers in comparison with healthy skin suggesting that low levels of this peptide contribute to poor wound healing in diabetic patients [26, 27].

On the other hand, hyperglycemia, both acute and chronic, has a profound effect on host defense response, innate and adaptative immune systems.

High concentration of glucose activates mitogen-activated protein kinases which influence transcription activity in the nucleus, upregulates TLR4 with increased NK-kappa β activation and IL-8 expression, and stimulates p62/PKC interaction which also results in NF-kappa β activation. These events regulate inflammatory responses and can alter both neutrophil and endothelial function.

Studies using both in vitro and in vivo methods have demonstrated defective neutrophil function in prolonged hyperglycemic states. Diabetic patients have higher susceptibility to infection and increased severity of infections compared to non-diabetic patients.

Chronic Hyperglycemic state negatively affects neutrophil respiratory burst capacity and monocytes proliferation irrespective of the phenotype of diabetes, the duration of the disease or insulin use.

Also produces changes in endothelial function that may be secondary to reduced nitric oxide. In vitro studies, high concentrations of glucose and AGEs decrease constitutive nitric oxide synthases.

Complement activation promotes the opsonization and phagocytosis of pathogens by macrophages and neutrophils. It can also cause direct lysis of microbes and the release of mediators (e.g., C3a and C5a), which direct neutrophil migration and chemotaxis.

Several studies have shown that elevated glucose levels affect the complement cascade system, blocking the complement fixation and reducing opsonization delay bacterial clearance [28].

The impact of a **diagnosis** of diabetes may lead to increased **stress** in patients and psychosocial stress affects the immune response, barrier function, wound healing and resistance to infection of healthy skin. Psychosocial stress results in a delay in barrier recovery and impairs the expression and the production of antimicrobial peptides, predisposing to cutaneous infection [29, 30].

Chronic psychosocial stress skews the immune response from a predominantly Th1 to a Th2 phenotype and disrupts barrier function via glucocorticoid induced inhibition of epidermal lipid synthesis, which consequently impairs LB formation and decreases the size and density of corneodesmosomes.

Cutaneous Barrier in Diabetics: Dermocosmetic Management

The aim of the dermocosmetic management of the CB in diabetic patients is to prevent and improve early stage of loss of integrity of the skin and reestablish normal hydration in order to mitigate the action of internal and external factors which influence the antimicrobial, antioxidant and ultraviolet radiation UVR protective functions. The therapeutic intervention involves a multidisciplinary approach: clinical, aesthetic and oncological dermatology.

It is essential to know the physiology of CB and skin ageing in diabetes mellitus in order to advise and provide proper treatments that will improve patient's quality of life.

Permeability Alteration

One of the most common skin manifestations of diabetes mellitus is xerosis (dry skin) which varies in severity and clinical symptomatology.

Skin barrier function, adequate cutaneous microcirculatory and autonomic nervous activity are mutually associated in healthy adults [31]. Several studies have shown that a deterioration of skin properties, an impaired cutaneous microcirculation function and an imbalance of autonomic nervous activity are observed in smokers and in patients with diabetes mellitus or Raynaud's phenomenon.

In diabetic patients with diabetic microangiopathy, there is an abnormal cutaneous perfusion caused by loss of cutaneous capillaries. Reduced skin blood flow (SkBF) recovery after cold stress and impaired responsiveness to local warming are thought to have a possible role in dry skin [32]. Diabetes and dry skin are a well documented associations and the presence of microvascular complications is related to its development in insulin dependent patients [33].

The term "dry skin" is used to refer to clinically dehydrated, rough and scaly skin. It happens when there is an alteration in the cornification process resulting in hyperkeratosis, scaling and abnormalities in the SC function. It may be seen in the entire cutaneous surface although it is mostly present in feet, pretibial areas and cheeks. Clinical manifestations include light roughness to major scaling with large plaques.

Xerosis is not only related to alterations of diabetes itself, but it is also linked to skin ageing process and others associated pathologies as well [34, 35]. Therefore,

Table 5.3 Differential diagnosis of xerosis

Malignancy	Linfoproliferative diseases
Autoinmune/infalmatory disease	Systemic lupus erythematosus Dermatomyositis Sarcoidosis Eosinophilic fascitis
Nutritional disease	Malnutrition Malabsorption (celiac disease/pancreatic insufficiency)
Metabolic disease	Diabetes Chronic renal failure Chronic hepatic dysfunction Hypothyroidism Hyperparathyroidism Hypopituitarism
Infectious disease	AIDS HTLV-I HTLV-II Leprosy
Neurologic	Sympathectomy
Medications	Statins Calcium channel blockers Cimetidine Nicotinic acid

people with diabetes have dry skin due to multifactorial origin [36]. Some of the most common causes of xerodermia are listed in Table 5.3.

It is important to point out the external factors that influence the degree of affectation such as use of medicines, environmental pollution, exposure to sun, diet, and smoking [37, 38].

Moisturizing and keratolytic agents are useful to treat dry skin. Diabetic patients with dry skin are specially predisposed to skin infections. That is why it is sometimes necessary to prescribe topical antibiotics [39].

Creams containing lipids and substances as urea are most commonly used [40, 41].

Lipids are divided according to their way of action in physiological and non-physiological [2].

Topical Treatment

Non Physiological Lipids

They are not usually found in LBs. They fill up extracellular spaces of SC. They are hydrophobic and block water movement and electrolytes.

These non-physiological lipids may quickly restore normal permeability of CB but only partially and without correcting the abnormality that originated it. Petrolatum (Vaseline), lanolin, bees wax, etc., are some examples of these.

Physiological Lipids

They are lipids or precursors that are usually found in LBs (cholesterol, free fatty acids and ceramides). These lipids are carried through SC to granular stratum cells where they mix with the pool of endogenous lipids and join the LBs (Fig. 5.2).

Ceramides make up 50% of intercellular lipids in the epidermis and are molecules often added to moisturizing creams [7].

Topical treatments with exogenous physiological lipids help reestablish both normal permeability of CB and antimicrobial function [42].

Antimicrobial peptides are packed into LBs to be released later into SC extracellular space. The availability of exogenous lipids leads to increase of production and release of these peptides.

A particularly interesting physiological lipid present in some creams for treatment of xerosis is N-palmitoylethanolamine. It acts at a cutaneous level as Cannabinoid Receptor agonist. These receptors play a role in the modulation of nociceptive symptoms. Its topical use has shown to be of great use in clinical studies to relieve chronic pruritus of various origins and in the treatment of postherpetic neuralgia [43, 44].

It may be useful to apply a mixture of physiological and non-physiological lipids as the response of physiological lipids is slow while non-physiological ones, such as petrolatum, result in partial improvement in permeability of CB almost at once.

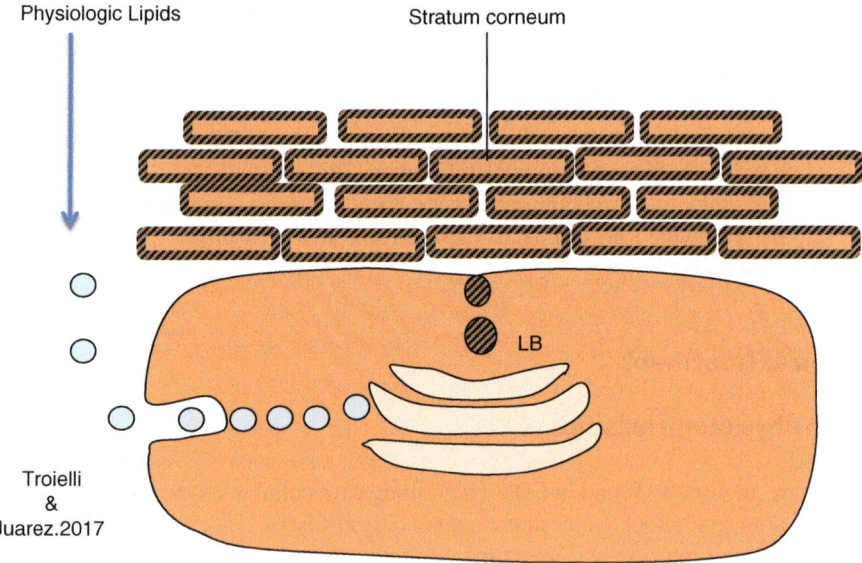

Fig. 5.2 Physiologic lipids traverse the stratum corneum, enter the nucleated cell layers, targeting the lamellar body (LB) secretory system (reproduced from Cutaneous Manifestations of Diabetes. Cohen Sabban E.N. 2017)

Topical Urea

Urea is an organic compound whose chemical structure is made up of a carbonyl group joined to two amino residues. Urea plays a very important physiological role in metabolism and excretion of nitrogenized products.

Topical urea is an effective therapeutic option in dry skin patients [45, 46].

Urea mechanism of action in the skin is still not fully understood. The studies suggest that the keratolytic and moisturizing effects of urea are due to the rupture of hydrogen bonds in the SC that leads to the rupture of the keratin molecules and increases the number of sites available for the unity of the water molecules. This aids restoration of altered CB and contributes to the scaling of normal skin [47].

There is evidence that urea also has antimicrobial properties, Grether et al. have shown that topical applications of urea at 20% improves the CB function and increases the expression of antimicrobial peptides in normal skin [45].

The urea uptake is followed by regulatory events such as expression of urea transporting elements and critical genes for the function of CB. These genes impact on the differentiation of keratinocytes, synthesis of lipids and production of antimicrobial peptides.

Urea is particularly interesting for use in diabetic patients as moisturizer and restorer. The ideal concentration is 20% (creams and ointments) and may be prescribed at 40% considering its keratolytic effect in patients with hyperkeratosis, e.g., plantar. In severe hyperkeratosis, the use under occlusion is recommended [48].

Urea shows excellent efficacy and safety profile although some patients may experience burning or stinging sensation during the first days of treatment [49].

Antioxidants and Sunscreens

Oxidative stress and action of AGEs are two processes that contribute to the impairment of CB function [20].

Besides, they are directly and indirectly related to the mechanisms that lead to photoageing and photocarcinogenesis which impact on the physical and mental health of patients.

Photoprotection diminishes ROS generated by UV radiation, partially prevents direct damage of cellular DNA, inflammation, immunosuppression and remodeling of extracellular matrix.

There is scientific evidence showing that combining sunscreens and topical antioxidants produce greater effect than the use of one of them on its own.

Antioxidants should be applied before sunscreen. Examples of most commonly used antioxidants are detailed in Table 5.4.

Sunscreens should have a broad spectrum protection, which means against UVB and UVA rays and Solar Protection Factor 30 or higher. Dry skin can be benefited with moisturizing sunscreens, as they contain lanolin, oils and dimethicone in their cream, lotion or ointment formulation. Otherwise, recommend patients to apply moisturizing cream.

Table 5.4 Commonly used antioxidants

Molecule	Role
Vitamin C	Suppresses UV production of free radicals
	Attenuates UV damage in the skin
	Promotes cutaneous wound healing
	Increase epidermal moisture content
Vitamin E	Suppresses lipid peroxidation
	Modulates photoaging
	Exhibit antiinflammatory roles
Polyphenols (phytochemical derivates) • Flavoniods: tea, soy, grapeseed • Non-flavonoids: grape, tea, polypodium leucotomos, nuts, peanuts	Antioxidants, anti-inflammatory and immunomodulatory action

Most broad spectrum formulas contain antioxidant ingredients.

Patients can be motivated to use daily sunscreen and antioxidants due to antiaging and cancer prevention benefits, so, explaining these advantages increases adherence to the treatment and improves the health care setting.

Pruritus

Pruritus is defined as an unpleasant sensation which results in scratching and may have an impact on a person's quality of life. It is a common symptom in diabetic patients caused by alteration of CB present in diabetes coupled to conditions associated to xerosis, like age, nephropathy, use of medicines (see Table 5.2). These conditions cause itching due to inflammation, dry skin, or xerosis.

Diabetic polyneuropathy is a very common cause of neuropathic pruritus. This type of pruritus flares when a nerve dysfunction occurs due to impairment or inflammation. Diabetic patients with neuropathy usually experience pain and/or itching in symmetrical distribution. Initially, it affects lower limbs and then extends to proximities. These symptoms have also been shown as chronic trunk pruritus and localized in scalp.

The management of this symptom is of the outmost importance, preventing the itch-scratch cycle. Scratching worsens the alteration already present in CB leading to chronic inflammation and infections.

Psychosocial Stress

Mental health in diabetic patients may be affected by psychological processes such as anger, denial, depression, stress, diabetic distress (stress generated by having the disease). These conditions alter the quality of life and impact patient's physical and mental health [50].

The skin responds to stress in two main ways: central and peripheral. The central way corresponds to hypothalamic pituitary adrenal (HPA) axis, the locus coeruleus-norepinephrine sympathetic adrenomedullary system. The peripheral equivalent refers to intracutaneous HPA axis and release of mediators from peripheral sensory and autonomic nerves. Activation of these two ways affects the cutaneous immune system, the CB function, healing and susceptibility to infections [29].

Studies carried out on animals and humans show that psychological stress alters the epidermal lipids synthesis. Recovery of CB function from any disturbance of the skin is delayed during periods of stress compared to periods of low stress. Moreover, it has been proven that psychosocial stress decreases the expression and release of epidermal AMP increasing the risk of infection.

Diet

A healthy diet contributes to adequate metabolic control of glycaemia and several associated risk factors and may also benefit the activity and physiology of CB.

A diet rich in natural antioxidants, low in AGEs and with adequate intake of water will maximize the effects of dermatology treatments.

Other estrategies

Diabetic patients must avoid cold air, low environmental humidity, and excessive contact with water (e.g., long baths) that impairs xerosis, particularly in winter time.

Frequent use of soap or products for body drying such as powders or gels contribute to the onset of xerosis and associated pruritus, therefore, the use of soaps with moisturizers or soap substitutes (syndet) are highly recommended.

Baths should not be longer than 10 min and taken only with warm water. It is convenient to apply moisturizing cream immediately after the bath and several times during the day to ensure proper moisturizing.

Low winter temperatures, dry weather and heating worsen xerosis, so the use of humidifiers may be useful.

Adequate therapy for the correct function of CB must include, besides moisturizing creams, the use of sunscreens and topical antioxidants in areas exposed to sunlight.

Conclusions

Alteration of CB in diabetes is due to diabetes per se and multiple factors such as ageing, physical and mental associated diseases, use of some drugs, and environmental insults.

It is crucial to preserve the integrity of CB of all diabetic patients not only of those with visible xerosis.

Patients must be taught to care for their skin and practice healthy habits to avoid xerosis and diminish damage from external factors.

This will reduce water loss and minimize the exposure to irritating and allergenic factors.

Symptoms such as pruritus and xerosis may alter quality of life and generate complications in the form of infections.

References

1. Del Rosso JQ, Levin J. The clinical relevance of maintaining the functional integrity of the stratum corneum in both healthy and disease-affected skin. J Clin Aesthet Dermatol. 2011;4(9):22–42.
2. Feingold KR, Elias PM. Role of lipids in the formation and maintenance of the cutaneous permeability barrier. Biochim Biophys Acta. 2014;1841(3):280–94.
3. Elias PM. Stratum corneum defensive functions: an integrated view. J Invest Dermatol. 2005;125(2):183–200.
4. Matsui T, Amagai M. Dissecting the formation, structure and barrier function of the stratum corneum. Int Immunol. 2015;27(6):269–80.
5. Feingold KR. Lamellar bodies: the key to cutaneous barrier function. J Invest Dermatol. 2012;132(8):1951–3. https://doi.org/10.1038/jid.2012.177.
6. Lodén M, Bárány E. Skin-identical lipids versus petrolatum in the treatment of tape-stripped and detergent-perturbed human skin. Acta Derm Venereol. 2000;80(6):412–5.
7. Meckfessel MH, Brandt S. The structure, function, and importance of ceramides in skin and their use as therapeutic agents in skin-care products. J Am Acad Dermatol. 2014;71(1):177–84.
8. Piérard GE, Piérard-Franchimont C, Scheen A. Critical assessment of diabetic xerosis. Expert Opin Med Diagn. 2013;7(2):201–7.
9. Park K. Role of micronutrients in skin health and function. Biomol Ther (Seoul). 2015;23(3):207–17.
10. Garibyan L, Chiou AS, Elmariah SB. Advanced aging skin and itch: addressing an unmet need. Dermatol Ther. 2013;26(2):92–103.
11. Ali SM, Yosipovitch G. Skin pH: from basic science to basic skin care. Acta Derm Venereol. 2013;93(3):261–7.
12. Demirseren DD, et al. Relationship between skin diseases and extracutaneous complications of diabetes mellitus: clinical analysis of 750 patients. Am J Clin Dermatol. 2014;15(1):65–70.
13. Kubo A, et al. The stratum corneum comprises three layers with distinct metal-ion barrier properties. Sci Rep. 2013;3:1731.
14. Watabe A, et al. Sweat constitutes several natural moisturizing factors, lactate, urea, sodium, and potassium. J Dermatol Sci. 2013;72(2):177–82.
15. Sakai S, et al. Functional properties of the stratum corneum in patients with diabetes mellitus: similarities to senile xerosis. Br J Dermatol. 2005;153(2):319–23.
16. Seirafi H, et al. Biophysical characteristics of skin in diabetes: a controlled study. J Eur Acad Dermatol Venereol. 2009;23(2):146–9.
17. Park HY, et al. A long-standing hyperglycaemic condition impairs skin barrier by accelerating skin ageing process. Exp Dermatol. 2011;20(12):969–74.
18. Lehman PA, Franz TJ. Effect of induced acute diabetes and insulin therapy on stratum corneum barrier function in rat skin. Skin Pharmacol Physiol. 2014;27(5):249–53.
19. Bosch R, et al. Mechanisms of photoaging and cutaneous photocarcinogenesis, and photoprotective strategies with phytochemicals. Antioxidants (Basel). 2015;4(2):248–68.
20. Rinnerthaler M, et al. Oxidative stress in aging human skin. Biomolecules. 2015;5(2):545–89.
21. Feldmeyer L, et al. The inflammasome mediates UVB-induced activation and secretion of interleukin-1β by keratinocytes. Curr Biol. 2007;17:1140–5.
22. Nestle FO. Skin immune sentinels in health and disease. Nat Rev Immunol. 2009;9(10):679–69.
23. Dana TG, Rayyan AK. Diabetic complications and dysregulated innate immunity. Front Biosci. 2008;13:1227–39.
24. He R, et al. IL-33 improves wound healing through enhanced M2 macrophage polarization in diabetic mice. Mol Immunol. 2017;90(2017):42–9.
25. Leal EC, et al. Substance P promotes wound healing in diabetes by modulating inflammation and macrophage phenotype. Am J Pathol. 2015;185(6):1638–48.
26. Gonzalez-Curiel I, et al. 1,25-dihydroxyvitamin D3 induces LL-37 and HBD-2 production in keratinocytes from diabetic foot ulcers promoting wound healing: an in vitro model. PLoS One. 2014;9(10):e111355.

27. Lan CC, et al. High-glucose environment inhibits p38MAPK signaling and reduces human β-defensin-3 expression [corrected] in keratinocytes. Mol Med. 2011;17(7–8):771–9.
28. Jafar N, et al. The effect of short-term hyperglycemia on the innate immune system. Am J Med Sci. 2016;351(2):201–11.
29. Hunter HJ, et al. The impact of psychosocial stress on healthy skin. Clin Exp Dermatol. 2015;40(5):540–6.
30. Chew BH, et al. Psychological aspects of diabetes care: effecting behavioral change in patients. World J Diabetes. 2014;5(6):796–808.
31. Nomura T, et al. Relationships between transepidermal water loss, cutaneous microcirculatory function and autonomic nervous activity. Int J Cosmet Sci. 2017;39(3):275–83.
32. Strom N, et al. Local sensory nerve control of skin blood flow during local warming in type 2 diabetes mellitus. J Appl Physiol. 2010;108:293–7.
33. Campos de Macedo GM, et al. Skin disorders in diabetes mellitus: an epidemiology and physiopathology review. Diabetol Metab Syndr. 2016;8(1):63.
34. Draelos Z. Aquaporins: an introduction to a key factor in the mechanism of skin hydration. J Clin Aesthet Dermatol. 2012;5(7):53–6.
35. Patel N, et al. Acquired ichthyosis. J Am Acad Dermatol. 2006;55(4):647–56.
36. Danby SG. Biological variation in skin barrier function: from A (atopic dermatitis) to X (xerosis). Curr Probl Dermatol. 2016;49:47–60.
37. Giménez-Arnau A. Standards for the protection of skin barrier function. Curr Probl Dermatol. 2016;49:123–34.
38. Saluja SS. A holistic approach to antiaging as an adjunct to antiaging procedures: a review of the literature. Dermatol Surg. 2017;43(4):475–84.
39. Piérard GE, et al. The skin landscape in diabetes mellitus. Focus on dermocosmetic management. Clin Cosmet Investig Dermatol. 2013;6:127–35.
40. Martini J, et al. Efficacy of an emollient cream in the treatment of xerosis in diabetic foot: a double-blind, randomized, vehicle-controlled clinical trial. J Eur Acad Dermatol Venereol. 2017;31(4):743–7.
41. Behm B. Impact of a glycolic acid-containing pH 4 water-in-oil emulsion on skin pH. Skin Pharmacol Physiol. 2015;28:290–5.
42. Seité S, et al. Importance of treatment of skin xerosis in diabetes. J Eur Acad Dermatol Venereol. 2011;25(5):607–9.
43. Ständer S, et al. Topical cannabinoid agonists. An effective new possibility for treating chronic pruritus. Hautarzt. 2006;57(9):801–7.
44. Phan NQ, et al. Adjuvant topical therapy with a cannabinoid receptor agonist in facial postherpetic neuralgia. J Dtsch Dermatol Ges. 2010;8(2):88–91.
45. Grether-Beck S, et al. Urea uptake enhances barrier function and antimicrobial defense in humans by regulating epidermal gene expression. J Invest Dermatol. 2012;132(6):1561–72.
46. Pan M, et al. Urea: a comprehensive review of the clinical literature. Dermatol Online J. 2013;19(11):20392.
47. Parker J. Moisturisers for the treatment of foot xerosis: a systematic review cita. J Foot Ankle Res. 2017;10:9.
48. Lodén M. Treatments improving skin barrier function. Curr Probl Dermatol. 2016;49:112–22.
49. Federici A, et al. Use of a urea, arginine and carnosine cream versus a standard emollient glycerol cream for treatment of severe xerosis of the feet in patients with type 2 diabetes: a randomized, 8 month, assessor-blinded, controlled trial. Curr Med Res Opin. 2015;31(6):1063–9.
50. American Diabetes Associaton. www.diabetes.org.

Cutaneous Markers of Diabetes Mellitus

6

Emilia Noemí Cohen Sabban

Cutaneous markers of Diabetes Mellitus (DM) are a heterogeneous group of dermatoses which, upon onset, force us to rule out an underlying DM. They may occur in any DM type, since no significant differences have been found between one type and the other.

But precisely some cutaneous markers may be the first manifestation of an undiagnosed DM and may even be years ahead of a DM diagnosis, as in the case of necrobiosis lipoidica or generalized granuloma annulare.

Instead, other cutaneous markers increase their incidence the longer the patient has been diagnosed with DM, such as diabetic dermopathy and spontaneous diabetic blisters [1].

It is important to know the long list of cutaneous markers of DM in order to suspect an underlying DM or to detect patients with a poorly controlled, long-standing disease, and refer them promptly.

Necrobiosis Lipoidica (NL)

It is a chronic granulomatous dermatosis most frequent among women between 30 and 40 years of age. It affects 0.3–1.2% of type 1 (T1DM) and 2 (T2DM) diabetic patients, while 90% of patients diagnosed with NL are diabetic.

In 60% of the cases, it occurs in patients with a diagnosis of DM, but due to the fact that NL may be the first sign of an undiagnosed DM, its onset requires the DM diagnosis to be checked on an annual basis [2] (Chart 6.1).

E.N. Cohen Sabban, M.D.
Dermatology Department, Instituto de Investigaciones Médicas A. Lanari,
University of Buenos Aires (UBA), Buenos Aires, Argentina
e-mail: emicohensabban@gmail.com

© Springer International Publishing AG 2018
E.N. Cohen Sabban et al. (eds.), *Dermatology and Diabetes*,
https://doi.org/10.1007/978-3-319-72475-1_6

Chart 6.1 Necrobiosis lipoidica

Frequency: 0.3 - 1.2%
Age: 25 to 40
Gender: 80% among women
Association with Diabetes: It may
be the first sign of an
undiagnosed DM.

Fig. 6.1 Necrobiosis
Lipoidica Initial lesion.
Erythematous nodule

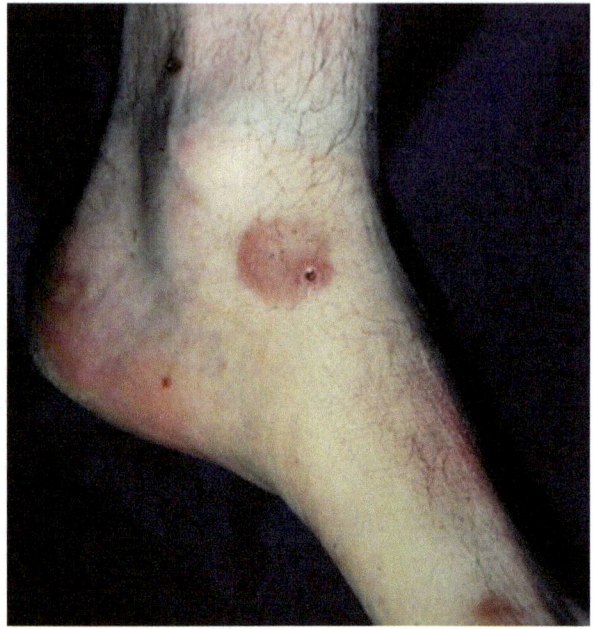

Although its etiology is unknown, it has been linked to microangiopathy, non-enzymatic glycation (NEG), platelet aggregation, etc. being vascular damage the most solid reason. In a recent multicenter study, involving a large number of diabetic patients with and without NL, it was not possible to prove such linkage; however, they found some of the metabolic consequences of hyperglycemia may play a significant role in the onset of NL [3].

Clinically, it starts with a small, well-defined erythematous nodule (Fig. 6.1), which gradually grows forming a flat, atrophic, yellowish plaque in the center (Fig. 6.2), through which dermal vessels may be seen. While borders are purplish-erythematous in color, they are the focus of lesion growth and remain raised (Figs. 6.3 and 6.4). Lesions may be single or multiple, unilateral or bilateral and are asymptomatic (Figs. 6.5, 6.6 and 6.7). During its course, which is generally chronic, it may become pigmented and once settled it virtually does not involve [4]. (Figs. 6.8, 6.9 and 6.10) They typically appear on the anterior and lateral surfaces of the legs (pretibial region) (Fig. 6.11), although they may also appear on the arms, trunk, face and scalp.

Fig. 6.2 Early lesion, slight peripheral elevation in the borders; there is no atrophy in the center yet, nor dermal vessels seen by transparency

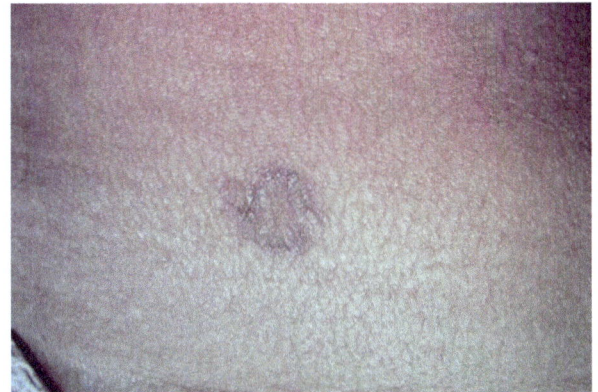

Fig. 6.3 Plaque of necrobiosis lipoidica with erythematous, raised borders with activity. There is no atrophy in the center yet

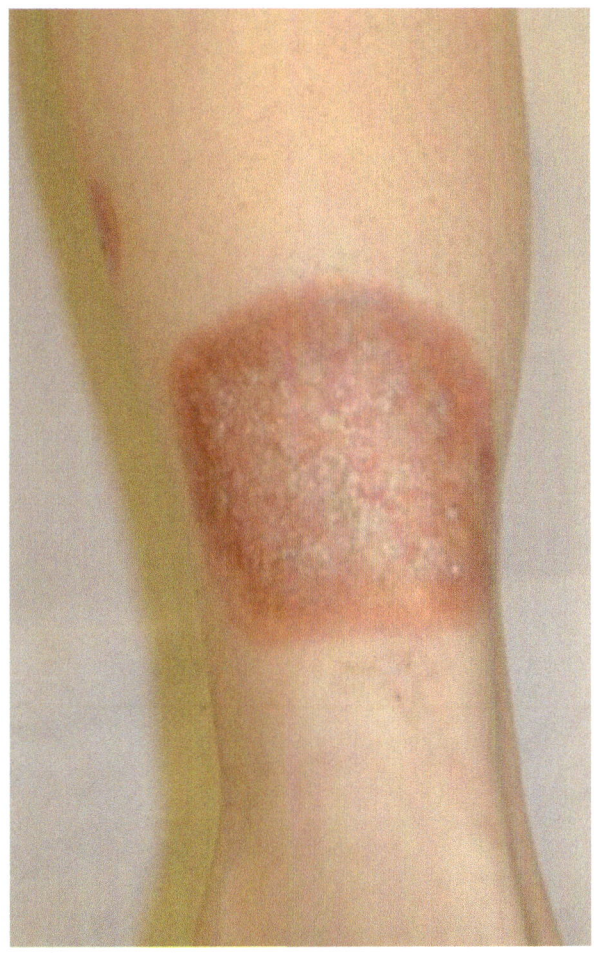

Fig. 6.4 Necrobiosis
Lipoidica

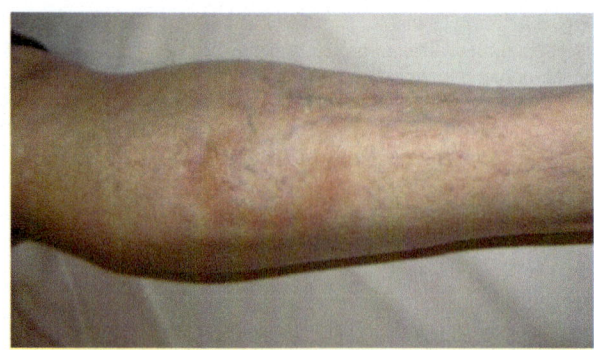

Fig. 6.5 Necrobiosis
lipoidica. Unilateral
atrophic plaque

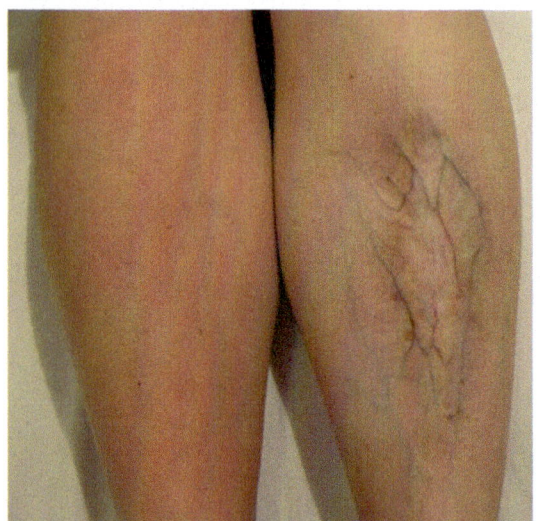

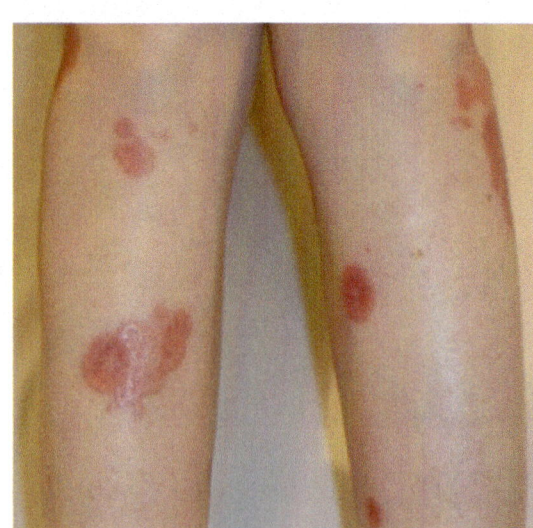

Fig. 6.6 Multiple and
bilateral plaques of
necrobiosis lipoidica

Fig. 6.7 Necrobiosis lipoidica. Multiple and bilateral plaques

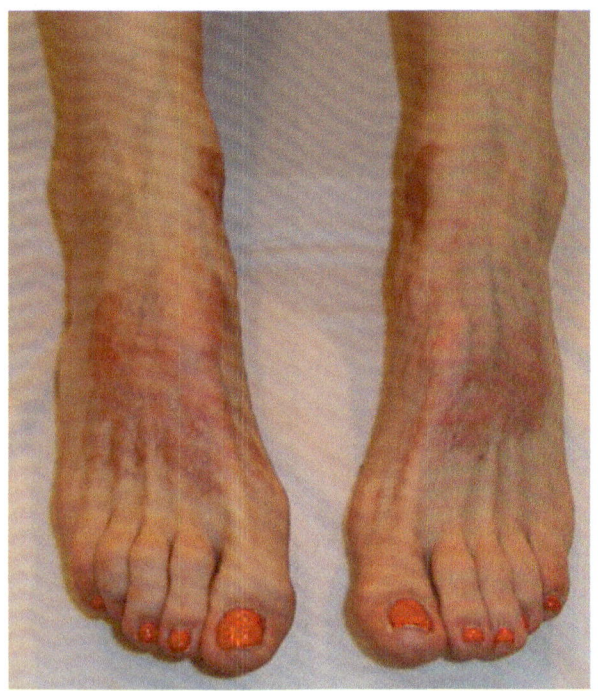

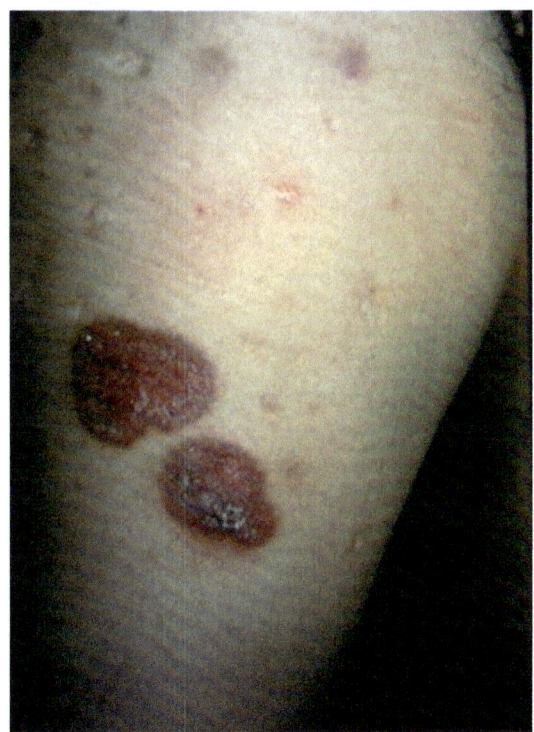

Fig. 6.8 Pigmented plaques of necrobiosis lipoidica

Fig. 6.9 Pigmented and
ulcerated plaques of
necrobiosis lipoidica

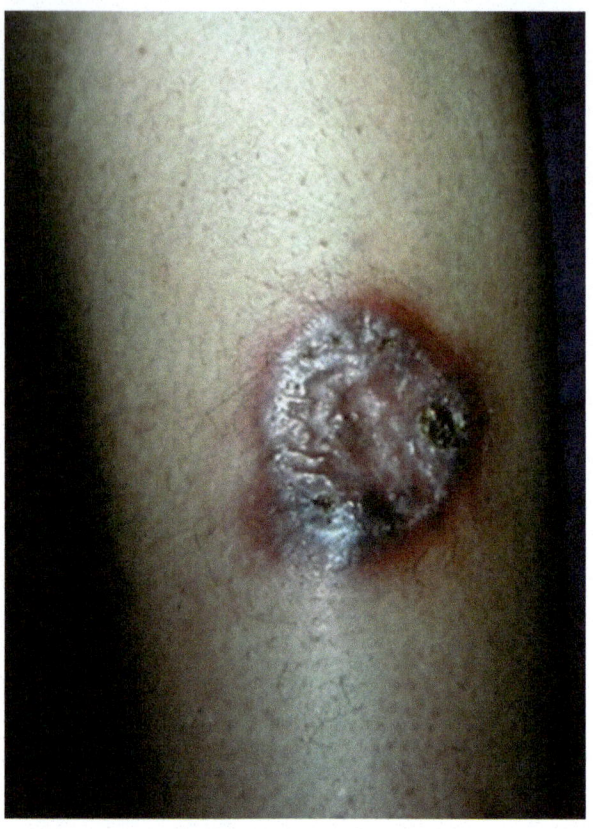

There are some clinical forms, among them, the "granuloma annular-like" variant is important because there are reports of the coexistence of both diseases in the same patient [5]. The ulcerated variant either spontaneously or from traumatism, comprises 15–35% of all NL and characteristically, it is painful (Fig. 6.12). It is a really therapeutic challenge, and sometimes is very frustrating [6, 7].

Microscopically it belongs to the group of diseases with a *"palisaded granuloma"* together with granuloma annulare, which has a similar clinical appearance (Figs. 6.13 and 6.14). The presence of extracellular lipids and the absence of mucin deposits in the central area are key clues for its differentiation [8, 9].

Dermoscopy may be useful to differentiate between NL and granuloma annulare (GA). NL presents a typical pattern made up, in most cases, of a prominent network of arborizing and hairpin vessels on a yellowish background, while GA has no distinctive pattern [10] (Fig. 6.15).

Taking into account the fact that it is a benign dermatosis, occurring in patients frequently polymedicated, the physician may take an expectant attitude. In order to prevent complications and promote ulcer healing, it is essential to change some lifestyle habits, such as quitting smoking and avoiding trauma and compression in case of lymphedema or venous stasis.

Fig. 6.10 Necrobiosis lipoidica. Pigmented plaque in which dermal vessels start to be seen due to the atrophy

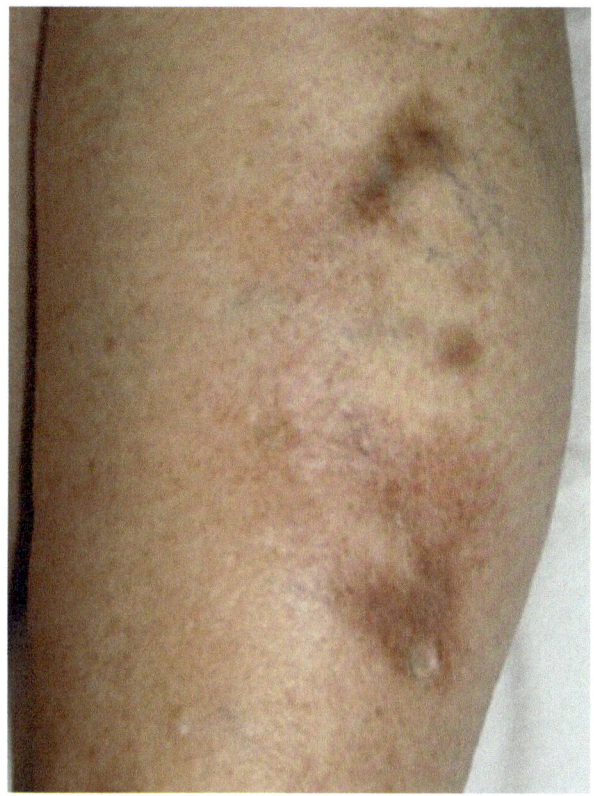

Fig. 6.11 Multiple pigmented plaques of necrobiosis lipoidica

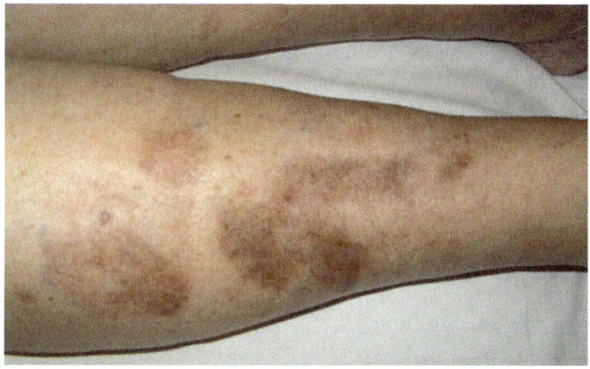

There is no efficient medical treatment for NL and while many cases with different degrees of therapeutic success have been reported, controlled, randomized research work including a significant number of patients is needed.

Corticosteroids are the cornerstone in the treatment of this dermatosis, due to their anti-inflammatory properties, topical with or without occlusion, intralesional (IL) or systemically for brief periods of time. If IL were the chosen modality,

Fig. 6.12 Ulcerated plaque of necrobiosis lipoidica with atrophic center

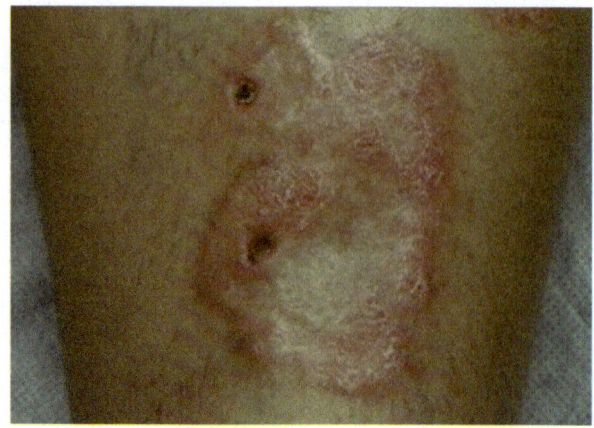

Fig. 6.13 Histopathological image of necrobiosis lipoidica with altered collagen fibers

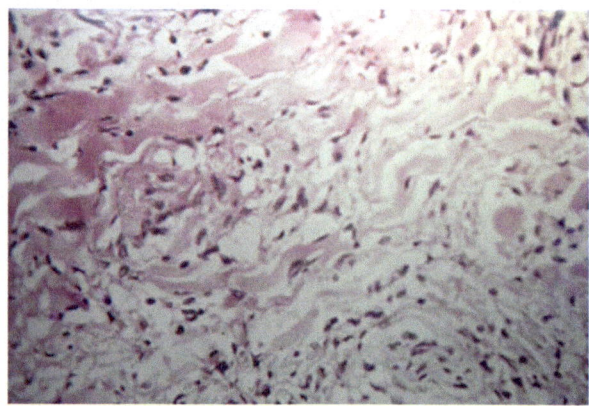

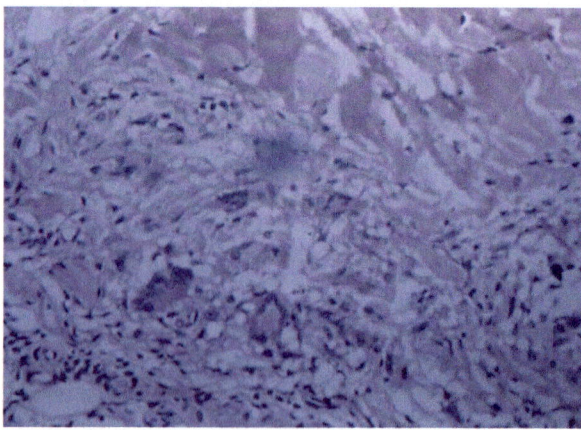

Fig. 6.14 At higher magnification; giant multinuclear cells that are part of the granuloma

Fig. 6.15 Dermoscopic pattern of necrobiosis lipoidica. Arborizing network of vessels on a yellowish background

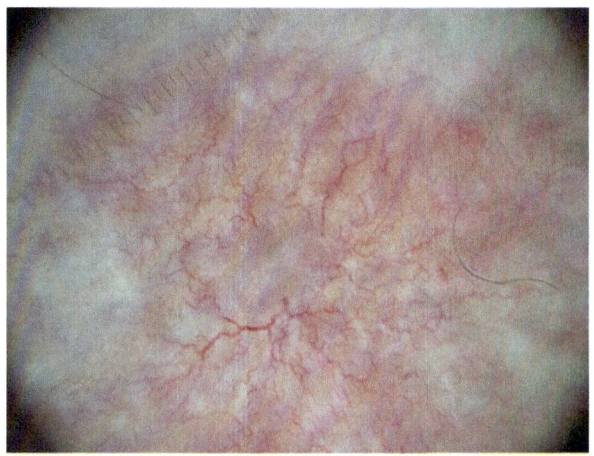

application must be done on the borders due to two reasons. One is that the central area is or will become atrophic and, therefore, these agents are contraindicated. Second, borders are the active part of the lesion and these agents reduce inflammation and prevent progression.

The hyperglycemic effect of systemic corticosteroids is well known; therefore, their indication to diabetic patients must be accompanied by a strict control of blood sugar levels, especially when they are to be applied on extensive areas or during long periods of time [11].

Among topical therapies, calcineurin inhibitors act inhibiting T cell activation and, consequently, interleukin (IL) production and proliferation, thus providing an anti-inflammatory and immunomodulating effect.

Another anti-inflammatory therapy is phototherapy, psoralen-UVA (PUVA) as well as UVA-1 which apparently is beneficial in the earlier stages of the disease [12].

Other options are drugs acting on hemostasis (vascular thrombosis), such as a combination of aspirin 40–80 mg/day and dipyridamole 200 mg/day that inhibit platelet aggregation and reduce blood viscosity; and Pentoxifylline, a methylxanthine, that also acts on red blood cell aggregation and reduces tumor necrosis factor alpha (TNF-α) production, thus improving blood flow. A dose of 400 mg 3 times/day is used [13].

Antimalarial drugs (such as hydroxychloroquine and chloroquine) inhibit chemotaxis of macrophages responsible for granuloma formation, although their effect is not immediate. Besides, chloroquine inhibits platelet aggregation thus preventing vascular occlusion [14, 15].

Fumaric acid esters inhibit inflammatory cytokines and prevent T lymphocytes proliferation. While results are encouraging, treatment starts with a low dose of 30 mg of dimethyl fumarate since it is poorly tolerated due to nausea, a dose-dependent side effect, and lymphopenia which may occur in almost half of the patients [16].

Cyclosporine is an immunosuppressant drug indicated for resistant ulcerated NL, because it inhibits IL-2 lymphocyte production thus preventing these cells proliferation and, consequently, the immune response. A dose of 2–4 mg/kg/day generates a fast improvement, closing ulcers in 2–4 months, but recurrence after discontinuation is the rule. Due to the fact that its adverse effects are related to nephrotoxicity, it is contraindicated in diabetic patients with a pre-existing nephropathy. Blood pressure, potassium levels, hemogram and renal function, among others, must be monitored. Mofetil mycophenolate is another immunosuppressant with a cytostatic effect on lymphocytes. Like cyclosporine, it is effective but recurrence is common once treatment is discontinued.

More recently, glitazones and photodynamic therapy have been used with some degree of success. Based on the involvement of TNF-α in granuloma formation, biologic anti TNF-α agents such as etanercept and infliximab have been used in NL cases refractory to other therapies [17].

Generalized Granuloma Annulare (GGA)

Generalized GA was defined as "affecting at least the trunk and either upper or lower, or both, extremities" [18] (Figs. 6.16, 6.17 and 6.18).

It is a dermatosis occurring in T1DM and T2DM patients, more frequently among adult women.

Clinically, it is made up of erythematous pink or skin colored papules coalescing to form annular, arcuate, polycyclic, well-defined plaques (Figs. 6.19, 6.20,

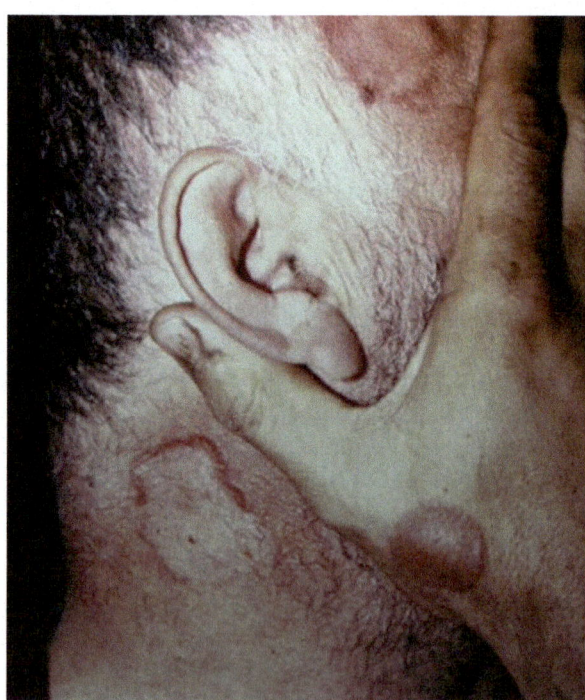

Fig. 6.16 Generalized granuloma annulare. Involvement of different areas of the body (face, neck, hands)

Fig. 6.17 Generalized granuloma annulare with severe damage in lower limbs

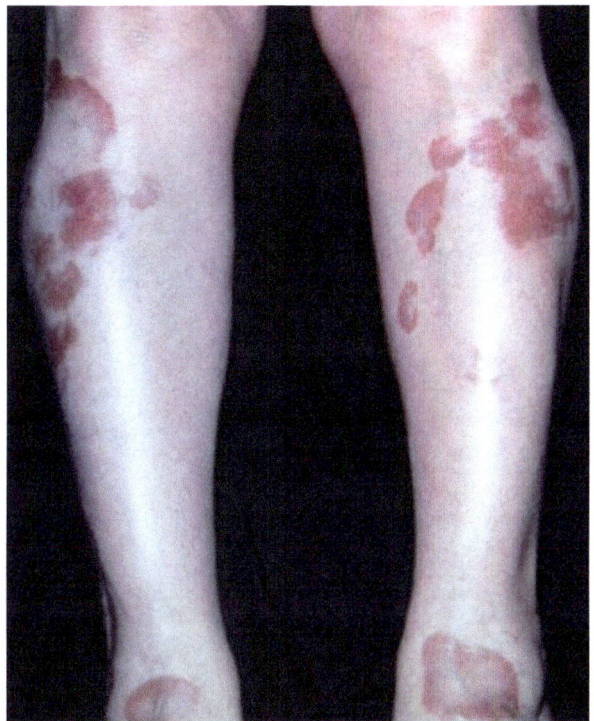

Fig. 6.18 Generalized granuloma annulare with severe damage in upper limbs

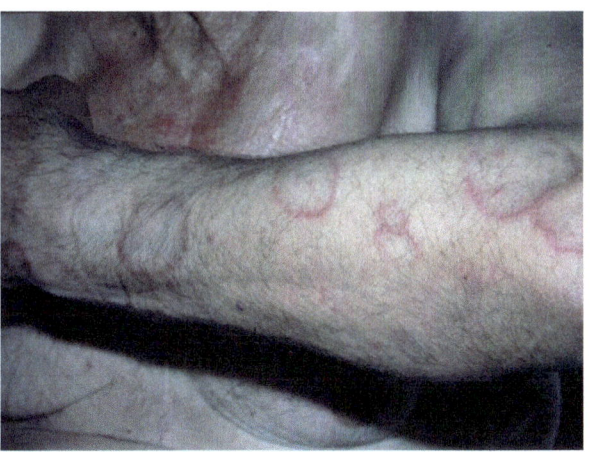

6.21, 6.22, 6.23 and 6.24). They are asymptomatic or slightly itchy; in its progression, there is no atrophy unlike what it happens with necrobiosis lipoidica [19] (Fig. 6.25). GGA constitutes 8.5–15% of all GA cases and is associated with DM. Unlike the localized form that tends to resolve spontaneously, the generalized form tends to last several years (Figs. 6.24 and 6.25).

Fig. 6.19 Multiple annular plaques of granuloma annulare in the dorsum of the hands

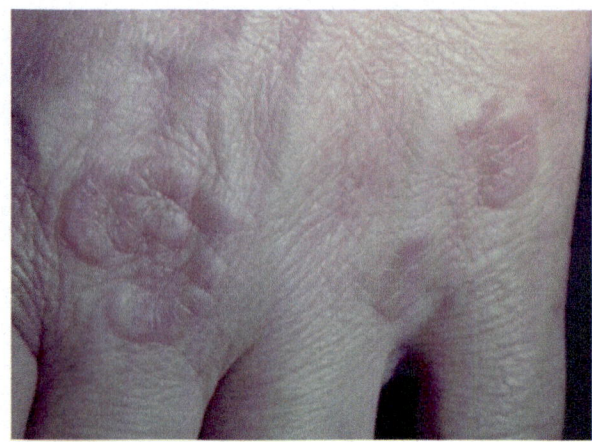

Fig. 6.20 Multiple annular erythematous plaques in a patient with generalized granuloma annulare

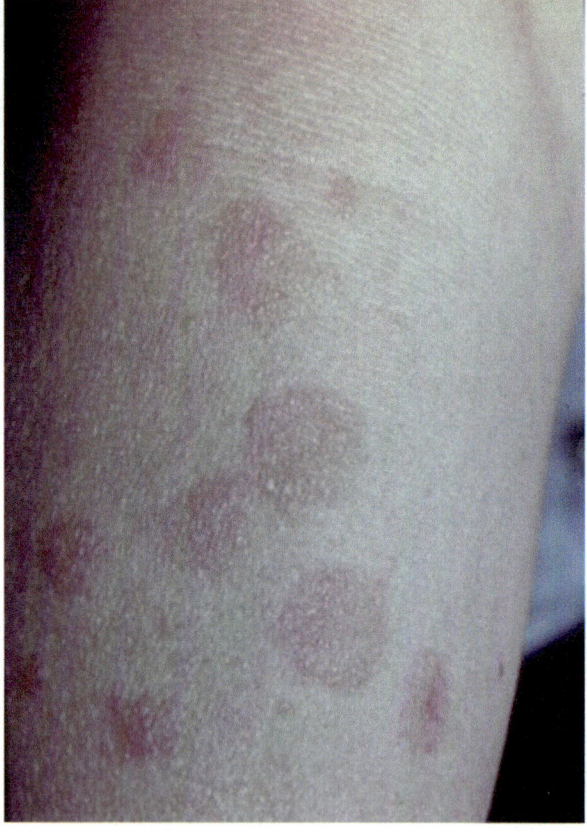

Although its etiology has not been determined, it has been postulated that delayed hypersensitivity to an unknown antigen may be the cause [20].

The histological clues are abundant mucin deposits, which leads to differentiated it from other granulomatous diseases such as NL, rheumatoid nodule and Sarcoidosis, coupled with a palisade granuloma or an interstitial distribution pattern [21].

Fig. 6.21 Bilateral annular plaques of granuloma annulare in the dorsum of the hands

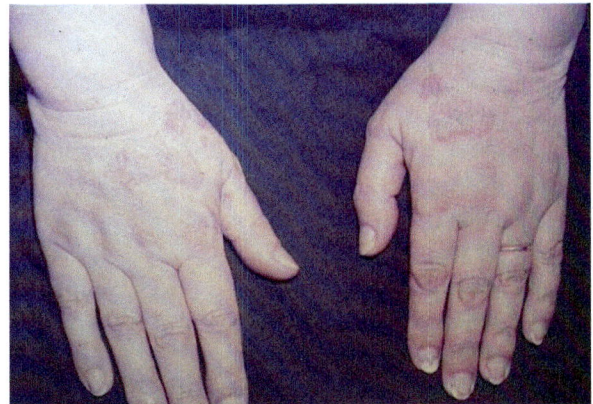

Fig. 6.22 Annular and arcuate plaques of granuloma annulare

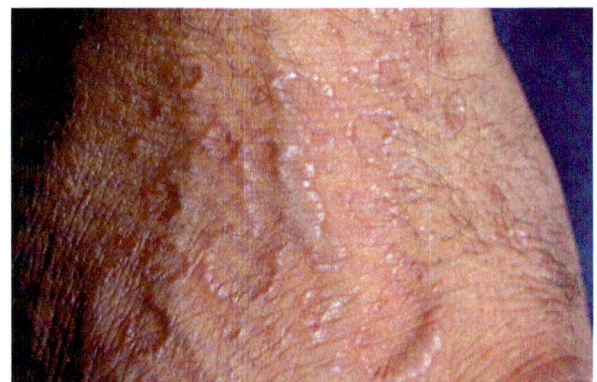

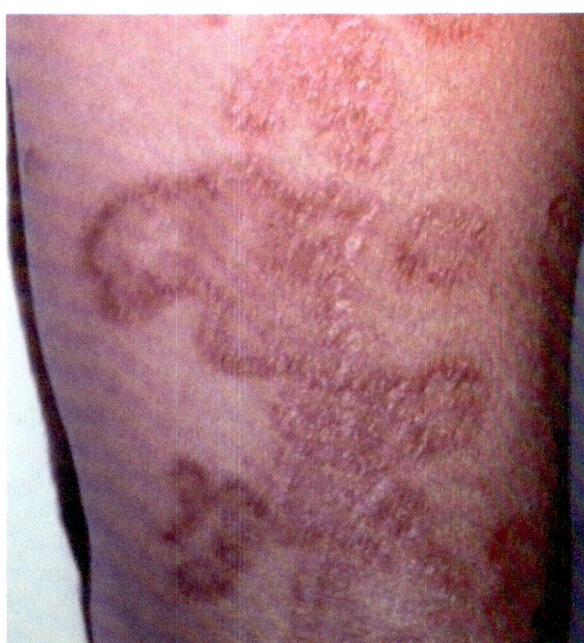

Fig. 6.23 Annular and polycyclic plaques formed by the coalescence of papules in the anterior surface of the leg

Fig. 6.24 Arcuate and polycyclic plaques of granuloma annulare in anterior trunk

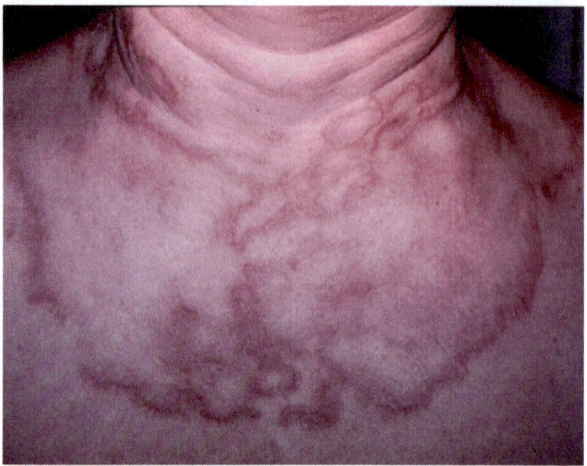

Fig. 6.25 Annular plaques with erythematous, raised borders. Note that there is no central atrophy

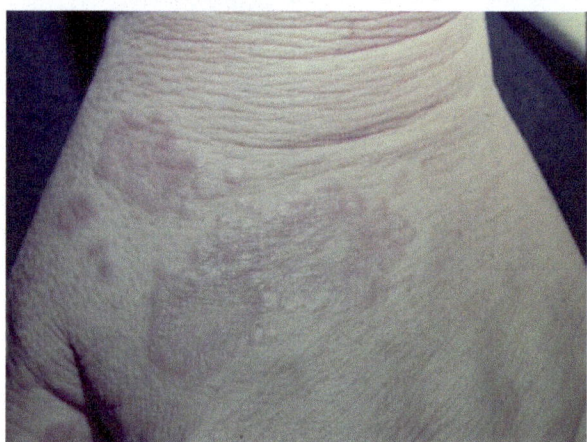

Chart 6.2 Generalized granuloma annulare

Frequency: Low
Age: 50
Gender: 2:1 F/M
Association with Diabetes: Up to 40% of GAG cases are associated with DM.

Dermoscopically, it does not have a distinct pattern like NL, most frequent findings were dotted or short linear vessels on a red and white background; and less frequently, absence of vessels on a white-yellowish background [22].

The selected therapeutic modality shall depend on the severity of the disease, comorbidities, probable adverse events and patient's preferences. Topical and IL corticosteroids are the first option. Other treatments include calcineurin inhibitors and cryotherapy [23].

While there is no successful systemic treatment for all GGA cases, corticosteroids and DDS (diaminodiphenyl sulfone) in doses of 100 mg/day would be the first choice [24].

Retinoids, pentoxifylline, antimalarial drugs, PUVA and photodynamic therapy (PDT) are some out of the long list of treatments for the generalized form [25]. Colchicine and potassium iodide alone or combined with nicotinamide, among others, are options more sporadically used and with a certain level of therapeutic success [26] (Chart 6.2).

Diabetic Dermopathy (DD)

Diabetic dermopathy (DD), also known under other denominations such as "pigmented pretibial patches" or "shin spots", occurs most frequently among T1 and T2 diabetic men of an average age of 50 years old (Fig. 6.26). Its incidence increases with age and DM duration [27].

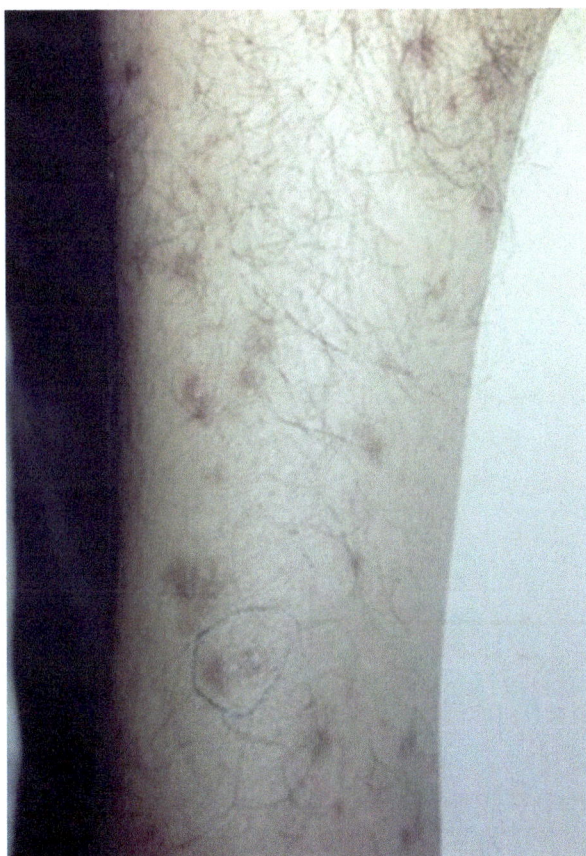

Fig. 6.26 Diabetic dermopathy. Smooth brown macules with no scales or crusts

While it has been described in up to 70% of diabetic patients, based on our observation, it was found only in 10% of patients. It is not a pathognomonic sign of DM, since 20% of patients are not diabetic.

It is clinically recognized as multiple, small macules whose brown coloration stems from the distribution of hemosiderin and, to a lesser degree, melanin in perivascular histiocytes [28] (Fig. 6.27). They are circular or oval, asymptomatic, well-demarcated macules with a smooth, soft surface, without scales or crusts (Figs. 6.28, 6.29 and 6.30). They are distributed bilaterally but are not symmetric, they are grouped or isolated and sometimes present a linear distribution; they do not disappear and do not improve with blood glucose control [29]. Some cases may evolve towards a slight atrophy which, together with their brownish color, have given it the old name of "circumscribed brown atrophy" [30] (Fig. 6.31).

Its pathogenesis is multifactorial: microangiopathy, inflammatory process and fibrosis are involved.

It has been negatively associated with DM microvascular complications (neuropathy, retinopathy and nephropathy) and with an increase in glycated hemoglobin

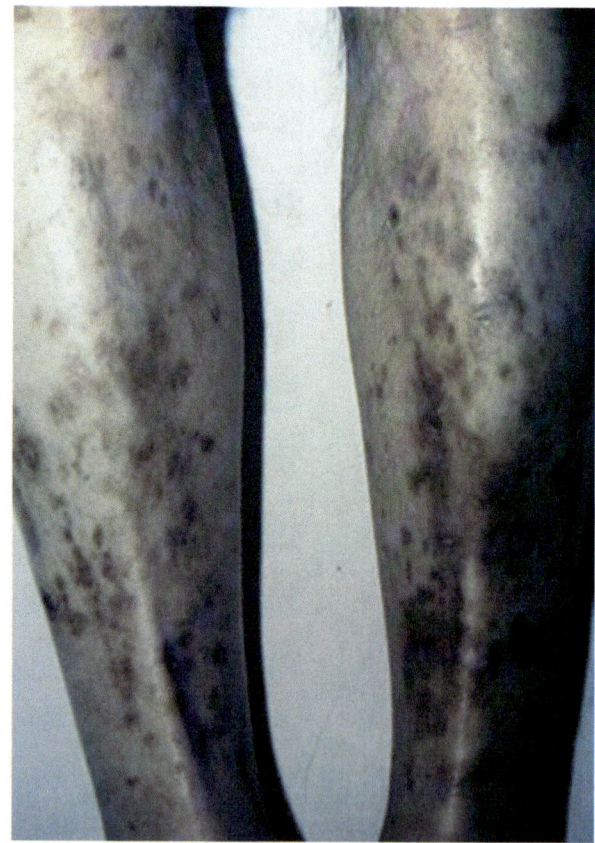

Fig. 6.27 Diabetic dermopathy, bilateral but no symmetrical involvement

Fig. 6.28 Pigmented
pretibial patches or
diabetic dermopathy

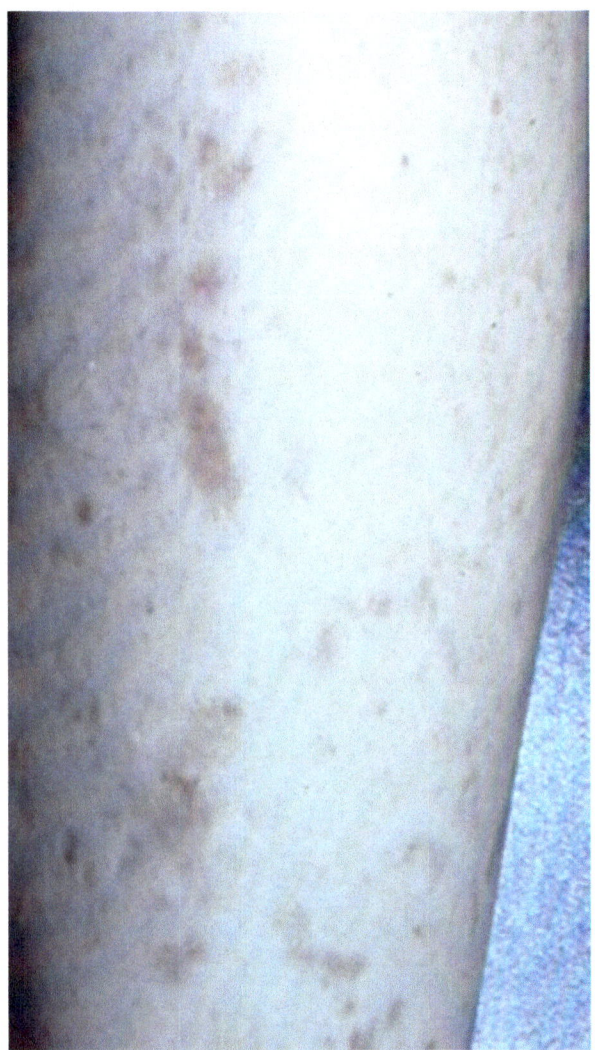

(HbA1c) and long-standing DM; therefore, the presence of DD must be deemed an alarming clinical sign [31, 32].

In general, it does not require treatment and also there is no effective treatment; some lesions resolve spontaneously [33] (Chart 6.3).

Bullosis Diabeticorum (BD)

It occurs only among diabetic patients; therefore, it is the only DM cutaneous marker deemed pathognomonic. Its incidence is very low, it occurs in less than 1% of patients and increases with age, and predominantly among male patients. Blisters

Fig. 6.29 Diabetic
dermopathy

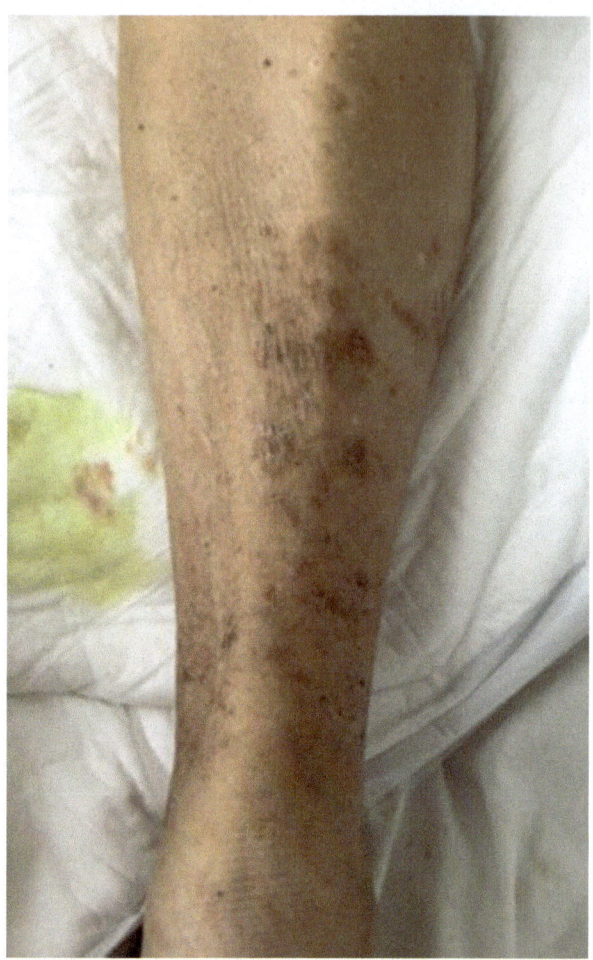

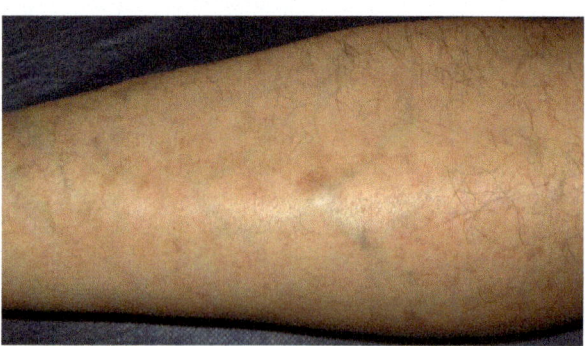

Fig. 6.30 Diabetic
dermopathy. Slight atrophy

Fig. 6.31 Diabetic dermopathy. The atrophy is notorious

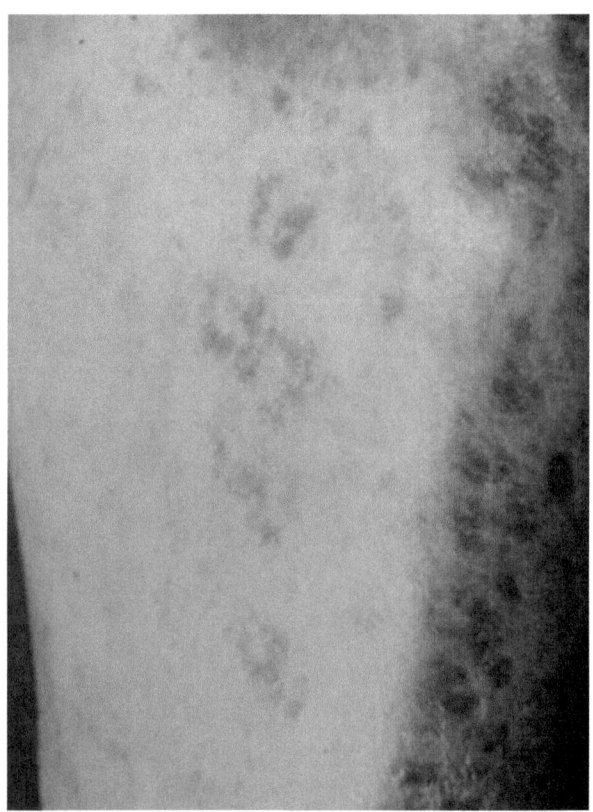

Chart 6.3 Diabetic dermopathy

Frequency: 10%
Age: the > age the > frequency
Gender: Widely predominant among men.
Association with Diabetes: Warning sign!

appear suddenly and generally overnight. In literature, they are not linked to trauma or friction; however, since most patients with BD also suffer peripheral neuropathy, this statement requires new research [34].

It has been proven that diabetic patients have a lower threshold for suction-induced blistering, which would partially explain the tendency of diabetic skin to blister formation, which in turn is partly due to cutaneous fragility resulting from diabetic angiopathy [35]. But also NEG of the basement membrane zone (BMZ) structures, such as the anchoring fibers keeping the dermis and epidermis together, is involved in its pathogenesis [36].

Blisters generally appear on the distal areas of the lower limbs, their content is serous or serohematic, they are painless and present no signs of inflammation. Most blisters are intraepidermal (without acantholysis); therefore, they tend to heal spontaneously and leave no scars (Figs. 6.32, 6.33, 6.34 and 6.35). More rarely, they are located under the dermoepidermal junction at the lamina lucida level of the BMZ. Direct and indirect immunofluorescence (IF) tests are negative [37, 38].

Complications such as ulceration and/or bacterial superinfection are infrequent; therefore, their brief duration plus their quick healing time without requiring

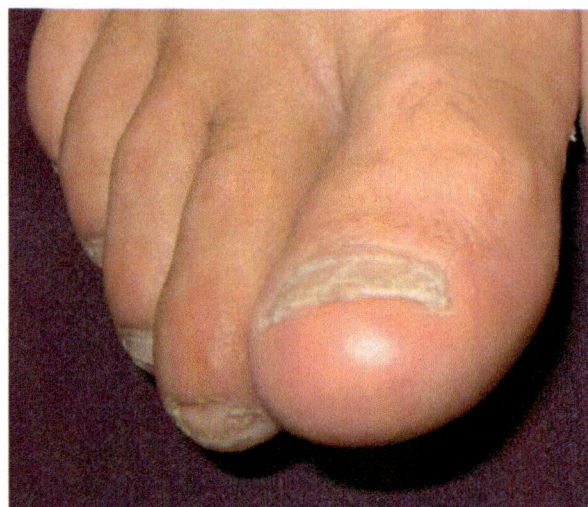

Fig. 6.32 Diabetic blister with serous content

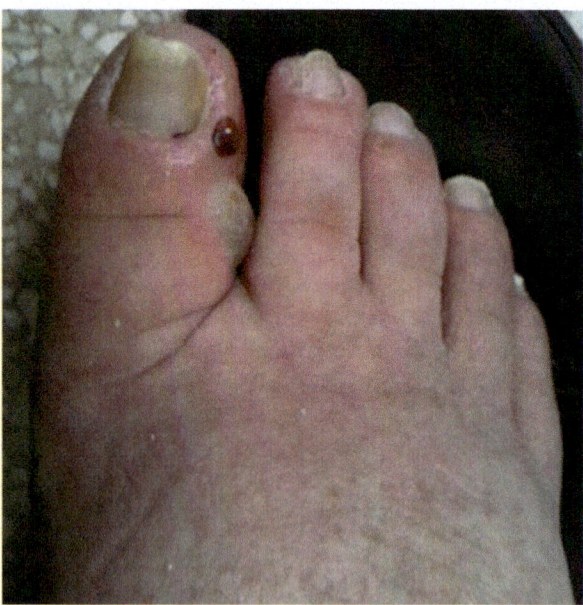

Fig. 6.33 Intact diabetic blister with serohematic content

Fig. 6.34 Diabetic blister

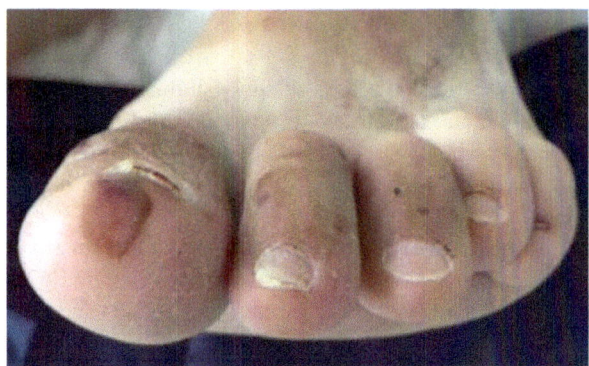

Fig. 6.35 Diabetic blister with hematic content in involution

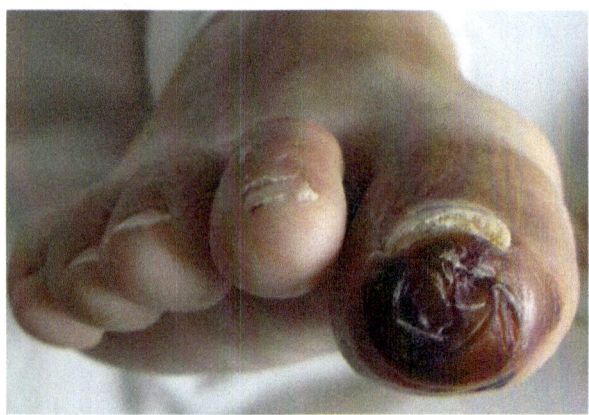

Chart 6.4 Bullosis diabeticorum

Frequency: Approximately 1%
Age: the > age the > frequency
Gender: 2:1 M/F
Association with Diabetes: Only pathognomonic marker, poor prognosis marker.

treatment would lead to consider it an insignificant sign. However, they are related to long-standing DM and microvascular complications such as neuropathy, so it is a poor prognosis marker [39].

Diagnosis in most cases is clinical and by exclusion; findings such as sterile blisters with negative cultures, normal blood and urine porphyrins levels and negative direct immunofluorescence are helpful [40].

Treatment is conservative, the blister roof must be kept intact and the fluid must be aspired with a sterile syringe in order to avoid superinfection. On the contrary, if blisters were complicated by ulceration, treatment must be aggressive and include a multidisciplinary approach [41] (Chart 6.4).

Xanthosis or Yellow Skin

This is the name given to a yellowish discoloration of the skin in palms and soles, nasolabial and axillary folds, compared to the sclera. While there are reports of it occurrence in 10% of diabetic patients, in our practice, it is an uncommon marker, that occurs mainly in adult patients, equally in both sexes [42] (Figs. 6.36, 6.37, 6.38, 6.39 and 6.40).

Its interrelationship with high levels of blood carotenes, whether due to a poor β carotene conversion into retinol, increase in serum lipids and a diet abundant in carotenoid-rich fruits and vegetables is controversial and carotenemia may be normal. It is also linked to the accumulation of non-enzymatic glycation end products (AGEs) that are brownish in color, produced by the NEG of skin proteins, such as collagen (collagen-AGE) [43–45]. Therefore, blood glucose levels control together with a suitable treatment may improve the skin yellowish discoloration [46] (Chart 6.5).

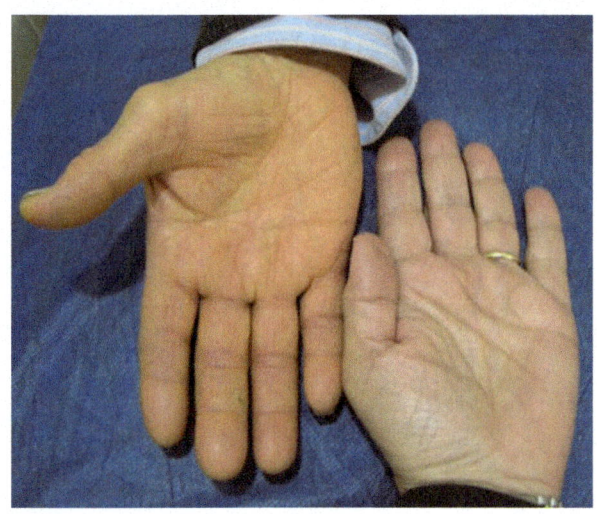

Fig. 6.36 Xanthosis. Patient's palm and control palm

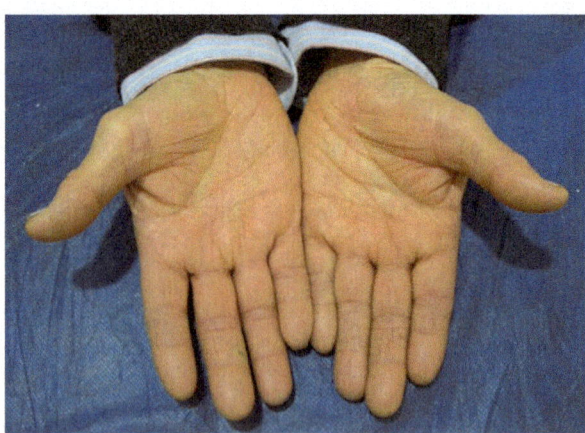

Fig. 6.37 Xanthosis. Both palms of the patient

Fig. 6.38 Xanthosis of both palms together with control palm

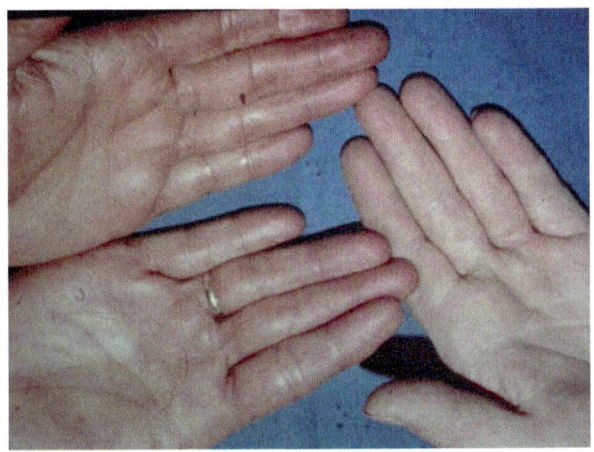

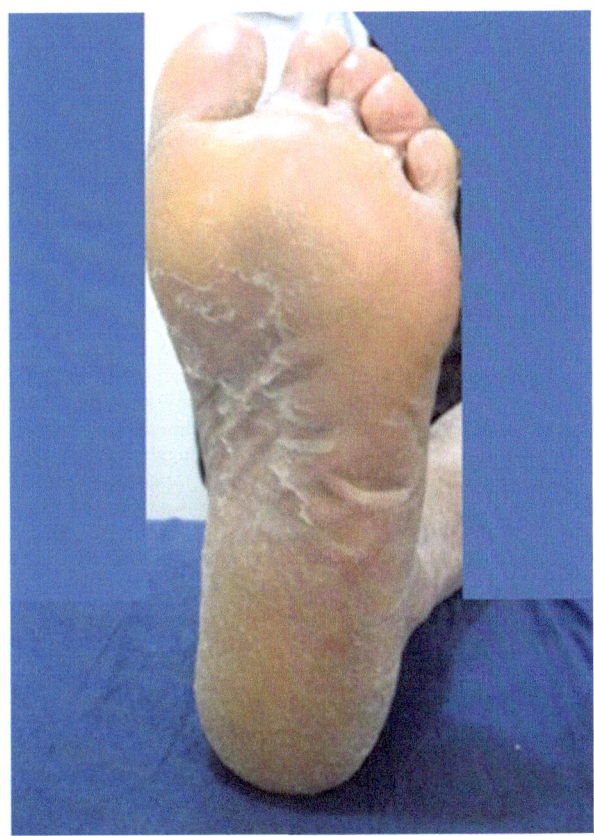

Fig. 6.39 Xanthosis affecting the plantar region

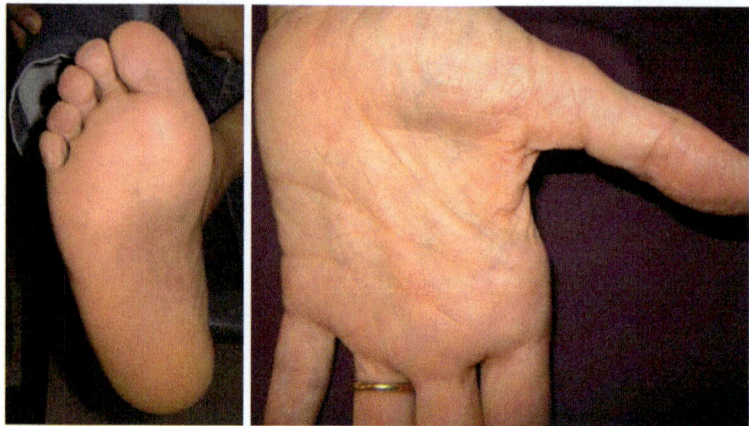

Fig. 6.40 Palmoplantar xanthosis of the same patient

Chart 6.5 Xanthosis

> Frequency: Unknown
> Age: Adults
> Gender: Equal for both genders
> Association with Diabetes: Linked to
> yellowish-brownish AGEs
> accumulation.

References

1. Farshchian M, Farshchian M, Fereydoonnejad M, Yazdanfar A, Kimyai-Asadi A. Cutaneous manifestations of diabetes mellitus: a case series. Cutis. 2010;86(1):31–5.
2. Sibbald C, Reid S, Alavi A. Necrobiosis lipoidica. Dermatol Clin. 2015;33(3):343–60.
3. Hammer E, Lilienthal E, Hofer SE, Schulz S, Bollow E, Holl RW, DPV Initiative and the German BMBF Competence Network for Diabetes Mellitus. Risk factors for necrobiosis lipoidica in Type 1 diabetes mellitus. Diabet Med. 2017;34(1):86–92.
4. Erfurt-Berge C, Seitz AT, Rehse C, Wollina U, Schwede K, Renner R. Update on clinical and laboratory features in necrobiosis lipoidica: a retrospective multicenter study of 52 patients. Eur J Dermatol. 2012;22(6):770–5.
5. Ianoşi SL, Tutunaru C, Georgescu CV, Ianoşi NG, Georgescu DM, Dănoiu S, Niculescu EC, Neagoe CD. Specific features of a rare form of disseminated necrobiosis lipoidica granuloma annulare type: a case report. Romanian J Morphol Embryol. 2014;55(4):1455–61.
6. Pătraşcu V, Giurca C, Ciurea RC, Georgescu CC, Ciurea ME. Ulcerated necrobiosis lipoidica to a teenager with diabetes mellitus and obesity. Romanian J Morphol Embryol. 2014;55(1):171–6.
7. Lozanova P, Dourmishev L, Vassileva S, Miteva L, Balabanova M. Perforating disseminated necrobiosis Lipoidica Diabeticorum. Case Rep Dermatol Med. 2013;2013:370361.
8. Hawryluk EB, Izikson L, English JC. Non-infectious granulomatous diseases of the skin and their associated systemic diseases: an evidence-based update to important clinical questions. Am J Clin Dermatol. 2010;11:171–81.
9. Travassos AR, Soares-De-Almeida L. Residents'corner February 2014. DeRmpath & Clinic: differential diagnosis in palisading non-infectious granulomas. Diagnosis: Case 1: Granuloma annulare. Case 2: Necrobiosis lipoidica. Eur J Dermatol. 2014;24(1):139–40.

10. Bakos RM, Cartell A, Bakos L. Dermatoscopy of early-onset necrobiosis lipoidica. J Am Acad Dermatol. 2012;66:e143–4.
11. Grillo E, Rodriguez-Muñoz D, González-Garcia A, Jaén P. Necrobiosis lipoidica. Aust Fam Physician. 2014;43(3):129–30.
12. Feily A, Mehraban S. Treatment modalities of necrobiosis lipoidica: a concise systematic review. Dermatol Rep. 2015;7:5749.
13. Wee E, Kelly R. Pentoxifylline: an effective therapy for necrobiosis lipoidica. Australas J Dermatol. 2017;58:65–8.
14. Kavala M, Sudogan S, Zindanci I, et al. Significant improvement in ulcerative necrobiosis lipoidica with hydroxychloroquine. Int J Dermatol. 2010;49:467–9.
15. Nguyen K, Washenik K, Shupack J. Necrobiosis lipoidica diabeticorum treated with chloroquine. J Am Acad Dermatol. 2002;46:S34–6.
16. Kota SK, Jammula S, Kota SK, Meher LK, Modi KD. Necrobiosis lipoidica diabeticorum: a case-based review of literature. Indian J Endocrinol Metab. 2012;16(4):614–20.
17. Reid SD, Ladizinski B, Kachiu L, Baibergenova A, Alavi A. Update on necrobiosis lipoidica: a review of etiology, diagnosis, and treatment options. J Am Acad Dermatol. 2013;69(5):783–91.
18. Dabski K, Winkelmann RK. Generalized granuloma annulare: clinical and laboratory findings in 100 patients. J Am Acad Dermatol. 1989;20:39–47.
19. Goucha S, Khaled A, Kharfi M, et al. Granuloma annulare. G Ital Dermatol Venereol. 2008;143(6):359–63.
20. Avitan-Hersh E, Sprecher H, Ramon M, Bergman R. Does infection play a role in the pathogenesis of granuloma annulare? J Am Acad Dermatol. 2013;68(2):342–3.
21. Piette EW, Rosenbach M. Granuloma annulare clinical and histologic variants, epidemiology, and genetics. J Am Acad Dermatol. 2016;75:457–65.
22. Lallas A, Zaballos P, Zalaudek I, Apalla Z, Gourhant JY, Longo C, Moscarella E, Tiodorovic-Zivkovic D, Argenziano G. Dermoscopic patterns of granuloma annulare and necrobiosis lipoidica. Clin Exp Dermatol. 2013;38:424–9.
23. Keimig EL. Granuloma annulare. Dermatol Clin. 2015;33(3):315–29.
24. Martín-Sáenz E, Fernández-Guarino M, Carrillo-Gijón R, et al. Efficacy of dapsone in disseminated granuloma annulare: a case report and review of the literature. Actas Dermosifilogr. 2008;99(1):64–8.
25. Piaserico S, Zattra E, Linder D, et al. Generalized granuloma annulare treated with methylaminolevulinate photodynamic therapy. Dermatology. 2009;218(3):282–4.
26. Pătraşcu V, Giurcă C, Ciurea RN, Georgescu CV. Disseminated granuloma annulare: study on eight cases. Romanian J Morphol Embryol. 2013;54(2):327–31.
27. Binkley GW. Dermopathy in diabetes mellitus. Arch Dermatol. 1965;92:106–7.
28. McCash S, Emanuel PO. Defining diabetic dermopathy. J Dermatol. 2011;38(10):988–92.
29. Murphy-Chutorian B, Han G, Cohen SR. Dermatologic manifestations of diabetes mellitus. A review. Endocrinol Metab Clin N Am. 2013;42(4):869–98.
30. Duhm G. Atrofia parda circunscrita pretibial y diabetes. Trabajo original 1 y 2 años de la docencia complementaria. UBA, Facultad de Medicina; 1970.
31. Brugler A, Thompson S, Turner S, Ngo B, Rendell M. Skin blood flow abnormalities in diabetic dermopathy. J Am Acad Dermatol. 2011;65(3):559–63.
32. Kiziltan ME, Benbir G. Clinical and nerve conduction studies in female patients with diabetic dermopathy. Acta Diabetol. 2008;45(2):97–105.
33. Morgan AJ, Schwartz RA. Diabetic dermopathy: a subtle sign with grave implications. J Am Acad Dermatol. 2008;58(3):447–51.
34. Lipsky BA, Baker PD, Ahroni JH. Diabetic bullae: 12 cases of a purportedly rare cutaneous disorder. Int J Dermatol. 2000;39(3):196–200.
35. Bernstein JE, Levine LE, Medenica M. Reduced threshold to suction-induced blister formation in insulin-dependent diabetes. J Am Acad Dermatol. 1983;8(6):790–1.
36. Zhang AJ, Garret M, Miller S. Bullosis diabeticorum: case report and review. N Z Med J. 2013;126(1371):91–4.
37. Domínguez-Borgúa A, Vide Sandoval-Cabrera D, Izaguirre-Gutiérrez VF, Gutiérrez-Sánchez CO. Diabetic blistering disease. Med Int Méx. 2014;30:468–73.

38. Gupta V, Gulati N, Bahl J, Bajwa J, Dhawan N. Bullosis diabeticorum: rare presentation in a common disease. Case Rep Endocrinol. 2014;2014:862912, 3 pages.
39. Craike P. Bullosis diabeticorum: a treatment conundrum. J Foot Ankle Res. 2011;4(Suppl 1):12.
40. Ghosh SK, Bandyopadhyay D, Chatterjee G. Bullosis diabeticorum: a distinctive blistering eruption in diabetes mellitus. Int J Diabetes Dev Ctries. 2009;29(1):41–2.
41. Cavalleiro de Macedo Mota AN, Solon Nery N, Barcaui CB. Case for diagnosis. An Bras Dermatol. 2013;88(4):652–4.
42. Haught JM, Patel S, English JC III. Xanthoderma: a clinical review. J Am Acad Dermatol. 2007;57:1051–8.
43. Ferringer T, Miller F. Cutaneous manifestations of diabetes mellitus. Dermatol Clin. 2002;20:483–92.
44. Huntley AC. Cutaneous manifestations of diabetes mellitus. Diabetes Metab Rev. 1993;9:161–76.
45. Julka S, Jamdagni N, Verma S, Goyal R. Yellow palms and soles: a rare skin manifestation in diabetes mellitus. Indian J Endocrinol Metab. 2013;17(Suppl1):S299–300. https://doi.org/10.4103/2230-8210.119625.
46. Lin J-N. Yellow palms and soles in diabetes mellitus. N Engl J Med. 2006;355:1486.

Thick Skin Syndrome

7

Emilia Noemí Cohen Sabban and Paula A. Friedman

Introduction

Diabetic patients show higher prevalence of rheumatic diseases as compared to general population due to the fact that Diabetes Mellitus (DM) affects all components of musculoskeletal system: muscles, bones and connective tissue [1, 2].

Different musculoskeletal disorders that involve hands and shoulders are described, including palmar flexor tenosynovitis, Dupuytren's contracture, carpal tunnel syndrome, Charcot arthropathy, reflex sympathetic dystrophy and shoulder's adhesive capsulitis. They can be painful and cause functional weakness (Figs. 7.1 and 7.2) [3, 4].

In the hand, DM produces the so-called "diabetic hand syndrome", being Limited joint mobility (LJM) the most frequent manifestation [5]. It is rather underexposed and underdiagnosed compared with other well-known manifestations of the disease. It's association with neuropathy and microvascular complications, should alert the physician about higher risk for the development of "Diabetic foot Syndrome" among other pathologies that can influence patients' health-related quality of life quite dramatically [6]. Prevalence of LJM increases with duration of DM, poor glycemic control, non-enzymatic glycation (NEG) and accumulation of advanced glycation end products (AGEs), increasing age and also in smokers [7, 8].

E.N. Cohen Sabban, M.D. (✉)
Dermatology Department, Instituto de Investigaciones Médicas A. Lanari,
University of Buenos Aires (UBA), Buenos Aires, Argentina
e-mail: emicohensabban@gmail.com

P.A. Friedman, M.D.
Dermatologist, Instituto de Investigaciones Médicas A. Lanari,
University of Buenos Aires, Buenos Aires, Argentina

© Springer International Publishing AG 2018
E.N. Cohen Sabban et al. (eds.), *Dermatology and Diabetes*,
https://doi.org/10.1007/978-3-319-72475-1_7

Fig 7.1 Dupuytren's
contracture

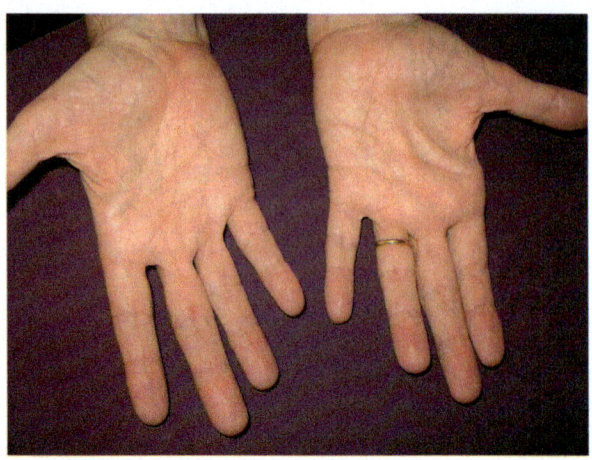

Fig. 7.2 Dupuytren's
contracture

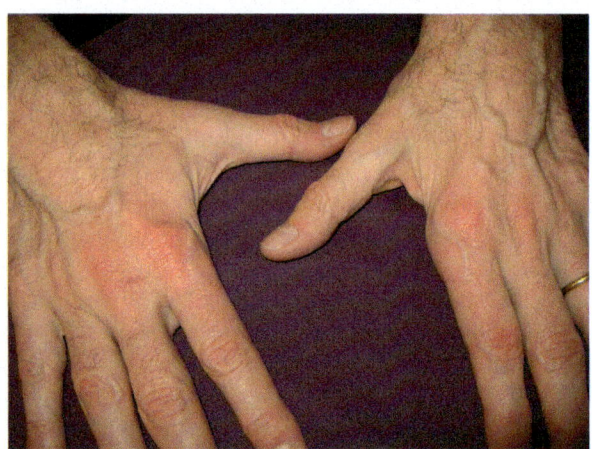

The thick skin syndrome includes four cutaneous manifestations: Finger pebbles (FP); Waxy skin (WS); Limited joint mobility (LJM); and Diabetic scleredema (DS) (Table 7.1) [9].

Finger Pebbles

Also known as Huntley's papules, FP consist of multiple tiny papules grouped on the extensor surface and lateral aspect of the fingers, on the knuckles of the metacarpophalangeal and interphalangeal joints, more frequently in the distal ones, and in the periungual region (Figs. 7.3, 7.4 and 7.5) [10, 11].

According to the literature, it is a very common finding that reaches up to 60–70% of diabetic patients, but in our experience, we do not find it so often. Moreover, it can happen in 20% of non-diabetic people, especially, manual workers. It is asymptomatic, and treatment is not required.

Table 7.1 Thick skin syndrome

	Finger pebbles	Waxy skin and limited joint mobility	Diabetic scleredema
Incidence	60%	30%	2.5%
Age	Infants/youth and adults	2 variants: child and youth and the most frequent adults	>40 years
Gender	Equal in both	Equal in both	4:1 male/female
Relationship with diabetes	80% in diabetic patients, 20% in non-diabetics	T1DM and T2DM	More in obese, long-standing and poorly controlled T2DM
Importance	Visual marker of skin thickening in DM	High risk of microvascular complications	Related to insulin resistance, retinopathy, HT, ischemic disease

DM diabetes mellitus, *T1DM* type 1 diabetes mellitus, *T2DM* type 2 diabetes mellitus, *HT* arterial hypertension

Fig. 7.3 Tiny papules, mostly located on the interphalangeal joint and periungual region

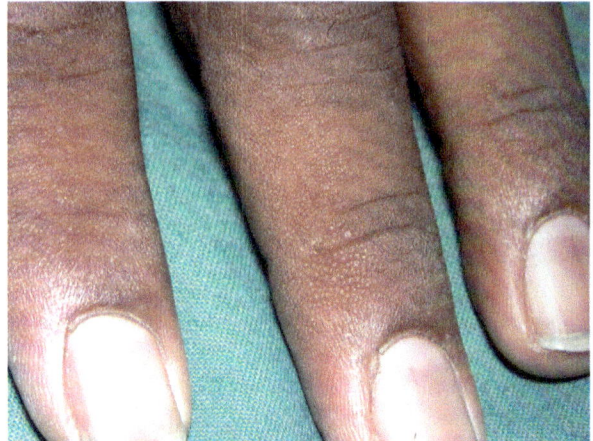

Fig. 7.4 Huntley's papules

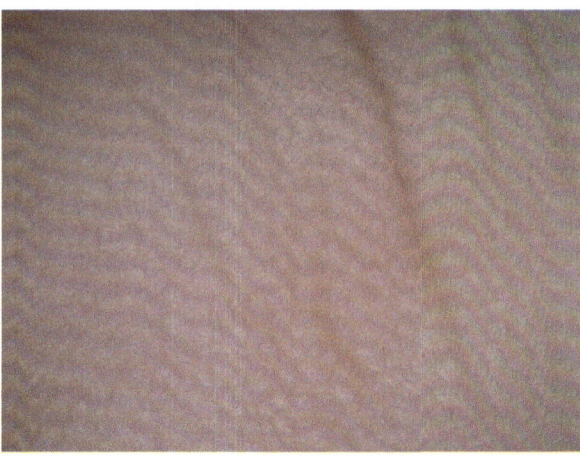

Fig. 7.5 Finger pebbles

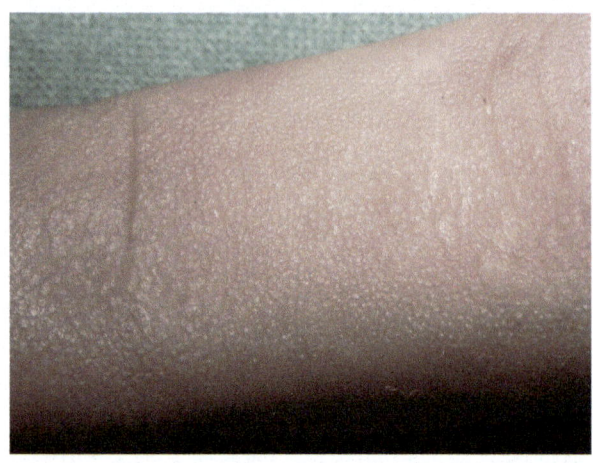

When it appears in diabetic patients, it is considered a visual marker of the thickening of the dorsum of the hands. It is associated with either type 1 DM (T1DM) or type 2 DM (T2DM) of both genders equally; although in Huntley's original description—later supported by other authors—it is more frequent in adults with T2DM. It has been suggested that the thickening is not only related to NEG of collagen fibers, but also to epidermal growth factors such as insulin-like growth factor (IGF-1) [12]. Finger pebbles are an early dermatologic sign of sclerodermiform alterations in hands [13].

The histologic features of FP are epidermal hyperplasia with a "church tower" aspect where orthokeratotic hyperkeratosis and regular acanthosis are evident; at the dermis level, we observe changes in the collagen fibers that are arranged vertically, papillomatosis and areas of angiogenesis along with insignificant perivascular infiltrates [14].

Saraiya et al. described an association between FP, acanthosis nigricans (AN) and cutaneous acrochordons in obese T2DM patients with insulin resistance (IR) and high levels of IGF-1 [15, 16]. FP are also associated to severe obesity in the context of IR without underlying DM, as in the reported case by Granel et al., whose patient suffers from Pickwick Syndrome (severe obesity, drowsiness, excessive appetite, hypoventilation, and sleep apnea) [17].

Waxy Skin

It is characterized by cutaneous changes over the dorsum of the hands and forearm due to the accumulation of dermal collagen of the skin. Under physical examination the skin is shiny and tight, difficult to fold, similar to scleroderma but with its own features, both in optical and electron microscopy. Clinical manifestations such as ulcers and Raynaud's phenomenon, capillaroscopic Scleroderma pattern, specific autoantibodies and other laboratory data are helpful in the differential diagnosis between both entities (Table 7.2) (Figs. 7.6 and 7.7) [18].

Table 7.2 Clues for the diagnosis of sclerodermiform changes in DM versus scleroderma

	DM	Scleroderma
Age	10–20 years	40–50 years
Gender	Equal	3:1 female/male
Diabetes	Type 1 and 2	There may be an abnormal glucose tolerance
Pain	No	Yes
Raynaud	No	Yes
Digital ulcers	No	Yes
Telangiectasia	No	Yes
Pigmentation	No	Yes
Capillaroscopy	Capillaries loss	SD pattern
Histology	Dermal collagen is thickened and hyalinized, spaces and clefts between fibers. Fat around eccrine sweat glands is preserved. No inflammatory reaction	Epidermal atrophy Homogenization of the dermis with loss of spaces between collagen bundles. Replacement of the periglandular fat by collagen

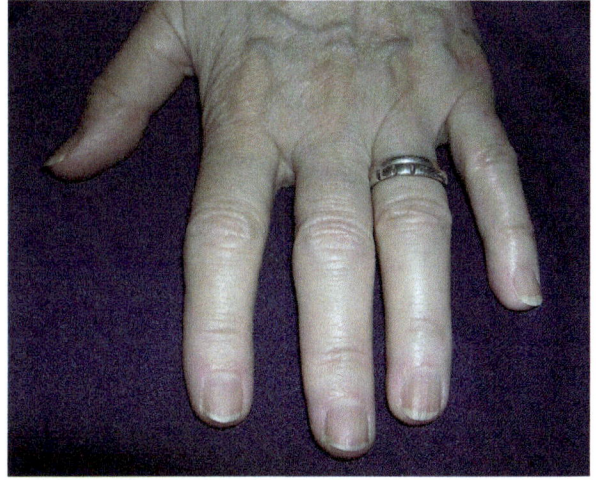

Fig. 7.6 Waxy skin. The skin is shiny and tight, difficult to fold

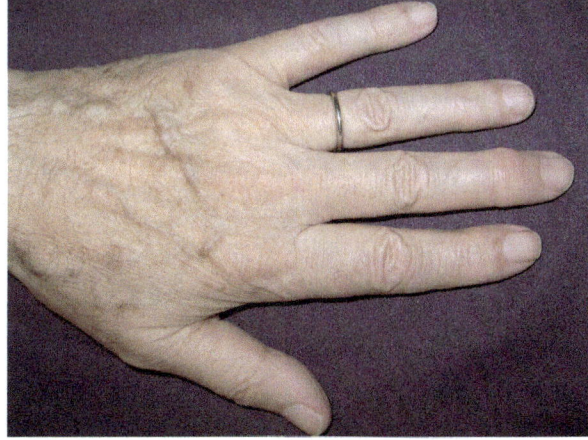

Fig. 7.7 Waxy skin at the phalanges. Limited joint mobility in an aerly stage. Normal aged and wrinkled skin of the patient at the back of the hand is observed

Waxy skin is more frequent in diabetic patients with LJM, in particular with those with moderate or severe involvement, than in diabetic individuals without that manifestation, which in turn, have thicker skin compared to non-diabetics. Histopathologically, dermoepidermal thickening with accumulation of collagen and loss of cutaneous appendages are characteristic features.

Limited Joint Mobility

LJM is caused by the thickening and stiffness of the periarticular connective tissue. It involves mainly the small joints of the hands and results in a severe finger contracture and the inability to extend the metacarpophalangeal and proximal and distal interphalangeal joints starting with the fifth and fourth fingers and expanding radially. It is painless and generally goes unnoticed until the deformity becomes so severe that it interferes with daily life with less grip strength and a notable difficulty to close the fingers into a fist and make fine movements (Figs. 7.8, 7.9, 7.10, 7.11, 7.12, 7.13, 7.14, 7.15, 7.16 and 7.17).

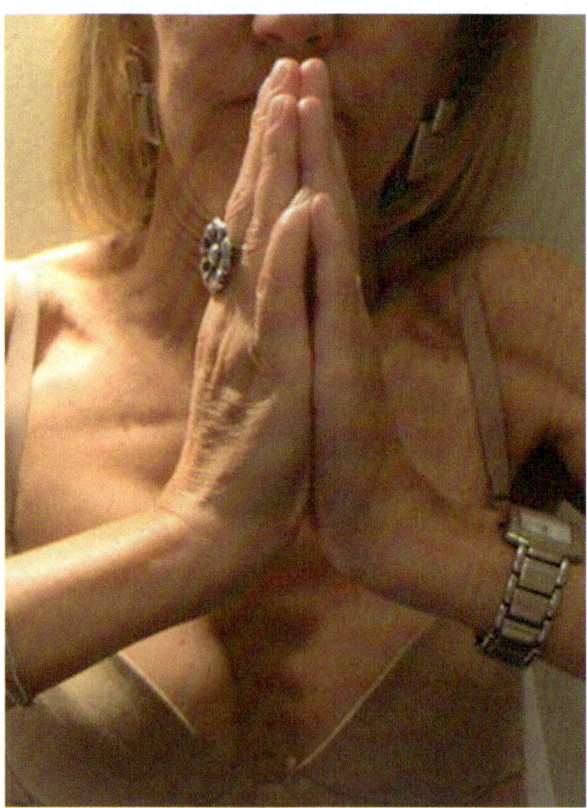

Fig. 7.8 Limited joint mobility of the fifth finger of both hands. Prayer sign

Fig. 7.9 Limited joint
mobility. Severe degree.
Prayer sign

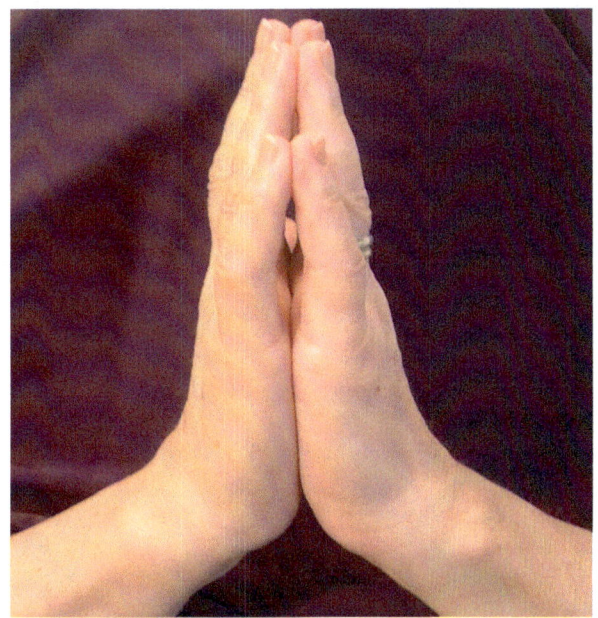

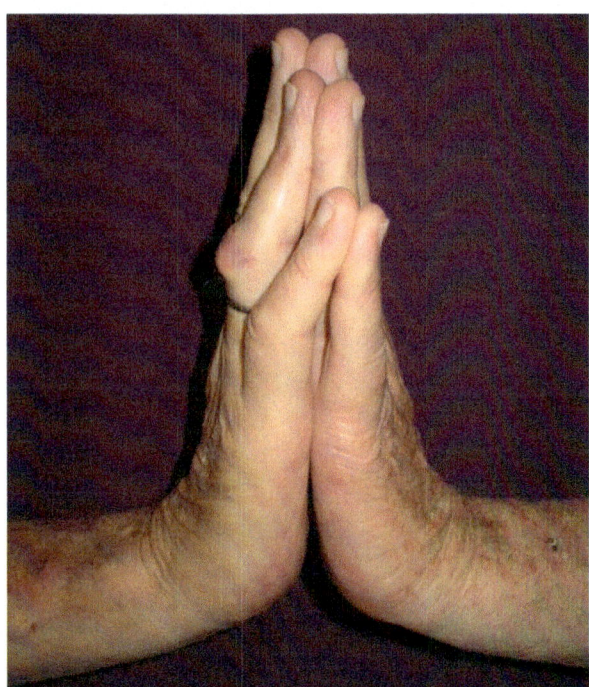

Fig. 7.10 Limited joint
mobility. Severe degree

Fig. 7.11 Limited joint mobility of the fifth fingers of both hands

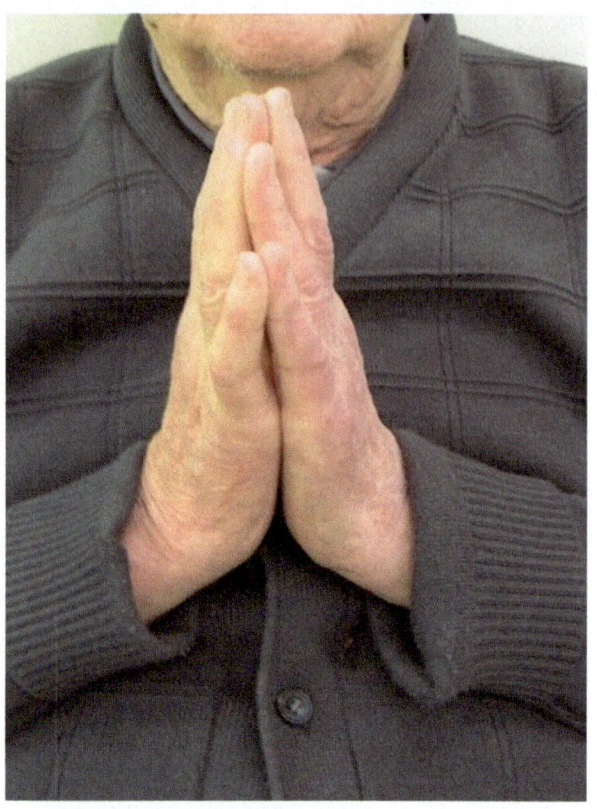

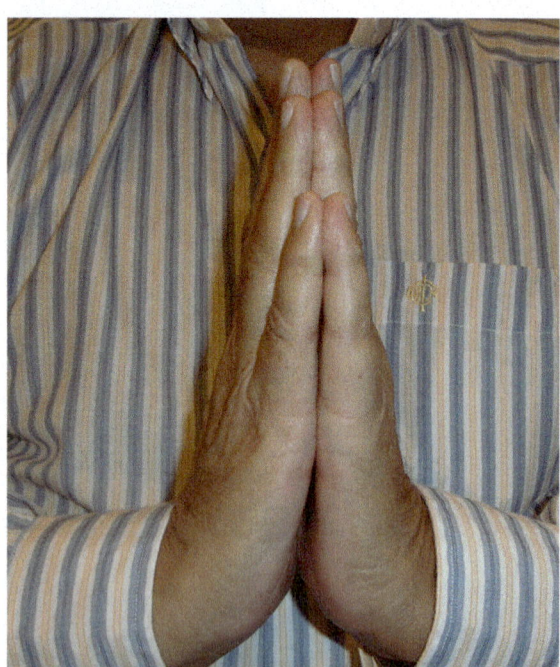

Fig. 7.12 Limited joint mobility of the fifth fingers of both hands

Fig. 7.13 Limited joint mobility of the fourth and fifth fingers of both hands

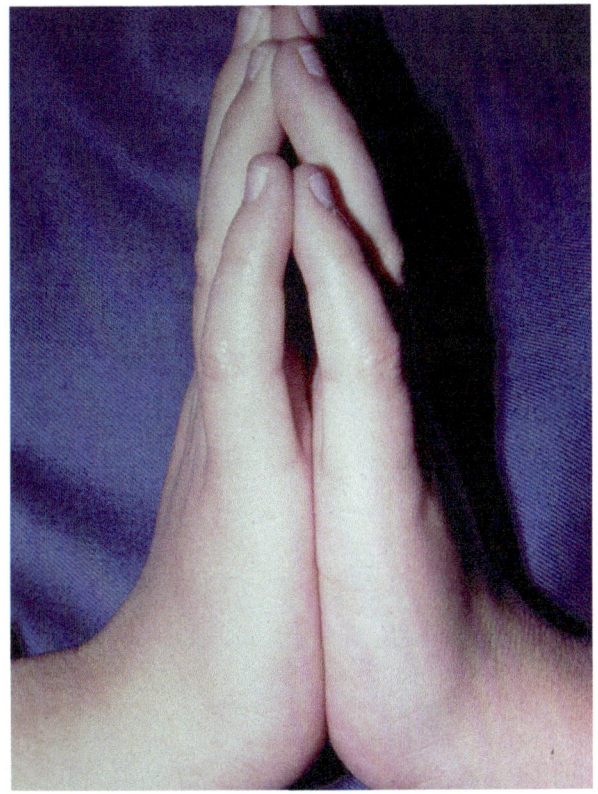

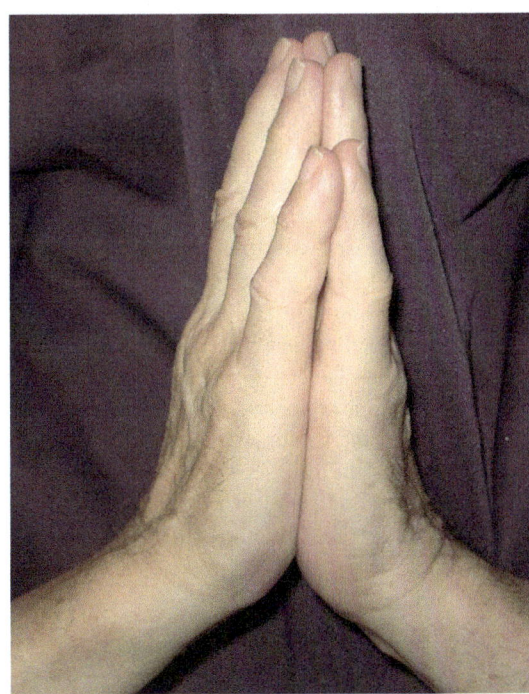

Fig. 7.14 Limited joint mobility. Prayer sign

Fig. 7.15 Limited joint
mobility. Severe degree

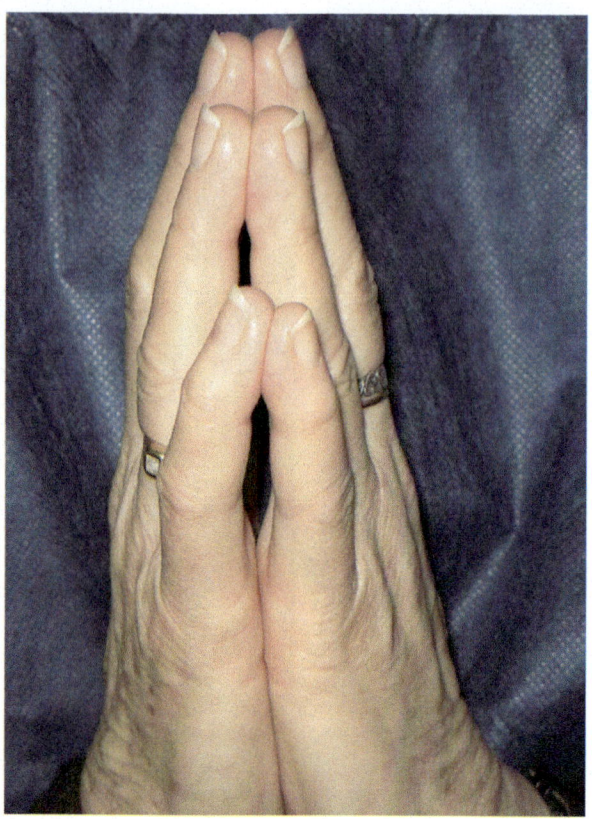

It is also known as cheiroarthropathy or "diabetic stiff hand syndrome" and has a prevalence of 30–40% of T1DM patients (8–50% of diabetic individuals); although it is also present in T2DM, both male and female equally.

Apart from the hands, other joints can be affected like wrists, elbows, knees, ankles, shoulders, the cervical and thoracolumbar spine, and other organs (lungs) [19]. Its original description on the 70s belongs to Rosembloom et al., where they reported three cases with long-lasting T1DM and LJM of the hands, wrists, elbows and ankles and in two of them along spinal column with other clinical features. X-rays did not show any joint disorders, which confirmed that the thickening was due to the thickening and stiffness of the periarticular tissue [20].

The main risk factor for the appearance of this disease is the DM duration [21]. There is a relationship between joint stiffness and increased NEG of periarticular collagen, cartilage and tendon, based on the proof that each increased unit of HbA1c from the beginning of the disease, corresponded to 46% of increase risk of developing LJM.

It is essential to emphasize that the presence of LJM in diabetic patients is an important marker of subsequent microvascular disease and can constitute a useful clinical tool for the identification of a subset of patients at high risk for developing early complications.

Fig. 7.16 Limited joint mobility. Severe degree

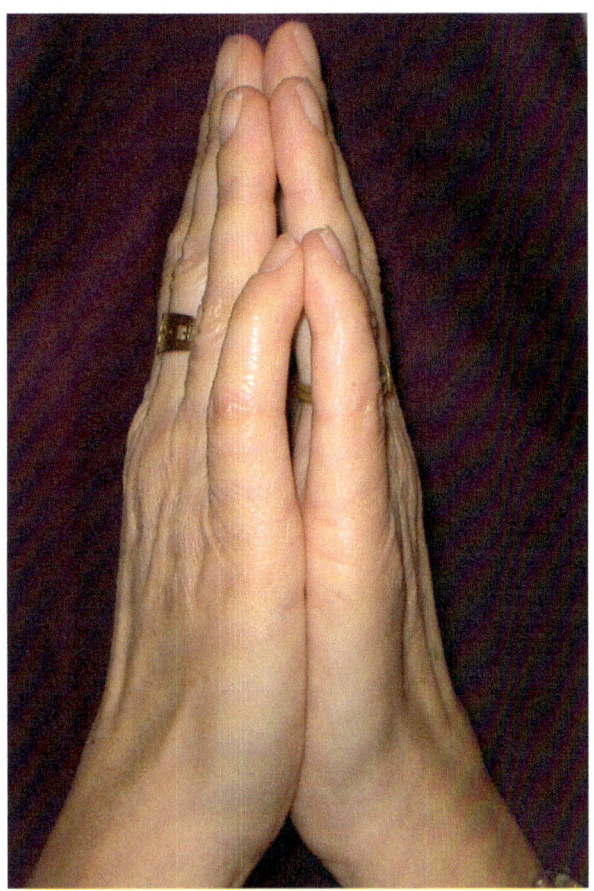

Some authors refer that LJM is an independent factor for the development of microvascular complications and increases the risk 3–5 times in these patients. A recent analysis found that in the presence of LJM, there is an 83% increase in the risk of developing microvascular complications after 16 years of having DM, as opposed to 25% of risk in the absence of LJM. Rosenbloom et al. observed that it is even more frequent in the case of the male gender, possibly due to a poor glycemic control, coronary heart and cerebrovascular disease. In women, it is related to early macrovascular complications [22].

In addition, LJM is associated with several disorders that should be taken into account such as higher risk of accidental falls—which is moderate according to balance assessment (19–20 s), and diabetic foot ulcers, due to an increase of the pressure on the metatarsophalangeal and submetatarsal joints plantar points [23, 24].

Thickening of the plantar fascia and the Achilles tendon, has also been described, more frequently in patients having LJM and peripheral neuropathy and correlated positively with the body mass index (BMI) [25]. Moreover, shoulder and hand's

Fig. 7.17 Limited joint mobility of the fifth and fourth fingers of both hands

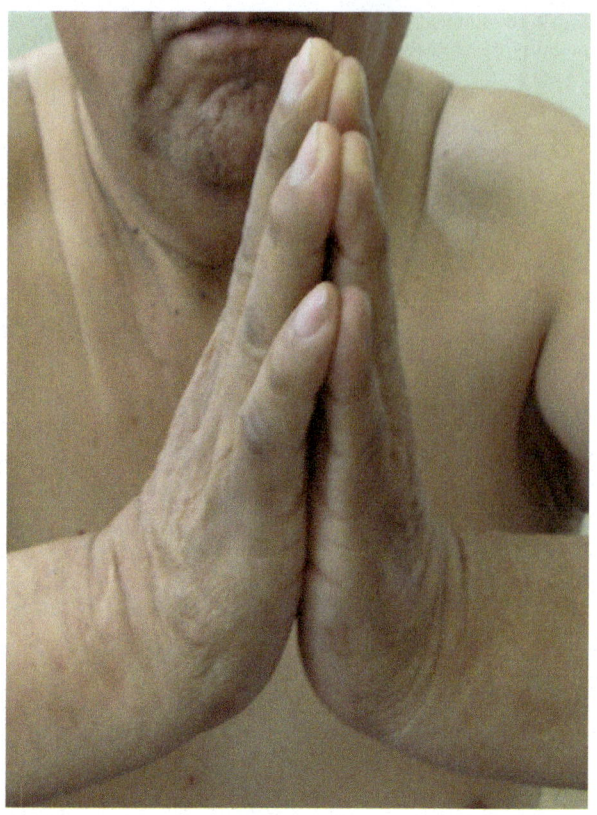

LJM may lead to upper extremity impairments compromising the strength and functionality of the upper extremity [26].

The degree of hand involvement has been classified into mild, when the limitation affects one or two proximal interphalangeal joints, one large joint or only metacarpophalangeal bilateral joints. Moderate limitation refers to three or more proximal interphalangeal joints or the joint of one finger and one large bilateral joint. Severe cases are constituted by the deformity of the hand at rest or involvement of the cervical spine. The progression of changes, since the initial detection of a mild limitation to moderate or severe condition varies, starting from 3 month to 4 years, with an average of 2 years. Fifty percent of young patients with DM for more than 5 years develop moderate or severe limitation.

There are simple tests that help in its recognition. One is the "prayer sign", where it is clearly impossible for the patient to oppose the palms together completely, without leaving a gap between the two; the magnitude will depend on the degree of the patient affectation. The other is the "table top sign" where the patient is not able to completely extend his/her hand on a table's surface: this makes the diagnosis of metacarpophalangeal contractures easier (Fig. 7.18) (Table 7.3) [27]. If both tests turn out positive, it is recommended to make a careful examination of each joint.

Fig. 7.18 Limited joint mobility. "table top sign": the patient is not able to completely extend his/her hand on a flat surface

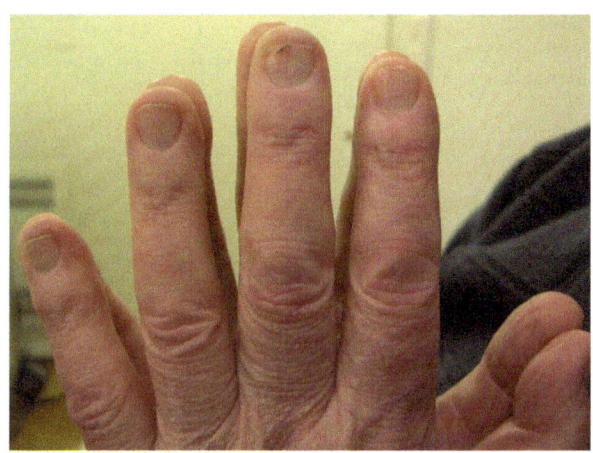

Table 7.3 Clinical signs for limited joint mobility (LJM)

Prayer sign	Table top sign
Evaluates the ability to oppose hands without leaving a space between them, allowing for the recognition of contractures in the metacarpophalangeal and interphalangeal proximal and distal joints	Determines the ability to completely extend palms on the table's surface, allowing the recognition of metacarpophalangeal joint contracture

Table 7.4 Degrees of severity of waxy skin and limited joint mobility

Degree 0	No changes
Degree I	Waxy skin, no contractures
Degree II	Contractures in the flexion of both little fingers
Degree III	Bilateral compromise of fingers and wrists
Degree IV	Bilateral compromise of other fingers
Degree V	Bilateral compromise of fingers, wrists and other joints

Brink-Starkman classification

Even though, the prayer sign and the table top sign are widely recognized in literature as diagnostic tools, they are not present in all cases as a rule. For subclinical forms of the disease, goniometry is used which in case of being positive, confirm the association between flexion restriction of small joints of the hands and microvascular complications in patients with DM [28]. In terms of severity assessment, two different classification are used (Tables 7.4 and 7.5) [29].

Cutaneous biopsy is rarely used for the diagnosis of this syndrome. Histopathological findings consist of a normal epidermis and an excess amount of thickened and hyalinized collagen fibers [30].

With regards to the natural evolution, after two decades of its acknowledgement, its incidence has experienced a substantial decrease, probably due to a better metabolic control. In 1998, the same physicians applying the same techniques they used

Table 7.5 Degrees of severity of waxy skin and limited joint mobility

Degree I	Waxy skin
Degree II	Contractures in the flexion of both little fingers
Degree III	Contractures in the flexion of other fingers
Degree IV	Bilateral compromise of wrists
Degree V	Compromise of other joints

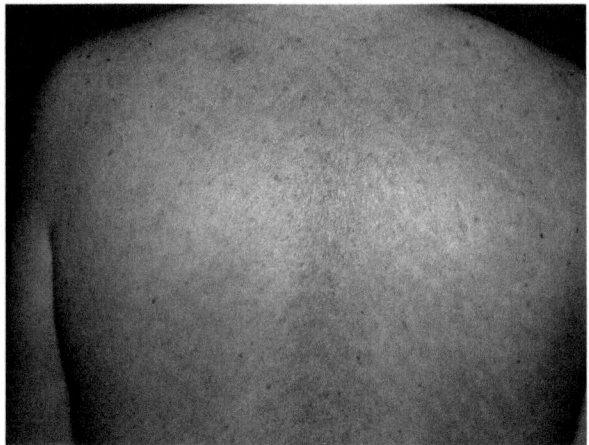

Fig. 7.19 Diabetic Scleredema. Thickness, diffuse, and symmetric skin induration of the upper back

in their description compared the initial findings and found that the frequency of LJM had decreased four times along with a dramatic decrease in other manifestations such as short stature. This important reduction in the frequency in kids and teenagers with DM over time was attributed to a better glycaemia and HbA1c monitoring and to new types and release systems of insulin [31, 32].

In the treatment of LJM, metabolic control is mandatory, in addition to physiotherapy and occupational therapy that can be helpful and yield variable results [33].

Diabetic Scleredema

It is a rare disorder that affects generally older than 40 year-old-male diabetic patients, with an approximate incidence of 2.5%. It is characterized by thickness and diffuse, asymptomatic and symmetric skin induration of the posterior neck and upper back, shoulders and arms, which confers an orange-peel appearance. Although less frequent, it may involve other parts of the body like the face, abdomen, thighs, and buttocks. In contrast to scleroderma, hands and feet are spared [34] (Fig. 7.19).

Nowadays three types of scleredema are described in literature: Type 1 is the classical form or scleredema adultorum of Buschke that mainly affects women and is typically preceded by an infectious process of upper airways most often due to Streptococcus which resolves spontaneously in contrast to Type 3, which is seen in

Table 7.6 Differences between scleredema diabeticorum and classical scleredema

	Scleredema diabeticorum	Classical scleredema
Gender	4:1 male/female	2:1 female/male
Age	Adults	
Previous infection	No	Yes; upper airways due to Streptococcus
Clinics	Insidious onset. Affects skin of the neck and upper back, although it may extend	Sudden onset. Affects skin of neck and upper back, localized in most of the cases
Retinopathy	Yes	No
Associations	Long standing T2DM, poorly controlled, Obese, insulin resistant patients. HT*, myocardial infarction	Rare
Evolution	Persistent	75% resolves spontaneously
Treatment	Generally unresponsive	None

HT arterial hypertension

long-standing and poor-controlled T2DM, the so-called Scleredema diabeticorum, which differs from the classical or type 1 Scleredema in its predominance in men, it is not preceded by any infectious process and does not resolve spontaneously, besides it is associated with insulin resistant state and obesity (Table 7.6).

In order to make a correct classification and diagnosis, physicians should take a comprehensive clinical history of the patient, laboratory tests with complete blood count, glycaemia, HbA1c levels, etc. and a skin biopsy to confirm the diagnosis [35].

Microscopically, thickened and irregularly distributed collagen fibers, separated by clear spaces in which mucin is deposited, evidenced with Alcian Blue stain, at the reticular dermis can be observed. Sometimes, the increase of the dermis thickness can reach up to four times its normal size. Moreover, subcutaneous fat can be replaced by collagen fibers [36].

Although there is considerable uncertainty about its pathogenesis, one possibility is that hyperglycemia would act as a stimulant for fibroblast proliferation and synthesis of extracellular matrix components. Another hypothesis is that a poor glycemic control may lead to an increase in NEG of the collagen fibers. The accumulation of AGE-modified collagen, which in turn are more resistant to collagenases degradation, is responsible for the skin induration [37–39].

The treatment of SD continues to be a challenge, lacking a gold standard and large placebo controlled trials. Most of the reported cases, achieved variable results. The first therapeutic step is the intensification of the metabolic control, although there is no consensus regarding the correlation between glycemic control and the improvement of SD.

Colchicine has been used in cases of SD, due to its anti-inflammatory properties and to its ability to prevent collagen synthesis [40]. Lin et al. reported a case of an association between SD and eccrine gland loss with the subsequent anhidrosis of the affected area. After 8 month of treatment with allopurinol 100 mg/day a mild relief was noted by the patient but without changes related to the lack of sweating [41].

Fig. 7.20 *Left*: Non-diabetic control patient. Wrinkles after immersion in the water. *Right*: Diabetic patient without wrinkles after immersion in the water

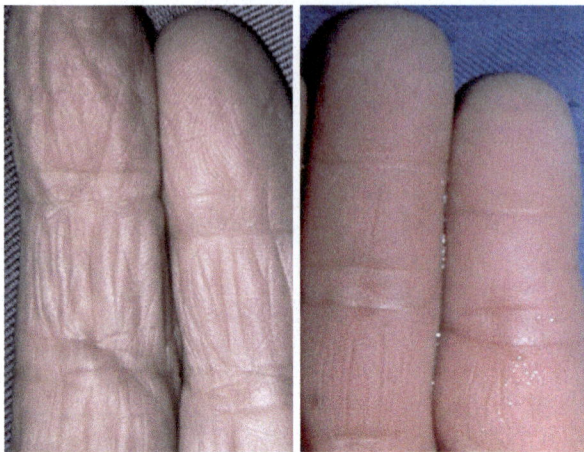

Immunosuppressant drugs like cyclosporine, corticosteroids (CST) and methotrexate (MTX) are other therapeutic options. It is believed that MTX, apart from interfering in the glycation process, can decrease the production of connective tissue or mucin by the fibroblasts and other cells that are involved [42]. Another therapeutic modality could be radiation therapy, psoralen combined with ultraviolet A (PUVA) (accumulative doses of UVA, 120 J/cm²). Shazzad et al. report a case of a patient with SD treated with a combination of PUVA and MTX with a good results [43]. Recently very good response have been reported with UVA1 phototherapy and intravenous immunoglobulin G (IVIG) [44–47].

In our experience, although the small number of patients with SD we have observed, cutaneous lesions didn't improve with a good glycemic control and the therapeutic response to the different modalities described, has been refractory.

As mentioned previously, the diagnosis of thick skin syndrome is basically clinical and there are non-invasive methods of detection like ocular inspection, palpation, the prayer sign and the table top sign. There is another way to check it, which is by detecting cutaneous wrinkles on the finger pads [48]. The patient's hands are submerged in warm water at 42 °C for 30 min. In diabetic patients, no wrinkles on the finger pads are observed, contrary to what happens in the general population (Fig. 7.20). The mechanism by which these wrinkles diminish, is unknown, but it is thought that the cause of the thickening of this part of the skin could be multifactorial and that sympathetic autonomic neuropathy with an increase in the deep tissue turgor, keratin NEG with an increase in the epidermal thickness, and the alteration of the blood flow through the finger pads, participate.

Conclusion

The thick skin syndrome includes several cutaneous manifestations. Many of them are associated with comorbidities, or in association with other syndromes and should be differentiated from other conditions such Scleroderma.

LJM is an often-missed Diabetes marker that in severe cases may interfere with daily life's routine. It's importance lies in the fact that it can be used as a surrogate sign for development of diabetic microvascular complications.

Moreover, it's association with higher risk of accidental falls, diabetic foot ulcers and upper extremity impairments have been reported many times in the literature.

Fortunately, there is an important decrease in its frequency due to a better glycaemia and HbA1c monitoring and the new types and release systems of insulin. Thus, metabolic control in patients with skin thick syndrome is mandatory.

References

1. Abate M, Schiavone C, Salini V, et al. Management of limited joint mobility in diabetic patients. Diabetes Metab Syndr Obes. 2013;6:197–207.
2. Singla R, Gupta Y, Kalra S. Musculoskeletal effects of diabetes mellitus. J Pak Med Assoc. 2015;65(9):1024–7.
3. Rosenbloom AL. Connective tissue disorders in diabetes. In: Defrongo RA, Ferrannini E, Keen H, Zimmet P, editors. International textbook F diabetes mellitus. 3rd ed. Wiley: Chichester; 2004.
4. Chen L-H, Li C-Y, Kuo L-C. Risk of hand syndromes in patients with diabetes mellitus: a population-based cohort study in Taiwan. Medicine. 2015;94(41):1575.
5. Schiavon F, Circhetta C, Dani L. The diabetic hand. Reumatismo. 2004;56(3):139–42.
6. Gerrits E, Landman G, Nijenhuis-Rosien L, et al. Limited joint mobility syndrome in diabetes mellitus: a mini review. World J Diabetes. 2015;6(9):1108–12.
7. Larkin ME, Barnie A, Braffett BH, Diabetes control and complications trial/epidemiology of diabetes Interventions and complications research group, et al. Musculoskeletal complications in type 1 diabetes. Diabetes Care. 2014;37(7):1863–9.
8. Nagesh VS, Kalra S. Type 1 diabetes: syndromes in resource-challenged settings. J Pak Med Assoc. 2015;65(6):681–5; 28.
9. Burner TW, Rosenthal AK. Diabetes and rheumatic diseases. Curr Opin Rheumatol. 2009;21(1):50–4.
10. Huntley C. Finger pebbles: a common finding in diabetes mellitus. J Am Acad Dermatol. 1986;14:612–7.
11. Libecco JF, Brodell RT. Finger pebbles and diabetes: a case with broad involvement of the dorsal fingers and hands. Arch Dermatol. 2001;137(4):510–1.
12. Singh R, Barden A, Mori T, et al. Advanced glycation end-products: a review. Diabetologia. 2001;44(2):129–46.
13. Cabo HA, Woscoff A, Casas JG. Empedrado digital: marcador temprano de engrosamiento cutaneo en pacientes diabeticos. Arch Argent Dermatol. 1988;48:185–9.
14. Guarneri C, Guarneri F, Borgia F, et al. Finger pebbles in a diabetic patient: Huntley's papules. Int J Dermatol. 2005;44:755–6.
15. Saraiya A, Al-Shoha A, Brodell RT. Hyperinsulinemia associated with acanthosis nigricans, finger pebbles, acrochordons, and the sign of Leser-Trelat. Endocr Pract. 2013;19(3):522–5.
16. Hollister DS, Brodell RT. Finger 'pebbles' A dermatologic sign of diabetes mellitus. Postgrad Med. 2000;107(3):209–10.
17. Granel B, Serratrice J, Mohamed H, et al. Pickwickian syndrome and vanishing finger pebbles. Arch Dermatol. 2001;137(4):508–10.
18. Tyndall A, Fistarol S. The differential diagnosis of systemic sclerosis. Curr Opin Rheumatol. 2013;25(6):692–9.
19. Shah KM, Clark RB, McGill JB, Lang CE, et al. Shoulder limited joint mobility in people with diabetes mellitus. Clin Biomech (Bristol, Avon). 2015;30(3):308–13.

20. Rosenbloom AL, Frias JL. Diabetes, short stature and joint stiffness—a new syndrome. Clin Res. 1974;22:92A.
21. Proubasta R. La mano diabética. Revista Iberoamericana de Cirugía de la mano. 2015;43(2):135.
22. Amin R, Bahu TK, Widmer B, et al. Longitudinal relation between limited joint mobility, height, insulin like growth factor I levels, and risk of developing microalbuminuria: the Oxford Regional Prospective Study. Arch Dis Child. 2005;90:1039–44.
23. Lopez-Martin I, Benito Ortiz L, Rodriguez-Borlado B, et al. Association between limited joint mobility syndrome and risk of accidental falls in diabetic patients. Semergen. 2015;41(2):70–5.
24. Mineoka Y, Ishii M, Tsuji A, et al. Relationship between limited joint mobility of the hand and diabetic foot risk in patients with type 2 diabetes. J Diabetes. 2017 Jun;9(6):628–33.
25. Craig ME, Duffin AC, Gallego PH, et al. Plantar fascia thickness, a measure of tissue glycation, predicts the development of complications in adolescents with type 1 diabetes. Diabetes Care. 2008;31(6):1201–6.
26. Shah KM, Clark BR, McGill JB, et al. Upper extremity impairments, pain and disability in patients with diabetes mellitus. Physiotherapy. 2015;101(2):147–54.
27. Rosenbloom AL, Silverstein JH. Connective tissue and joint disease in diabetes mellitus. Endocrinol Metab Clin N Am. 1996;25:473–83.
28. Pandey A, Usman K, Reddy H, et al. Prevalence of hand disorders in type 2 diabetes mellitus and its correlation with microvascular complications. Ann Med Health Sci Res. 2013;3(3):349–54.
29. Starkman H, Brink S. Limited joint mobility (LJM) of the hand in patients with diabetes mellitus. Diabetes Care. 1982;5:534–6.
30. Liu T, McCalmont TH, Frieden IJ, et al. The stiff skin syndrome: case series, differential diagnosis of the stiff skin phenotype, and review of the literature. Arch Dermatol. 2008;144(10):1351–9.
31. Infante JR, Rosenbloom AL, Silverstein JH, et al. Changes in frequency and severity of limited joint mobility in children with type 1 diabetes mellitus between 1976–78 and 1998. J Pediatr. 2001;138:33–7.
32. Rosenbloom AL. Limited Joint mobility in childhood diabetes: discovery, description, and decline. J Clin Endocrinol Metab. 2013;98:466–73.
33. Del Rosso A, Matucci Cerinic M, De Giorgio F, et al. Rheumatological manifestations in diabetes mellitus. Curr Diabetes Rev. 2006;2(4):455–66.
34. Rebora A, Rongioletti F. Mucinoses. In: Bolognia JL, Jorizzo JL, Rapini RP, editors. Dermatology. London: Mosby; 2003. p. 647–58.
35. Salazar-Nievas M, Crespo-Lora V, Rubio-Lopez J, et al. Cutaneous indurated plaque on the abdomen associated with diabetes mellitus. Aust Fam Physician. 2013;42(12):876–7.
36. Beers WH, Ince A, Moore TL. Scleredema adultorum of Buschke: a case report and review of the literature. Semin Arthritis Rheum. 2006;35(6):355–9.
37. Tran K, Boyd KP, Robinson MR, et al. Scleredema diabeticorum. Dermatol Online J. 2013;19(12):20718.
38. Gruson LM, Franks A Jr. Scleredema and diabetic sclerodactyly. Dermatol Online J. 2005;11(4):3.
39. Yaqub A, Chung L, Rieger KE, et al. Localized cutaneous fibrosing disorders. Rheum Dis Clin N Am. 2013;39(2):347–64.
40. Sapadin AN, Fleischmajer R. Treatment of scleroderma. Arch Dermatol. 2002;138:99.
41. Lin I-C, Chiu H-Y, Chan J-Y, Lin S-J. Extensive scleredema adultorum with loss of eccrine glands. J Am Acad Dermatol. 2014;71(3):99–101.
42. Doğramacı AC, Inan MU, Atik E, et al. Scleredema diabeticorum partially treated with low-dose methotrexate: a report of five cases. Balkan Med J. 2012;29(2):218–21.
43. Shazzad MN, Azad AK, Abdal SJ. Scleredema diabeticorum—a case report. Mymensinghmed J. 2015;24(3):606–9.
44. Janiga J, Ward DH, Lim HW. UVA-1 as a treatment for scleredema. Photodermatol Photoimmunol Photomed. 2004;20(4):210–1.
45. Kroff EB, de Jong EM. Scleredema diabeticorum case series: successful treatment with UV-A1. Arch Dermatol. 2008;144(7):947–8.

46. Kroft E, Berkhof N, van der Kerkhof P, et al. Ultraviolet A phototherapy for sclerotic skin diseases: a systematic review. J Am Acad Dermatol. 2008;59(6):1017–30.
47. Martin C, Requena L, Manrique K, et al. Scleredema diabeticorum in a patient with type 2 diabetes mellitus. Case Rep Endocrinol. 2011;560:560273. https://doi.org/10.1155/2011/560273.
48. Clark C, Pentland B, Ewing D, et al. Decreased skin wrinkling in diabetes mellitus. Diabetes Care. 1984;7(3):224–7.

Insulin Resistance and Acanthosis Nigricans

8

Federico Reissig

Insulin resistance is related to impaired cell signal transduction, i.e. insulin receptor function and complex postreceptor events in the cells. To a certain extent, the defect is genetically determined. However, the role of external factors such as nutrition or lifestyle has been increasing.

Insulin resistance is considered to be a key feature present in the Metabolic syndrome.

Insulin resistance and related metabolic conditions are becoming increasingly frequent, and a substantial proportion of apparently healthy people are reported to be insulin resistant.

The Insulin resistance syndrome refers to the cluster of abnormalities and related physical outcomes that occur more commonly in insulin resistant individuals. Given tissue differences in insulin dependence and sensitivity, manifestations of the insulin resistance syndrome are likely to reflect the composite effects of excess insulin and variable resistance to its actions [1].

There are many causes of insulin resistance (see Table 8.1), however overweight and obesity are the most common.

The presentation of insulin resistance depends on the type and stage of the insulin-resistant state. Most patients have one or more clinical features of the insulin-resistant state. Many patients do not develop overt diabetes despite extreme insulin resistance.

Patients may present with the following:

- Metabolic syndrome—(see diagnostic criteria—Table 8.2) [2]
- Obesity (most common cause of insulin resistance) or history or excessive body weight

F. Reissig
Diabetes Division, Hospital de Clínicas "José de San Martín", Buenos Aires, Argentina
e-mail: federeissig@gmail.com

© Springer International Publishing AG 2018
E.N. Cohen Sabban et al. (eds.), *Dermatology and Diabetes*,
https://doi.org/10.1007/978-3-319-72475-1_8

Table 8.1 Causes of insulin resistance

1. Obesity/overweight (especially excess visceral adiposity)
2. Excess glucocorticoids (Cushing's syndrome or steroid therapy)
3. Excess growth hormone (acromegaly)
4. Pregnancy, gestational diabetes
5. Polycystic ovary disease
6. Lipodystrophy
7. Autoantibodies to the insulin receptor
8. Mutations of insulin receptor
9. Mutations of the peroxisome proliferators' activator receptor γ (PPAR- γ)
10. Mutations that cause genetic obesity
11. Hemochromatosis

Table 8.2 Metabolic syndrome diagnostic criteria

Central obesity (defined as waist circumference ≥94 cm for Europid men and ≥80 cm for Europid women, plus any two of the following four factors:
• Raised TG level: ≥150 mg/dL, or specific treatment for this lipid abnormality
• Reduced HDL cholesterol: <40 mg/dL in males and <50 mg/dL in females, or specific treatment for this lipid abnormality
• Raised blood pressure: systolic BP ≥130 or diastolic BP ≥85 mmHg, or treatment of previously diagnosed hypertension
• Raised fasting plasma glucose (FPG) ≥100 mg/dL, or previously diagnosed type 2 diabetes

TG triglycerides, *BP* blood pressure

- Type 2 diabetes mellitus, IGT (impaired glucose test) or IFG (impaired fasting glucose).
- History of biochemical abnormalities, such as dyslipidemia.
- History of hypertension.
- Symptoms related to macrovascular disease (e.g., stroke, coronary artery disease, peripheral vascular disease)
- History of Polycystic ovary syndrome (PCOS).

Numerous definitions of the metabolic syndrome have been suggested since the original described by Reaven in 1988. According to the current definition the metabolic syndrome is diagnosed if at least three of the following five Criteria are present: abdominal obesity measured by waist circumference, hypertension, hypertriglyceridemia, hyperglycemia and high LDL cholesterol.

Laboratory Studies

Routine laboratory measurements in the evaluation of patients with insulin resistance syndrome include the following:

- Plasma glucose level (fasting and oral glucose tolerance test)
- Hb A1c (Glycohemoglobin level), used to assess chronic hyperglycemia.

- Fasting insulin level—A measure of the degree of insulin resistance in many patients with insulin resistance syndrome
- Lipid profile (fasting total cholesterol, low-density lipoprotein [LDL], high-density lipoprotein [HDL], cholesterol, triglyceride)—Insulin resistance syndrome characterized by elevated LDL-B levels (small, dense, pattern B), high triglyceride levels, and reduced HDL-C levels
- Electrolyte levels (BUN [blood urea nitrogen], creatinine, and uric acid levels)—Hyperuricemia is common and is often considered a component of the metabolic syndrome.
- Microalbuminuria is a marker of endothelial dysfunction.
- Homocysteine (H[e])—An elevated level is a risk factor for atherosclerosis, which predicts macrovascular disease—levels are regulated by insulin.
- Plasminogen activator inhibitor (PAI)-1—An elevated level is associated with insulin resistance syndrome and is correlated with obesity, waist-to-hip ratio, hypertension, fasting and postprandial insulin levels, fasting glucose levels, and elevated triglyceride and LDL levels [3]. An increased PAI-1 level signifies impaired fibrinolysis.

Insulin sensitivity can be assessed through the following methods:

- Fasting insulin level—This provides an indirect assessment of insulin sensitivity, a useful measure in patients with insulin-resistance.
- Euglycemic insulin clamp technique—Plasma glucose levels are held constant, with variable glucose infusion. Biochemical responses that are surrogate estimates of insulin resistance, such as glucose disposal and anti-lipolysis, are determined. This method is considered the criterion standard.
- The latter tests are more accurate, but they are not routinely used in clinical practice.
- Homeostatic model assessment for insulin resistance (HOMA-IR) and quantitative insulin sensitivity check index (QUICKI)—These are the most widely used simple indices for assessing insulin resistance in clinical research and practice. Both indices are based on fasting glucose and insulin measurements; they differ mainly in the log transformation of these variables in QUICKI [4].
- HOMA-IR is derived from the product of the insulin and glucose values divided by a constant, that is, calculated by using the following formula: fasting glucose (mg/dL) × fasting insulin (μU/mL)/405 (for SI units: fasting glucose (mmol/L) × fasting insulin (μU/L)/22.5). A value greater than 2.7 indicates insulin resistance.
- QUICKI is derived by calculating the inverse of the sum of the logarithmically expressed values of fasting insulin and glucose: 1/[log(fasting glucose) + log(fasting insulin)]. It measures insulin sensitivity, which is the inverse of insulin resistance. A value of less than 0.339 indicates insulin resistance.
- They both compensate for fasting hyperglycemia, and the results for the indices correlate reasonably well with the euglycemic clamp technique. Some investigators believe that QUICKI is superior to HOMA-IR, for instance in reproducibility, but the two indices correlate very well [5].
- A recent study suggests fasting insulin sensitivities are not better than routine clinical variables in predicting insulin sensitivity among black Africans [6].

Table 8.3 Comparison of acanthosis nigricans (AN) severity in terms of homeostatic model assessment insulin resistance (HOMA-IR)

	Insulin resistance	Metabolic syndrome		
Index	Cut-off value[a]	Cut-off value[b]	Sensibility (95%CI)	Sensibility (95%CI)
HOMA1-IR	2.7	2.3	76.8 (72.1–80.5)	66.7 (63.3–70.0)
HOMA2-IR	1.8	1.4	79.2 (74.7–82.8)	61.2 (57.6–64.6)

CI confidence interval
[a]The 90th percentile in the healthy group
[b]The optimal cut-off value verified in ROC analysis

The homeostatic model assessment (HOMA) is a validated method to measure insulin resistance from fasting glucose and insulin. The original model HOMA1-IR, first published by Mattews et al. in 1985 [4], has been widely used, especially in epidemiological and clinical studies. Recently, the model was updated with some physiological adjustments to a computer version (HOMA2-IR) [7].

Cut-off values of HOMA1-IR and HOMA2-IR indexes to identify insulin resistance and metabolic syndrome (Table 8.3).

Physical Examination

1. Central obesity, is a strong marker of insulin resistance syndrome. Waist or waist-to-hip ratio, height, weight, and body mass index (BMI) may indicate insulin resistance syndrome. This notion was supported by an Argentinian study that found waist circumference and BMI to be the anthropometric indexes that best correlate with the presence of insulin resistance [8].
2. Varying degrees of hirsutism or virilization may be present in women with Polycystic ovary syndrome (PCOS).
3. Others findings:
   Premature arcus cornealis—Deposits of cholesterol and phospholipids
   Xanthelasma—Indicates that lipid status should be investigated
   Lipemia retinalis—Retinal vessels with milky, chylomicron-rich plasma commonly observed in acute, uncontrolled diabetes
   Skin xanthomata—Eruptive xanthomas found most commonly on the buttocks
   Tendon xanthomata—Usually over the patellar and Achilles tendon
4. Acanthosis nigricans (AN) is common in patients with insulin resistance syndrome; it has been reported in nearly one tenth of women evaluated for PCOS.

In the benign form of AN, the factor is probably insulin or an insulin like growth factor (IGF) that incites the epidermal cell proliferation due to the effect of high circulating levels of insulin on insulin like growth factor (IGF) receptors in the skin. Other proposed mediators include other tyrosine kinase receptors (epidermal growth factor receptor [EGFR] or fibroblast growth factor receptor [FGFR]).

At high concentrations, insulin may exert potent proliferative effects via high-affinity binding to IGF-1 receptors. In addition, free IGF-1 levels may be elevated in obese patients with hyperinsulinemia, leading to accelerated cell growth and differentiation [9].

Table 8.4 The neck severity of Acanthosis Nigricans

Neck severity description
0 Absent: not detectable on close inspection
1 Present: clearly present on close visual inspection, not visible to the casual observer, extent not measurable
2 Mild: limited to the base of the skull, does not extend to the lateral margins of the neck (usually <7.62 cm in breadth)
3 Moderate: extending to the lateral margins of the neck (posterior border of the sternocleidomastoid) (usually 7.62–15.24 cm), should not be visible when the participant is viewed from the front
4 Severe: extending anteriorly (>15.24 cm), visible when the participant is viewed from the front

Insulin and IGF-1 levels are affected by hepatitis C infection and both of them may be implicated in the pathogenesis of acrochordons and AN through their proliferative and differentiating properties [10].

This skin disorder is characterized by brown hyperpigmentation, hyperkeratosis, and papillomatosis and it is a clinical marker that has been linked to surrogate markers of insulin resistance in adults [11].

It can develop in various parts of the body, including the neck, axillae, knees, elbows, and inguinal folds.

AN severity was evaluated based on the neck severity scale (Table 8.4) designed by Burke et al. [12].

The Fig. 8.1 shows the relation between AN and obesity/metabolic syndrome in the childhood [13].

Others Forms of Acanthosis Nigricans

Despite the acanthosis related to insulin resistance and obesity, there are other eight types of acanthosis nigricans described.

Syndromic Acanthosis Nigricans

Syndromic acanthosis nigricans is the name given to AN that is associated with a syndrome. In addition to the widely recognized association of AN with insulin resistance, acanthosis nigricans has been associated with numerous syndromes (see the Table in Pathophysiology). The type A syndrome and type B syndrome are special examples.

The type A syndrome also is termed the hyperandrogenemia, insulin resistance, and acanthosis nigricans syndrome (HAIR-AN syndrome). This syndrome is often familial, affecting primarily young women (especially black women). It is associated with polycystic ovaries or signs of virilization (e.g., hirsutism, clitoral hypertrophy). High plasma testosterone levels are common. The lesions of acanthosis nigricans may arise during infancy and progress rapidly during puberty.

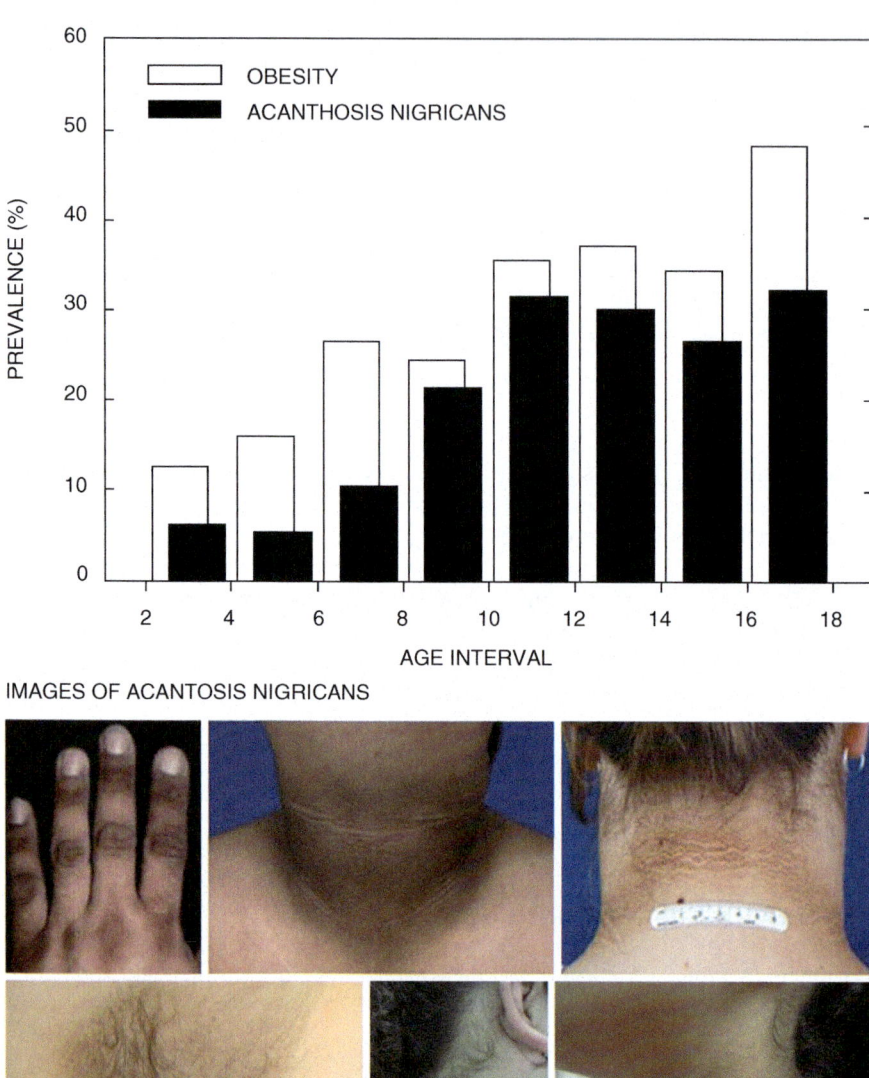

Fig. 8.1 Relation between acanthosis nigricans (AN) and obesity in children

The type B syndrome generally occurs in women who have uncontrolled diabetes mellitus, ovarian hyperandrogenism, or an autoimmune disease such as systemic lupus erythematosus, scleroderma, Sjögren syndrome, or Hashimoto thyroiditis. Circulating antibodies to the insulin receptor may be present. In these patients, the lesions of acanthosis nigricans are of varying severity.

Acral Acanthosis Nigricans (Acralacanthotic Anomaly)

It occurs in otherwise healthy patients. It is most common in dark-skinned individuals (African American descent), lesions being prominent over the dorsal aspects of hands and feet.

Unilateral Acanthosis Nigricans

It is a rare form of AN, inherited as an autosomal dominant trait. Lesions are unilateral along lines of Blaschko and may become evident during infancy, childhood, or adulthood. Lesions occur over the face, scalp, chest, abdomen, especially periumbilical area, back and thigh. Lesions can enlarge gradually before stabilizing or regressing. Unilateral nevoid AN is not related to endocrinopathy.

Generalized Acanthosis Nigricans

Generalized AN is rare and has been reported in pediatric patients without underlying systemic disease or malignancy [14].

Familial Acanthosis Nigricans

Familial AN is a rare genodermatosis that seems to be transmitted in an autosomal dominant fashion with variable phenotypic penetrance. The lesions typically begin during early childhood but may manifest at any age. Familial AN often progresses until puberty, at which time it stabilizes or regresses.

Drug-Induced Acanthosis Nigricans

Drug-induced AN, although uncommon, may be due to several medications, including nicotinic acid, insulin, systemic corticosteroids, fusidic acid, protease inhibitors, estrogens and methyltestosterone. Nicotinic acid has been most widely associated with AN, developing on abdomen and flexor surfaces and resolving within 4–10 weeks of discontinuation [15]. Fibroblast growth factor receptor ligands such as palifermin may cause drug-induced AN [16].

The lesions of AN may regress following discontinuation of the offending medication.

Malignant Acanthosis Nigricans

Malignant AN, which is associated with internal malignancy, is the most worrisome AN variant, because the underlying neoplasm is often an aggressive cancer (see the Table in Pathophysiology).

Acanthosis nigricans has been reported with many kinds of cancer, but, by far, the most common underlying malignancy is an adenocarcinoma of gastrointestinal origin, usually a gastric adenocarcinoma. In an early study of 191 patients with malignant AN, 92% had an underlying abdominal cancer, of which 69% were gastric. Another study reported 94 cases of malignant AN, of which 61% were secondary to a gastric neoplasm.

Malignant AN in pediatric patients has been described with gastric adenocarcinoma, Wilms tumor, and osteogenic sarcoma.

In 25–50% of cases of malignant AN, the oral cavity is involved. The tongue and the lips most commonly are affected, with elongation of the filiform papillae on the dorsal and lateral surfaces of the tongue and multiple papillary lesions appearing on the commissures of the lips. Oral lesions of AN seldom are pigmented.

Tripe palms may show altered dermatoglyphs due to alteration of epidermal rete ridges.

Malignant AN is clinically indistinguishable from the benign forms; however, one must be more suspicious if the lesions arise rapidly, are more extensive, are symptomatic, or are in atypical locations.

Regression of AN has been seen with treatment of the underlying malignancy, and reappearance may suggest recurrence or metastasis of the primary tumor.

Mixed-Type Acanthosis Nigricans

Mixed-type acanthosis nigricans refers to those situations in which a patient with one of the above types of AN develops new lesions of a different etiology. An example of this would be an overweight patient with obesity-associated AN who subsequently develops malignant AN.

Differential Diagnoses

- Epidermal naevus
- Confluent and reticulated papillomatosis of Gougerot-Carteaud
- Dowling-Degos disease (reticular pigmented flexural anomaly)
- Atopic Dermatitis
- Becker Melanosis
- Candidiasis
- Dermatologic aspects of Addison disease
- Dermatologic manifestations of Hemochromatosis
- Dermatologic manifestations of Pellagra
- Erythrasma
- Giant melanocytic nevi
- Ichthyosis hystrix
- Linear epidermal nevus
- Lichen simplex chronicus

- Mycosis fungoides
- Plaque Parapsoriasis
- Pemphigus vegetans

Another marker of insulin resistance are the acrochordons. An association with type 2 diabetes mellitus has been observed [17].

A study of 118 research subjects with acrochordon reported an incidence of 40.6% of either overt type 2 diabetes mellitus or impaired glucose tolerance. Reports exist suggesting that the mechanism is through the effect of insulin and glucose starvation [18]. The previous study showed no correlation between the location, size, color, or number of acrochordons with impairment of glucose tolerance.

They are smalls, softs, commons, benign usually pedunculated neoplasm, that are found particularly in persons who are obese. They are also a marker of increased risk of atherosclerosis and cardiovascular disease [19].

It is usually skin colored or hyperpigmented, and it may appear as surface nodules or papillomas on healthy skin. Most acrochordons vary in size from 2 to 5 mm in diameter, although larger acrochordons up to 5 cm in diameter are sometimes evident. The most frequent localizations are the neck and the axillae, but any skin fold, including the groin, may be affected.

Acrochordons are frequently present in patients with metabolic alteration as the Fig. 8.2 shows [20].

METABOLIC ALTERATION	PERCENTAGE
INSULIN RESISTANCE	71,3
DIABETES MELLITUS	49,3
OBESITY	51,3
PRE DIABETES	18

IMAGES OF ACROCHORDONS

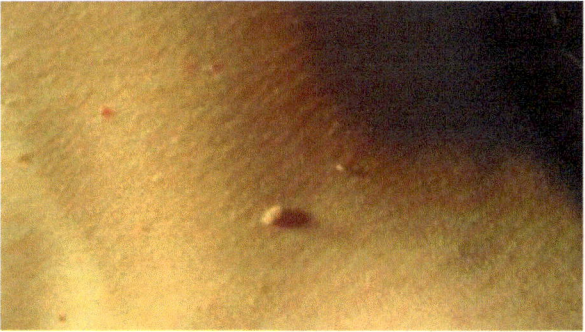

Fig. 8.2 Acrochordon: skin colored, soft, usually pedunculated benign neoplasm

Differential Diagnoses

Also, consider the following:

• Pedunculated seborrheic keratosis
• Nodular exophytic (polypoid) melanoma
• Pseudosarcomatous polyp

References

1. Reaven G. The metabolic syndrome or the insulin resistance syndrome? Different names, different concepts, and different goals. Endocrinol Metab Clin North Am. 2004;33:283–303.
2. Anderson PJ, Critchley JAJH, Chan JCN, et al. Factor analysis of the metabolic syndrome: obesity vs insulin resistance as the central abnormality. Int J Obes. 2001;25:1782.
3. De Taeye B, Smith LH, Vaughan DE. Plasminogen activator inhibitor-1: a common denominator in obesity, diabetes and cardiovascular disease. Curr Opin Pharmacol. 2005;5(2):149–54.
4. Muniyappa R, Lee S, Chen H, Quon MJ. Current approaches for assessing insulin sensitivity and resistance in vivo: advantages, limitations, and appropriate usage. Am J Physiol Endocrinol Metab. 2008;294(1):E15–26.
5. Antuna-Puente B, Faraj M, Karelis AD, et al. HOMA or QUICKI: is it useful to test the reproducibility of formulas? Diabetes Metab. 2008;34(3):294–6.
6. Sobngwi E, Kengne AP, Echouffo-Tcheugui JB, Choukem S, Sobngwi-Tambekou J, Balti EV, et al. Fasting insulin sensitivity indices are not better than routine clinical variables at predicting insulin sensitivity among Black Africans: a clamp study in sub-Saharan Africans. BMC Endocr Disord. 2014;14:65.
7. Levy JC, Matthews DR, Hermans MP. Correct homeostasis model 5.assessment (HOMA) evaluation uses the computer program. Diabetes Care. 1998;21(12):2191–2.
8. Hirschler V, Ruiz A, Romero T, Dalamon R, Molinari C. Comparison of different anthropometric indices for identifying insulin resistance in schoolchildren. Diabetes Technol Ther. 2009;11(9):615–2.
9. Higgins SP, Freemark M, Prose NS. Acanthosis nigricans: a practical approach to evaluation and management. Dermatol Online J. 2008;14(9):2.
10. El Safoury OS, Shaker OG, Fawzy MM. Skin tags and acanthosis nigricans in patients with hepatitis C infection in relation to insulin resistance and insulin like growth factor-1 levels. Indian J Dermatol. 2012;57:102–6.
11. Burke JP, Hale DE, Hazuda HP, Stern MP. A quantitative scale of acanthosis nigricans. Diabetes Care. 1999;22:1655–9.
12. Burke JP, Hale DE, Hazuda HP, Stern MP. A quantitative scale of acantosis nigricans. Diabetes Care. 1999;22:1655–9.
13. Ice CL, Murphy E, Minor VE, Neal WA. Metabolic syndrome in fifth grade children with acanthosis nigricans: results from the CARDIAC project. World J Pediatr. 2009;5(1):23–30.
14. Gönül M, Kiliç A, Cakmak SK, Gül U, Ekiz OD, Ergül G. Juvenile generalized acanthosis nigricans without any systemic disease. Pediatr Int. 2009;51(4):595–7.
15. Sinha S, Schwartz RA. Juvenile acanthosis nigricans. J Am Acad Dermatol. 2007;57(3):502–8.
16. Lane SW, Manoharan S, Mollee PN. Palifermin-induced acanthosis nigricans. Intern Med J. 2007;37(6):417–8.
17. Goyal A, Raina S, Kaushal SS, Mahajan V, Sharma NL. Pattern of cutaneous manifestations in diabetes mellitus. Indian J Dermatol. 2010;55(1):39–41.

18. Mathur SK, Bhargava P. Insulin resistance and skin tags. Dermatology. 1997;195(2):184.
19. Sari R, Akman A, Alpsoy E, Balci MK. The metabolic profile in patients with skin tags. Clin Exp Med. 2009;10(3):193–7.
20. Guerra C, et al. Metabolic diseases associated with acrochordons. Folia Dermatol Peru. 2006;17(2):60–4.

Fungal Infections in Diabetics

9

Alexandro Bonifaz, Aline Armas-Vázquez,
and Andrés Tirado-Sánchez

Introduction

Diabetes mellitus (DM) is the most common endocrine disorder, affecting 8.3% of the worldwide population, is strongly associated with the development of fungal infections and diseases connected with skin manifestations. Diabetes-associated skin diseases are often seen in clinical practice, among these cutaneous infections are involved. Cutaneous infections occur most commonly in type 2 (T2DM) than in type 1 diabetes (T1DM) [1–3]; and can be a cause of morbidity or mortality.

The risk of infection in DM is related to the hyperglycemic environment developing microcirculation change, reduced phagocytosis due to neutrophil role damage, weakened leukocyte adherence, delayed chemotaxis, depression of the antioxidant system and humoral immunity. Moreover, there is a lack of C4 in diabetics, leading to a polymorphonuclear dysfunction and reduced cytokine response [4, 5].

Glucose levels in healthy individuals' skin are similar to the serum levels, however in diabetic patients these levels are higher (40%); this was described many years ago and it was named glycohistechia (glucohistechia), and it is related to the higher concentrations of glucose in the skin, the higher risk for infections [6, 7].

The prevalence rate of infectious diseases among diabetic patients is 55–61%, and includes candidiasis, dermatophytosis (tineas) and bacterial infections. Saprophytic fungi prefer low pH environments, which is noted during diabetic ketoacidosis (DKA) and thrive in hyperglycemia.

Usually fungal infections associated with DM are prevalent on the interdigital spaces, external genital skin and folds [2, 8]. Early diagnosis and effective treatment, both play an important role in proceeding to the therapy of mycotic infections.

A. Bonifaz (✉) • A. Armas-Vázquez • A. Tirado-Sánchez
Dermatology Service, Mycology Department, Hospital General de México,
"Dr. Eduardo Liceaga", Ciudad de México, México
e-mail: a_bonifaz@yahoo.com.mx

© Springer International Publishing AG 2018
E.N. Cohen Sabban et al. (eds.), *Dermatology and Diabetes*,
https://doi.org/10.1007/978-3-319-72475-1_9

This chapter comprises the most frequent mycotic and pseudomycoses or bacterial (actinomycetes) infections in diabetic patients; diseases directly related to the pathophysiology of this disease and include: (1). Superficial mycoses: dermatophytosis or tinea and candidiasis; (2) Deep mycoses: mucormycosis, Majocchi's granuloma; and (3) Pseudomycoses: erythrasma and actinomycosis.

Superficial Mycoses

Dermatophytosis

They are several conditions affecting the stratum corneum (SC) related to keratinophilic fungi called dermatophytes and fall into three genera *Trichophyton*, *Microsporum* and *Epidermophyton*, belonging to diverse origins as: anthropophilic, zoophilic and geophilic group.

Most studies comparing controlled and uncontrolled diabetic population and healthy individuals, failed to show a difference between the most common tinea (pedis and corporis tineas and onychomycosis), however, most agree that fungal infections are more extensive, and develop faster and some such as feet and nails favor secondary bacterial infections, leading to diabetic foot syndrome in uncontrolled patients [3, 9–13].

Tinea Pedis and Tinea Corporis

The main etiological agent for tinea pedis is *Trichophyton rubrum* in approximately 70%, followed by *Trichophyton interdigitale* (formerly *T. mentagrophyyes* var. *interdigitale*); the remaining etiologic agents (20% approximately), include other species like *Epidermophyton floccosum*, which comprises 5% of those cases. It occurs in three clinical forms: interdigital (most frequent) presenting with scales, maceration and erythema; hyperkeratotic with extensive areas of hyperkeratosis with small vesicles in the dorsum of the foot and soles. Occasionally mixed clinical forms can be seen. Patients with tinea pedis may present some complications, the most common are: contact dermatitis, secondary bacterial infections (impetigo) and hypersensitivity (Ides). In few chronic cases, a syndrome of "two feet, one hand" can be seen. Undoubtedly, the most important aspect of tinea pedis is that its chronicity leads to onychomycosis [9, 10, 13, 14].

There are no clear reports pointing that tinea corporis is more common in diabetics, but the phenomenon of glycohistechia, could help developing rapid and extended cases, and thus, if chronic, may evolve to deep tinea.

KOH direct examination (10%) is a helpful tool to diagnose tinea; the diagnostic findings include thin hyphae and dermatophytes isolation in Sabouraud dextrose agar media with and without antibiotics, confirm the etiologic agent [9, 13].

In limited cases, any topical antimitotic, especially imidazoles, ciclopirox and terbinafine can be used. However, for extensive cases, itraconazole should be added at doses of 200–300 mg/day or terbinafine at 250 mg/day for 3–4 weeks [12, 14].

Onychomycosis

Similar to tinea corporis, onychomycosis due to dermatophytes is not more frequent in diabetic patients than in healthy population, however its clinical manifestations are more generous and its presentation is faster than these subjects. There are few studies pointing out a slight predominance in diabetics, especially with persistent hyperglycemia and high glycosylated hemoglobin levels [15–18]. Akkus et al. [17], reported that tinea pedis and onychomycosis develop more often among diabetic patients with poor glycemic control and peripheral vascular disease, resulting in the highest incidence of foot ulcers [17].

The clinical types of onychomycosis among diabetics are similar to healthy subjects; the most frequent clinical form is subungual distal onychomycosis, which rapidly spreads until total dystrophic onychomycosis is reached. The first one starts at the free edge and advances to the base or nail matrix and by progressing the fungus gives way to the total dystrophic onychomycosis, which is the most destructive form of the nail, presenting severe pachyonychia, loss of brightness and consistency of the nail plate. To a lesser extent, there are: lateral, proximal and superficial white onychomycosis [9, 15, 16]. Like the feet, the main etiological agents are *T. rubrum*, followed by *T. interdigitale*.

Clinical symptoms of onychomycosis include onycholysis, hyperkeratosis, brittleness, paronychial inflammation, and color change; dystrophic nails look thick, brittle and discolored, often with a yellow shade. The nail plate may be separated from the nail bed (onycholysis). Characteristic is paronychial inflammation of the nail edge surrounding skin. The most severe clinical manifestation of the disease is total dystrophic onychomycosis. Nails can be very painful and make walking difficult.

An example of the importance of DM-associated onychomycosis is observed in the study of Arenas et al., in a survey of more than 12,000 patients in whom the main predisposing factor was DM in 22%, followed by hypertension in 16% [18].

It is noteworthy that onychomycosis can also be caused by non-dermatophyte molds, this is often seen in diabetic patients, and the most isolated species are *Aspergillus* spp., *Scopulariopsis brevicaulis* and *Fusarium* spp., among others. These fungi develop clinical manifestations similar to the dermatophytes, but their treatment is different [19–21].

Vascular insufficiency, impaired wound healing, and compromised immunologic state predispose to secondary fungal and bacterial infections (paronychia, cellulitis). Diabetic patients with peripheral neuropathy and sharp edged nails are more likely to cause abrasion injuries, what affect in decreased quality of life and is a risk factor for other foot disorders and limb amputation. Erosion of the nail bed and hyponychium can progress osteomyelitis of underlying bone.

Fungal foot infections occur in one-thirds of patients and increase the risk of developing diabetic foot syndrome (a major reason of disability and mortality in diabetic subjects), particularly men. The most common pathogens are: yeast and dermatophytes and the most frequent dermatophyte is *Trichophyton rubrum*.

Direct examination with KOH (10%) and simple biopsies are useful to diagnose onychomycosis. For dermatophytes: thin hyphae are sometimes observed with arthroconidia, and when dealing with non-dermatophyte: molds, structures characteristic of fungi can be observed as aspergillary heads or conidia of various forms. Cultures should be performed with Sabouraud dextrose agar media with and without antibiotics; the criterion for considering mold as an etiological agent is with at least three isolates [14, 20].

The two most commonly used treatments are terbinafine and itraconazole, the first one is commonly suggested for dermatophytes and the later for dermatophytes and molds. The administration can be continuous or pulsed doses and is usually added for 3–4 months. Terbinafine is used at doses of 250–500 mg/day and itraconazole 200–400 mg/day.

Topical therapy in the form of solutions or varnishes (amorolfine, ciclopirox, efinaconazole) is accompanying with oral or in patients where systemic therapy is contraindicated [14, 15, 22].

It is important to note that diabetic patients are often under various treatments and thus drug interactions must be considered; itraconazole is metabolized at the cytochrome P-450 (3A4) level and may interact with oral hypoglycemic agents and other drugs developing a risk of severe hypoglycemia, whereas terbinafine has different pharmacokinetic (1A2) and thus minimal interactions [14, 22].

Another contraindication of itraconazole in diabetic patients is congestive heart failure because of its negative inotropic effect. Given the high prevalence of heart disease in diabetics, it is important to take this precaution [22, 23] (Fig. 9.1).

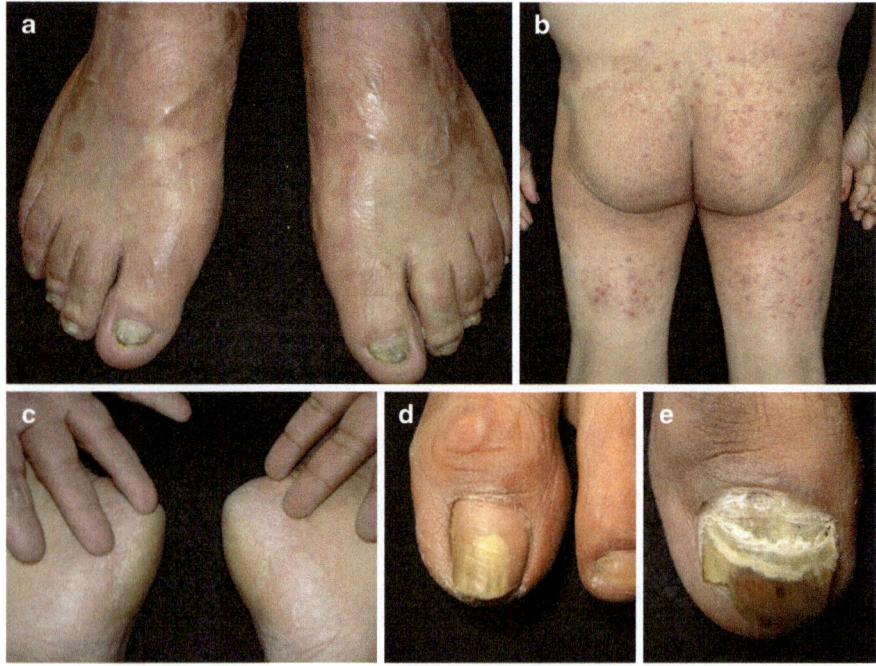

Fig. 9.1 (**a**) Dorsal and interdigital tinea pedis and distal subungual onychomycosis. (**b**) Extensive tinea corporis and micronodular lesions of Majocchi granuloma. (**c**) Two-foot and one hand syndrome, (**d**) Distal subungual onychomycosis, (**e**) Total dystrophic onychomycosis

Candidiasis

The risk of this infection increases with hyperglycemia, which favors *Candida* spp. growth. It is not uncommon that these could be the first manifestation of DM. There is an explanation for which *Candida* colonization is frequent in Diabetes: increased serum glucose restricts neutrophil role and their capacity to phagocyte *Candida* species T1DM patients. Other factors that increase *Candida* colonization are older age, abnormal HbA1c, the use of antibiotics 14 days previous and history of *Chlamydia*. T1DM and T2DM female patients may be equally likely to get *Candida*, but those with T1DM may be less able to clear it. A better glucose control may reduce the risk of *Candida* colonization. *C. albicans* is more often seen among T1DM patients, while in T2DM, the most common agent is *C. glabrata*. The most common clinical forms include vulvovaginal and balanoposthitis candidiasis and angular stomatitis [2, 4, 24, 25].

Vulvovaginal Candidiasis

Candida species are responsible for vulvovaginal candidiasis (representing 25% of vulvovaginal infections). Predominant species are *Candida albicans*, *Candida glabrata* and *Candida tropicalis*. The incidence of infection affects 70–75% of women. The prevalence is higher among sexually active, young women. Women with uncontrolled, severe T2DM are more prone to be infected.

Antibiotic use, hyperglycemia, diabetes type and HbA1c level are recognized as risk factors for vulvovaginal candidiasis.

It is a frequent and recurrent infection; clinically, vulvovaginal candidiasis can be asymptomatic or can clinically manifest with acute pruritus, cottage-cheese-like vaginal discharge, vaginal soreness, irritation, vulvar burning, dyspareunia, external dysuria, slight odor, erythema and swelling of the labia and vulva. Vaginal mucosa is also erythematous. The cervix can be involved and it is possible to extend to the labia majora and minora or to the inguino-crural region [14, 25].

It is present almost in every woman with DM, followed by a period of glycosuria. The rate of vaginal colonization with *Candida* sp. increases in people with DM. To the source of infection belongs to intestinal reservoir, sexual transmission and vaginal relapse (persisting).

Identification of the type of infection and classification of its degree of severity can assist in the selection of appropriate therapy. Microscopic examination of vaginal secretion and culturing confirm the diagnosis. There is a possibility to use PCR detection test. In women and adolescent girls with recurrent vulvovaginal candidiasis may be a marker of DM and thus, a glucose tolerance test is recommended [1, 24, 25].

Balanoposthitis

Balanitis is an inflammation of the glans of the penis, while posthitis is an inflammation of the prepuce. In males with diabetes, the most common etiological agent of balanoposthitis is *Candida albicans,* and it is often seen in uncircumcised males. Usually in diabetics this is not sexually transmitted, that is why all males with this entity should be screened for DM. In some countries like India, DM is mostly diagnosed by dermatologists [14, 26]. Clinically presents as a pruritic erythematous rash with small papules, erosions or dry dull areas with glazed appearance and preputial fissuring. In elderly and no sexually active patients, itch and erythema of prepuce is more common, rather than in young sexually active patients that presents with itching, burning and increased smegma collection.

With the store of advanced glycation end products, an undermine production of collagen and extracellular organization, lowered hydroxyproline content and superoxide dismutase activity is observed, leading to preputial fissures [26, 27].

Oral Candidiasis

DM is a predisposing factor of oral candidiasis, especially pseudomembranous candidiasis. It clinically presents as median rhomboid glossitis, central papillary atrophy, atrophic glossitis, pseudomembranous candidiasis, denture stomatitis or angular cheilitis.

The most frequent form associated with DM is pseudomembranous type, which presents with creamy and whitish, erythematous pseudomembranous plaques; its common symptoms include burning and pain.

Oral cavity is also affected, mostly with *Candida albicans, C. krusei* and *C. glabrata* in that order. Also, non-albicans species and other yeasts (*Pichia, Trichosporon, Geotrichum*), can be identified in the oral cavity of patients with poorly controlled diabetes, being prone to frequent and severe fungal infections. This is related to the production of extracellular enzymes such as proteinase and phospholipase [1, 5, 14]; also, the poor glycemic control is associated with high concentration of glucose in blood and saliva, which can be a nutrient for fungi. These mechanisms, as well as the presence of removable prostheses or cigarette smoking, increase the risk of fungal infections in Diabetes [28].

Untreated candidiasis can lead to serious, even fatal complications or be a cause of chronic hyperplastic candidiasis, known as candidal leukoplakia.

Cutaneous Candidiasis and Onychomycosis

Cutaneous forms of candidiasis are characterized by intertriginous lesions (large and small folds) composed of erythematous-squamous plaques, with fissures or erosions, vesicles, pustules and with small satellite plates. The most common symptoms are itching and, occasionally burning. It is commonly associated with Diabetes and obesity [29–33].

Candida onychomycosis is less frequent than dermatophytosis, mostly seen on fingernails (85%). It is often associated with DM and post-trauma (manicure and pedicure), as well as excess moisture in the hands. It occurs in two clinical forms: Perionyxis or paronychia; it arises on the proximal or lateral fold and displays with inflammation around the nail (perionyxis) and with pain, the nails are opaque, and usually a single nail is affected. The second form is onycholysis, it starts at the free edge, with detachment of the nail plate, and the nail becomes opaque and striated and may have yellow or green shades. Both forms can be markers of DM, mostly uncontrolled [33–36] (Fig. 9.2).

In order to diagnose cases of cutaneous candidiasis and onychomycosis, direct examinations with KOH (10%) are carried out, where psedohyphae and blastoconidia (yeasts) are observed. Isolation of the various *Candida* species is achieved in

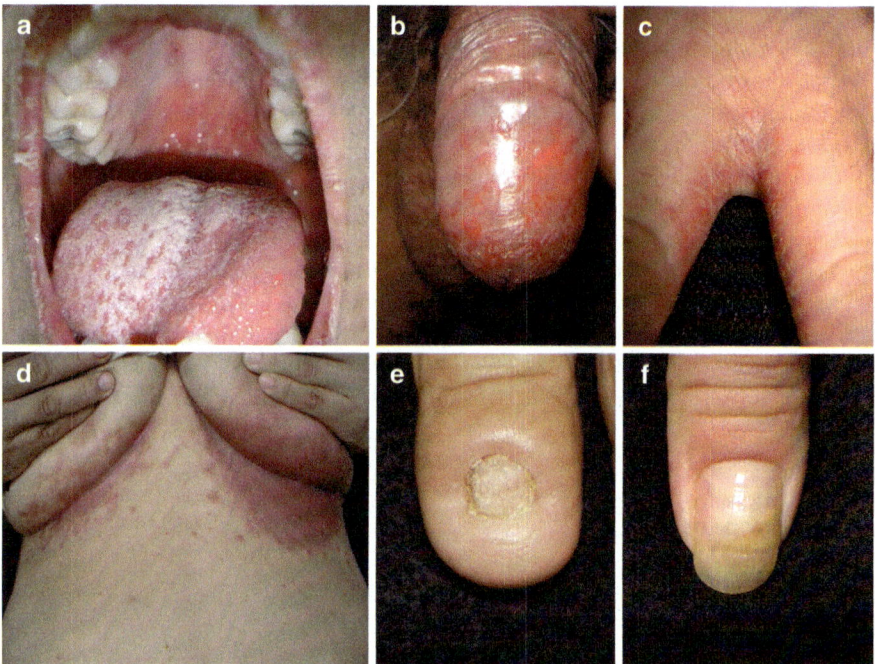

Fig. 9.2 (**a**) Pseudomembranous candidiasis, (**b**) balanitis, (**c**) candidal intertrigo, (**d**) submammary candidiasis with satellite lesions, (**e**) candidal paronychia, (**f**) candidal onycholysis

Sabouraud dextrose agar media without antibiotics, however, the most useful are chromogenic like CHROMcandida®, and identifying species is performed by mycological, biochemical and molecular tests. It is important to classify species because it determines the treatment [14].

The incidence of oral candidiasis can be reduced by appropriate prophylaxis, like patient education, avoiding tobacco use; proper glycemic control and oral hygiene, soaking the denture in 0.1% hypochlorite solution or clorhexidine solution, or even white vinegar (dilution 1:20) may be useful for prophylaxis.

The regiment of drugs depends on culture identification, affected part of body, severity of infection, earlier management and patient immune status. In limited cases, any topical antimycotic, imidazoles or ciclopirox can be used. Topical therapy is also advised to patients with need of systemic treatment (intolerance or resistance to local application), due to the possibility of lowering dose and duration of systemic preparations, in order to reduce the incidence of adverse effects and drug interactions.

For oral mucosal or oral cases, oral triazoles such as fluconazole should be used at doses of 150–300 mg/day, usually in single doses and occasionally, more doses are required. Alternative options include itraconazole 200–400 mg/day for 3–7 days depending on the response and in the case of fluconazole resistance; posaconazole, voriconazole and caspofungin are also effective options.

For vulvovaginal candidiasis, itraconazole (400 mg, single-dose: 200 mg in the morning and 200 mg in the evening), has good efficacy and safety. In the case of limited response, the managing should be prolonged to 5–7 days. The common side effect is burning sensation. Fluconazole can be an option; however, only 33% of diabetic women with vulvovaginitis candidiasis achieve the success in treating with fluconazole (single dose 150 mg). It is associated with high prevalence of *C. glabrata* in diabetic population.

In diabetic patients, the modifications to insulin doses are needed for a period of oral infection to avoid infection related hyperglycemia; also, the drug interaction with hypoglycemic agents can be essential in diabetic population.

Terbinafine has mild activity against *Candida* sp., therefore it is not recommended for *Candida* infections. Identification of the species and susceptibility tests are very useful because some species may have resistance to the various antimycotics. Sensitivity test results can be helpful in choosing the most effective treatment; however, the mostly common reason of poor response to antibiotic is non-compliance [14, 26, 29, 34].

Deep Mycoses

Mucormycosis

Is an invasive fungal infection caused by *Mucorales* (Subphylum *Mucoromycotina)*, being *Rhizopus arrhizus* the most common etiological agent, followed by *Mucor circinelloides* and *Lichtheimia corymbifera*. These is the most serious condition and men are more affected than women (ratio 6:4) [1, 37, 38].

The decompensated or ketoacidotic DM is undoubtedly the most important cause for developing mucormycosis, especially the rhinocerebral form, in our experience this association represents 80% of cases. The proposed mechanism for this association is related to the metabolic decontrol, and thus the free serum iron ions (Fe^{2+}) that stimulates the infection; these are favored by the acid pH (6.8–7.3), as well as with the mucorals, have a ketone enzymatic system-reductase, which is active in acidosis and hyperglycemia and degrades ketone bodies; also, diabetic patients have a lower defensive activity, mainly in neutrophils response to infection.

Also, deferoxamine (iron chelator), acts as siderophore inducing fungal growth and adhesion, promoting development of *Mucorales* in hemodialysis [37–39].

In our experience, most cases of mucormycosis, are associated with T2DM, but cases in children are usually observed more often in T1DM or juvenile DM, which is also the one that usually and easily decompensates. In a study reported by our group, 50% of the cases in children and adolescents were rhinocerebral type associated with T1DM [39].

There are many clinical forms of mucormycosis: rhinocerebral, pulmonary, cutaneous, gastrointestinal, disseminated, and miscellaneous type. The most frequent form is the rhinocerebral one, and it has an important association with DKA or simply uncontrolled DM in about 33–88% of cases, this is because systemic acidosis creates the proper environment for growing and spreading *Rhizopus* [24, 37–40]. The pulmonary form is associated with neutropenia. Clinically begins with a palpebral fistula and then areas of necrosis mostly in the nasal cornets and palate ulceration. A classic triad has been described: paranasal sinusitis, ophthalmoplegia with blindness and one-sided proptosis with cellulitis. The mortality rate is high (85–90%) due to a rapid progression and/or a late diagnosis [1, 5, 37, 38].

Secondary skin manifestations are the most frequent and associated with rhinocerebral cases (up to 70%). It begins with unilateral and periorbital edema; Erythematous nasal mucosa, there is palatine involvement in one third of the cases formed by necrotic ulcers of rapid development, usually located in hard palate. From the eyelid fistula, there is usually a single, fetid, seropurulent fistula at the level of the eyelid, which becomes a necrotic area, sometimes of great extent, at the eyelid, nasal septum and close skin.

The primary cutaneous type is seen in patients with DM in 10–15% of cases. The majority of cases originate from trauma that inoculate the fungus, those associated with DM present more in sites of catheters or venipuncture (by adhesive bands), even grafting. The episode of sinusitis not responding to short-term antibacterial therapy should be considered as mucormycosis. Its main manifestation includes necrotic lesions with well-limited bedspreads of brownish or black color and ulcers of necrotic background, indurated and that drain exudate fetid blackish. There are also cases associated with injuries due to motor vehicle accidents, earthquakes, or burns, which usually occur in immunocompetent patients, but when they are associated with diabetics their development is faster, most of them manifested as necrotic lesions, cellulitis and fasciitis [14, 41] (Fig. 9.3).

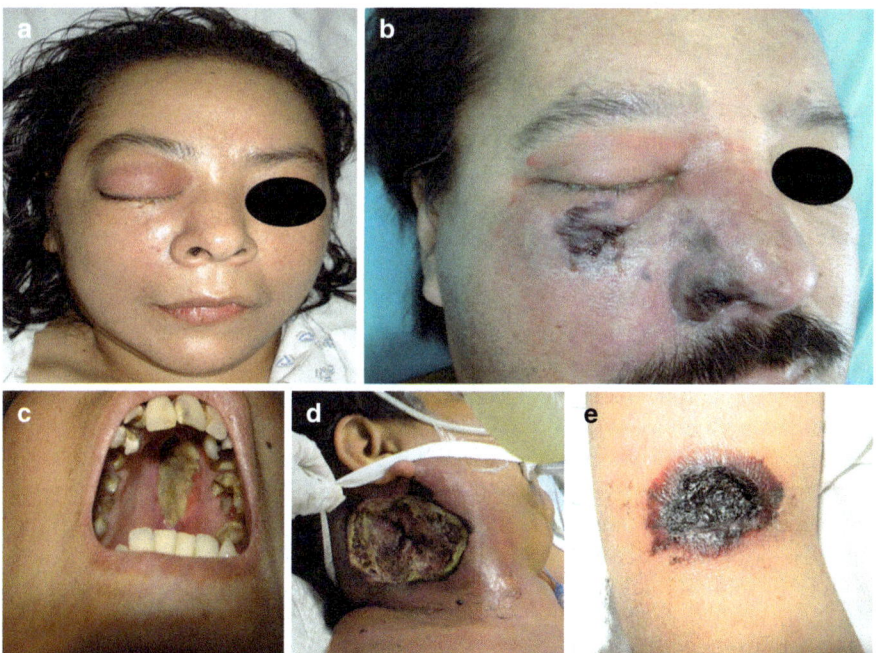

Fig. 9.3 (**a**) Rhinocerebral mucormycosis, with eyelid edema, (**b**) Mucormycosis rhinocerebral with extensive necrosis, (**c**) palatine ulcer, (**d**) Primary cutaneous mucormycosis after car accident (Courtesy Guevara E), (**e**) Mucormycosis in a venoclysis zone

An early diagnosis is crucial for a better prognosis. Initially, a direct examination is required, with KOH 10–20%, showing the characteristic broad, coenocytic, branched, hyaline hyphae.

Repeat cultures should be performed on Sabouraud dextrose agar. Colonies are white-gray, hairy, and cottony, with rapid development (3–5 days) and their identification is based on their reproduction forms and can be completed by molecular biology.

Treatment begins with reversal of triggering causes as DKA, metabolic acidosis or uncontrolled DM. First line treatment is a combination therapy with amphotericin B in the liposomal presentation (5–7 mg/kg/day) (lipid 3–5 mg/kg/day) [38] or desoxycholate at a dose of 0.25–0.75 mg/kg/day, up to 1–1.5 mg/kg/day in severe cases, added to oral posaconazole (600–800 mg/day) or caspofungin (70 mg/day as load dose followed by 50 mg/day), and extensive surgical debridement to remove necrotic tissue if needed. Systemic therapy is recommended for 4–6 weeks. The protocols with additional regiment of rifampicin or tetracycline aren't recommended because of lack of studies.

Survival rates decrease if the treatment is started 6 days or more after the beginning or diagnosis of the disease. The mortality of diabetic patients with mucormycosis is 44%; however, increases more than 80% with intracranial involvement, with death occurring before 2 weeks from early onset. Aggressive debridation or surgical treatment can decrease death rate [6, 24, 37, 38, 41].

Majocchi's Granulomas (MG)

It is a deep dermatophytosis, caused by various dermatophytes, especially antropophilic ones of the genus *Trichophyton*; this infection initiates as a superficial process that deepen the dermis and sometimes to other structures. For developing, there must be previous tinea (mainly tinea pedis and onychomycosis) and the two most frequent predisposing factors include Diabetes and topical or systemic steroids (or both). It is estimated that at least half of the cases are associated with poorly controlled or decompensated DM. Clinically, MG present more often on lower limbs (60%); upper limbs and trunk are less commonly affected. The disease develops a chronic herpetic form indistinguishable from tinea corporis, which evolves to the classic, nodular phase, formed by 0.5–3 cm, violet, painful nodules with hard consistency by palpation; they can become ulcerated. Deepening the dermatophytes into the skin occurs in patients with an immune response change, but not in immunosuppressed ones, because the immune response is necessary for pathogenesis [42, 43] (Fig. 9.1).

It is necessary to perform a biopsy for diagnosing MG; suppurative and sometimes tuberculoid granuloma is reported, consisting of lymphocytes and histiocytes and it is possible to note filaments and spores inside the hair follicles, especially with PAS (Periodic Acid of Schiff) staining. Isolating the dermatophyte completes the diagnosis. These patients have a weak response to intradermal antigen (trichophytin) [24, 42–44].

Long-term high doses of oral antifungals achieves successful responses in most cases. Terbinafine at 500 mg/day and itraconazole 400 mg/day with a minimum of one month are usually preferred. As mentioned above; it is important to oversee drug interactions, mainly for itraconazole [14, 22, 24].

Pseudomycoses

Erythrasma

It is a chronic superficial infection caused by *Corynebacterium minutissimum*, a coriniform actinomycete, which mainly affects large folds (axillary and groin) and interdigital spaces, in the form of erythematous-squamous plaques. It is an opportunistic infection; the main predisposing factors are hyperhidrosis, obesity and DM [33, 45–47].

It is often located in axillary, inguinocrural, submammary and intergluteal fold and the interdigital spaces of feet, in the form of erythematous plaques, which turn pale brown, covered by a thin scale, mostly asymptomatic and occasionally with mild pruritus. In chronic cases associated with obesity and DM, the clinical picture appears with maceration, fissures, and lichenification of the skin. There is an extensive presentation of erythrasma called "tropical", observed in obese black women or in patients with uncontrolled DM. In general, erythrasma must be clinically distinguished from tinea and candidosis [33, 45–47] (Fig. 9.4).

Laboratory diagnosis can be useful, remarking a coral red fluorescence that emits with a Wood's lamp, however the most useful test is a Gram staining of the scaling maceration, where Gram-positive thin filaments, microsiphonated (1 μm wide) and its isolation is achieved in rich culture media (blood agar, chocolate agar) where thin filamentous structures with diphtheria- and bacillary-like forms are observed. Biopsies are useful for diagnosis; a slight inflammatory process is observed, and bacteria can be seen as filaments and coccoid forms restricted to the SC [14, 45].

Oral erythromycin at doses of 1 g/day for a week is the treatment of choice for extensive or recurrent cases; clarithromycin and chloramphenicol are also useful. For the limited cases, topical therapy such as erythromycin, fusidic acid, mupirocin, clindamycin and garamycin may be effective and Whitfield (salicylic + benzoic acid) ointment is also useful. Some imidazoles (bifonazole, miconazole, sertaconazole) have good action although not as effective as antibacterial; the latter are important when the diagnosis is not correct and diagnosis of superficial mycosis (candidiasis or tinea) is suspected [14, 47].

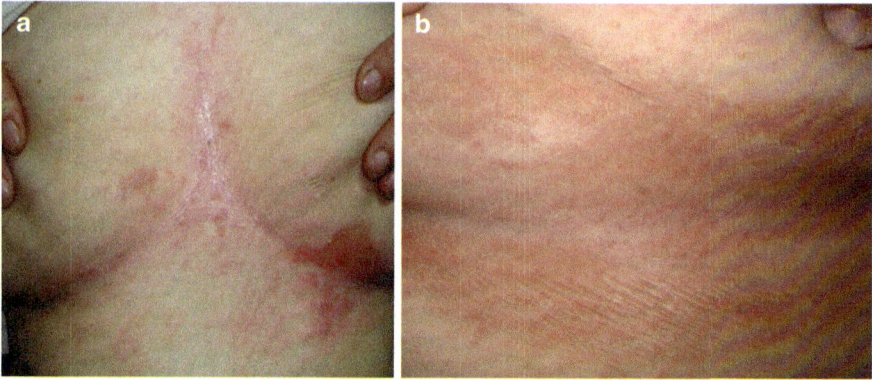

Fig. 9.4 (**a**) Erythrasma in submamary region, (**b**) Intertrigo of erythrasma

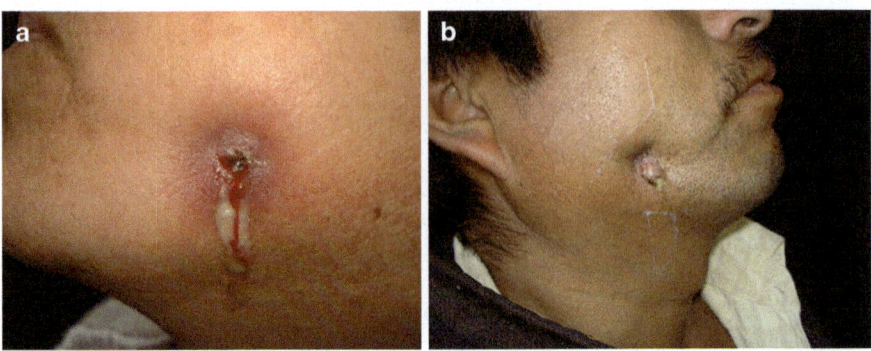

Fig. 9.5 (a) Cervical actinomycosis with extensive exudate, (b) cervico-facial actinomycosis

Actinomycosis

It is a chronic granulomatous disease, produced by several opportunistic, anaerobic or microaerophilic actinomycetes, especially *Actinomyces israelii*. It is characterized by causing volume increase, deformation of the affected area, with abscesses and fistulae, draining purulent exudate containing the parasitic forms called "grains". It is located in the cervicofacial region (most common clinical form in 75% of cases), thoracic, and abdominal [14, 24, 48–50].

In general, the etiological agents are anaerobic or microaerophilic actinomycetes, non-alcohol-acid-resistant, being part of the oral cavity microbiota, as well as amygdala crypt, large intestine and vaginal mucosae (with intrauterine devices).

The predisposing causes for the cervicofacial form include lack of oral hygiene, dental caries and periodontal diseases. DM is an adjacent factor. In a recent report conducted by our group [49], actinomycosis can be associated with DM in up to 45% of cases (Fig. 9.5).

The laboratory diagnosis is done by watching "grains" (similar to those of sulfur), which are yellowish compact masses of several varying in sizes (50–30,000 μm) microfilaments; cultures must be done in anaerobiosis, for example gas "pack" or in special liquid media for anaerobiosis (thioglycollate and Brewer's gel), form suspended colonies composed of Gram positive thin filaments, microsiphoned and with cocoid and bacillary forms. The biopsy is useful for diagnosis, it is often reported a suppurative granuloma and basophilic, multilobulated grains, often with cleaves in the margin [14].

The treatment of choice for actinomycosis is based on penicillin at high doses, i.e. up to 30–50 million units. Amoxicillin/clavulanate, as well as sulfamethoxazole trimethoprim, tetracycline, clindamycin, and imipenem/cilastatin are also useful options [14, 49, 50] (Table 9.1).

Table 9.1 Mycosis and pseudomycosis associated with diabetes mellitus

Mycosis/pseudomycosis	Etiological agent (main)	Clinical manifestation (main)	Laboratory diagnosis	Treatment
Dermatophytosis				
Tinea pedis and corporis	*Trichophyton rubrum*	Interdigital and plaques	Hyphae	Topical azoles
Onychomycosis	*Trichophyton rubrum*	Erythematous squamous with border / DSO, TDO	Hyphae and arthroconidia	Terbinafine and itraconazole
Majocchi's granuloma	*Trichophyton rubrum*	Nodular and ulcerative	Biopsy: granuloma with hyphae and conidia	Terbinafine and itraconazole
Candidiasis				
Oral	*C. albicans*	Pseudomembranous	Pseudohyphae with blastoconidia	Topical imidazoles, triazoles: fluconazole and itraconazole
Vulvovaginal	*C. albicans* and *C. glabrata*	Vaginitis with leukorrhea		
Cutaneous	*C. albicans*	Intertrigo		
Onychomycosis	*C. albicans* and *C. parapsilosis*	Paronychia & onycholysis		
Erythrasma	*Corynebacterium minutissimum*	Intertrigo	Gram positive thin filaments	Erythromycin
Mucormycosis				
Primary cutaneous	*Rhizopus sp., Saksenaea sp.* and *Apophysomyces sp.*	Necrotic lesions with erythema and eschar	Broad, coenocytic hyphae	Amphotericin B + surgery
Secondary cutaneous	*Rhizopus arrhizus* and *Lichtheimia sp.*	Palpebral fistula, necrotic lesions and palate ulceration	Broad, coenocytic hyphae	Amphotericin B + posaconazole + surgery
Actinomycosis	*Actinomyces israelii*	Cervical with increase in volume and fistules	Microsiphonated grains	Penicilin Amoxicillin/clavulanic acid

C Candida, DSO distal subungual onychomycosis, *TDO* total dystrophic onychomycosis

Conclusions

Particular attention must be given to patients with Diabetes mellitus because of high incidence of fungal infections among these patients. The prevalence of mycosis in diabetics is a serious mortality cause. The problem may be minimalized by proper use of prophylaxis and regular communication with patient. To avoid treatment-resistance every case of mycosis must be precisely diagnosed, with an adequate adherence to the treatment by the patient. Adjusting an adequate treatment based on agent sensitivity, severity of the patient's condition and comorbidity will be of vital importance in the prognosis and future complications that this group of patients may develop.

References

1. Mendes AL, Miot HA, Junior HV. Diabetes mellitus and the skin. An Bras Dermatol. 2017;92:8–20.
2. Duff M, Demidova O, Blackburn S, et al. Cutaneous manifestations of diabetes mellitus. Clin Diabetes. 2015;33:40–8.
3. Skorepová M. Mycoses and diabetes. Vnitr Lek. 2006;52:470–3.
4. Namazi MR, Yosipovitch G. Diabetes mellitus. In: Callen JP, Jorizzo JL, Bolognia JL, editors. Dermatological signs of internal disease. 4th ed. Philadelphia: Elsevier año; 2009. p. 189–98.
5. Casqueiro J, Casqueiro J, Alves C. Infections in patients with diabetes mellitus: a review of pathogenesis. Indian J Endocrinol Metab. 2012;16:S27–36.
6. Saul A, Martínez G. La Piel: en: Saul A. Lecciones de dermatología. 16 edición ed. Cd. De México: McGraw-Hill; 2014. p. 1–18.
7. Neumann E. Glycohistechia in psoriasis prior to and following medication of peroral antidiabetics. Dermatologica. 1960;120:120–5.
8. Campos de Macedo GM, Nunes S, Barreto T. Skin disorders in diabetes mellitus: an epidemiology and physiopathology review. Diabetol Metab Syndr. 2016;8:63.
9. Romano C, Massai L, Asta F, Signorini AM. Prevalence of dermatophytic skin and nail infections in diabetic patients. Mycoses. 2001;44(3–4):83–6.
10. García-Humbría L, Richard-Yegres N, Pérez-Blanco M, Yegres F, Mendoza M, Acosta A, Hernández R, Zárraga E. Superficial mycoses: comparative study between type 2 diabetic patients and a non-diabetic control group. Investig Clin. 2005;46:65–74.
11. Tosti A, Hay R, Arenas-Guzmán R. Patients at risk of onychomycosis—risk factor identification and active prevention. J Eur Acad Dermatol Venereol. 2005;19(Suppl 1):13–6.
12. Ozcan D, Seçkin D, Demirbilek M. In vitro antifungal susceptibility of dermatophyte strains causing tinea pedis and onychomycosis in patients with non-insulin-dependent diabetes mellitus: a case-control study. J Eur Acad Dermatol Venereol. 2010;24:1442–6.
13. Papini M, Cicoletti M, Fabrizi V, Landucci P. Skin and nail mycoses in patients with diabetic foot. G Ital Dermatol Venereol. 2013;148:603–8.
14. Bonifaz A. Micología médica básica. 5ª edición ed. Cd. de México: McGraw-Hill; 2015.
15. Oz Y, Qoraan I, Oz A, Balta I. Prevalence and epidemiology of tinea pedis and toenail onychomycosis and antifungal susceptibility of the causative agents in patients with type 2 diabetes in Turkey. Int J Dermatol. 2017;56:68–74.
16. Manzano-Gayosso P, Hernández-Hernández F, Méndez-Tovar LJ, Palacios-Morales Y, Córdova-Martínez E, Bazán-Mora E, López-Martinez R. Onychomycosis incidence in type 2 diabetes mellitus patients. Mycopathologia. 2008;166(1):41–5.
17. Akkus G, Evran M, Gungor D, Karakas M, Sert M, Tetiker T. Tinea pedis and onychomycosis frequency in diabetes mellitus patients and diabetic foot ulcers. A cross sectional—observational study. Pak J Med Sci. 2016;32:891–5.

18. Arenas R, Bonifaz A, Padilla MC, Arce M, Atoche C, Barba J, et al. Onychomycosis. A mexican survey. Eur J Dermatol. 2010;20:611–4.
19. Wijesuriya TM, Kottahachchi J, Gunasekara TD, Bulugahapitiya U, Ranasinghe KN, Neluka Fernando SS, Weerasekara MM. Aspergillus species: an emerging pathogen in onychomycosis among diabetics. Indian J Endocrinol Metab. 2015;19:811–6.
20. Bonifaz A, Cruz-Aguilar P, Ponce RM. Onychomycosis by molds. Report of 78 cases. Eur J Dermatol. 2007;17:70–2.
21. Hwang SM, Suh MK, Ha GY. Onychomycosis due to nondermatophytic molds. Ann Dermatol. 2012;24:175–80.
22. Cathcart S, Cantrell W, Be E. Onychomycosis and diabetes. J Eur Acad Dermatol Venereol. 2009;23:1119–22.
23. Zane LT, Chanda S, Coronado D, Del Rosso J. Antifungal agents for onychomycosis: new treatment strategies to improve safety. Dermatol Online J. 2016;22(3.) pii: 13030/qt8dg124gs.
24. Edwards JE Jr, Tillman DB, Miller ME, et al. Infection and diabetes mellitus. West J Med. 1979;130:515–21.
25. de Leon EM, Jacober SJ, Sobel JD, et al. Prevalence and risk factors for vaginal *Candida* colonization in women with type 1 and type 2 diabetes. BMC Infect Dis. 2002;2:1.
26. Kalra S, Chawla A. Diabetes and balanoposthitis. J Pak Med Assoc. 2016;66:1039–41.
27. Verma SB, Wollina U. Looking through the cracks of diabetic candidal balanoposthitis. Int J Gen Med. 2011;4:511–3.
28. Fernandez-Martinez RF, Jaimes-Aveldañez A, Hernández-Pérez F, et al. Oral *Candida spp* carriers: its prevalence in patients with type 2 diabetes mellitus. An Bras Dermatol. 2013;88:222–5.
29. Dorko E, Baranová Z, Jenca A, Kizek P, Pilipcinec E, Tkáciková L. Diabetes mellitus and candidiases. Folia Microbiol (Praha). 2005;50:255–61.
30. Asokan N, Binesh VG. Cutaneous problems in elderly diabetics: a population-based comparative cross-sectional survey. Indian J Dermatol Venereol Leprol. 2017;83:205–21.
31. Martin ES, Elewski BE. Cutaneous fungal infections in the elderly. Clin Geriatr Med. 2002;18:59–75.
32. Scheinfeld NS. Obesity and dermatology. Clin Dermatol. 2004;22:303–9.
33. Mahajan S, Koranne RV, Sharma SK. Cutaneous manifestation of diabetes mellitus. Indian J Dermatol Venereol Leprol. 2003;69:105–8.
34. Jayatilake JA, Tilakaratne WM, Panagoda GJ. Candidal onychomycosis: a mini-review. Mycopathologia. 2009;168(4):165–73.
35. Abad-González J, Bonifaz A, Ponce RM. Onicomicosis por Candida asociada con diabetes mellitus. Dermatologia. Rev Mex. 2007;51:135–41.
36. Araiza-Santibánez J, Tirado-Sánchez A, González-Rodríguez AL, Vázquez-Escorcia RM, Ponce-Olivera RM, Bonifaz A. Onychomycosis in the elderly. A 2-year retrospective study of 138 cases. Rev Med Hosp Gen Méx. 2016;79(1):5–10.
37. Bonifaz A, Tirado-Sánchez A, Calderón L, et al. Cutaneous mucormycosis: mycological, clinical, and therapeutic aspects. Curr Fungal Infect Rep. 2015;9(4):229–37. https://doi.org/10.1007/s12281-015-0236-z.
38. Perusquía-Ortiz AM, Vázquez-González D, Bonifaz A. Opportunistic filamentous mycoses: aspergillosis, mucormycosis, phaeohyphomycosis and hyalohyphomycosis. J Dtsch Dermatol Ges. 2012;10:611–21.
39. Bonifaz A, Tirado-Sánchez A, Calderón L, et al. Mucormycosis in children: a study of 22 cases in a Mexican hospital. Mycoses. 2014;57 Suppl 3:79–84.
40. Chow V, Khan S, Balogun A, et al. Invasive rhino-orbito-cerebral mucormycosis in a diabetic patient—the need for prompt treatment. Med Mycol Case Rep. 2014;23:5–9.
41. Di Carlo P, Pirrello R, Guadagnino G, et al. Multimodal surgical and medical treatment for extensive rhinocerebral mucormycosis in an elderly diabetic patient: a case report and literature review. Case Rep Med. 2014;2014:527062.
42. Bonifaz A, Tirado-Sánchez A, Ponce-Olivera RM. Granuloma de Majocchi. Gac Med Mex. 2008;144:427–33.

43. Erbagci Z. Deep dermatophytoses in association with atopy and diabetes mellitus: Majocchi's granuloma tricophyticum or dermatophytic pseudomycetoma? Mycopathologia. 2002;154:163–9.
44. Tirado-Sánchez A, Ponce RM, Bonifaz A. Majocchi granuloma. (Dermatophytic granuloma): updated therapeutic options. Curr Fungal Infect Rep. 2015;9:204–12.
45. Montes LF, Dobson H, Dodge BG, Knowles WR. Erythrasma and diabetes mellitus. Arch Dermatol. 1969;99:674–80.
46. Ahmed I, Goldstein B. Diabetes mellitus. Clin Dermatol. 2006;24(4):237–46.
47. Holdiness MR. Management of cutaneous erythrasma. Drugs. 2002;62:1131–41.
48. de Andrade AL, Novaes MM, Germano AR, Luz KG, de Almeida Freitas R, Galvão HC. Acute primary actinomycosis involving the hard palate of a diabetic patient. J Oral Maxillofac Surg. 2014;72:537–41.
49. Boyanova L, Kolarov R, Mateva L, Markovska R, Mitov I. Actinomycosis: a frequently forgotten disease. Future Microbiol. 2015;10:613–28.
50. Bonifaz A, Tirado-Sánchez A, Calderón L, Montes de Oca G, Torres-Camacho P, Ponce RM. Treatment of cutaneous actinomycosis with amoxicillin/clavulanic acid. J Dermatol Treat. 2017;28:59–64.

Daniel Stecher

Epidemiology

Diabetes is a chronic disease whose complications imply a high impact on the population, both from the point of view of the patients' health, and the social and economic costs it represents for the health system. The CDC reported that diabetes affected 9.4% of the population [1]. In Argentina, the National Survey of Risk Factors conducted in 2013 by the Health Ministry showed a prevalence of 9.8% [2].

Within the complications of this disease, the diabetic foot represents one of the most fearsome. It is estimated that 15% of diabetic patients will develop an ulcer of the foot, between 15 and 30% will require some type of amputation which is preceded in 60% of cases by an infected ulcer [3, 4]. The rate of amputations in the United States in people with diabetes is 4.6/1000 [3] .whereas a study on amputations in the city of Buenos Aires, Argentina, showed that it is 50.7% [5]. In addition to the costs that these complications represent and the difficulties for the social and labor reinsertion of the amputated person, the mortality associated with amputations is 70% at 5 years [3].

Definition

The presence of an infection must be considered in any diabetic patient with foot injuries accompanied by any of the following features: erythema, edema, heat, flushing, swelling, purulent secretion, devitalized or friable tissues and necrosis. Particular attention should be paid to the presence of factors associated with infection such as recurrent ulcers or more than 30 days of evolution, history of

D. Stecher, M.D.
Infectious Diseases Division, Facultad de Medicina, Universidad de Buenos Aires,
Ciudad Autónoma de Buenos Aires, Argentina
e-mail: dstecher@intramed.net

© Springer International Publishing AG 2018
E.N. Cohen Sabban et al. (eds.), *Dermatology and Diabetes*,
https://doi.org/10.1007/978-3-319-72475-1_10

amputation or peripheral vascular disease, traumatic injuries due to walking bare-foot and renal failure. Other elements to evaluate are loss of sensation of protection (see section on pathogenesis) and ulcers with positive bone probe tests (see section osteomyelitis) [3].

Pathogenesis

The pathogenesis of diabetic foot infections involves one or more risk factors being neuropathy the most important. This is responsible for the loss of the "feeling of protection" so the patient does not perceive traumatic injuries such as those produced by inappropriate footwear [6]. As a consequence, a deformity of the foot with biomechanical alteration of the load is produced, which results in the formation of calluses that evolve towards the formation of ulcers. Peripheral arterial disease, present in 50% of diabetics with foot ulcers, contributes to delay the healing of ulcers. The lack of sensitivity causes the ischemia to be manifested asymptomatically. Although a small proportion of patients may present exclusively ischemic ulcers, most of the time the mechanism is neuroischemic. Diabetic microangiopathy is not currently considered a primary factor in the generation of ulcers or delayed healing [4].

Diagnosis

Clinical Evaluation

The evaluation of the foot should take into account the characteristics of the ulcers (location, diameter, depth, presence and type of secretion, and presence of erythema at the edges). Other clinical manifestations to consider are the presence of cellulitis, necrosis and crepitus.

Ulcers located in the plant or areas of bone deformity usually correspond to a neuroischemic mechanism whereas those located at the edges of the foot or extremity of the fingers are usually pure ischemic.

In order to avoid the excessive use of antimicrobials, the infected and uninfected ulcers should be differentiated. Non-infected ulcers, with no secretion or cellulitis around the ulcers, are considered uninfected whereas those with larger diameter and depth with purulent secretion and/or peripheral cellulitis should be considered as infected [3, 4] (Fig. 10.1).

The clinical evaluation allows classifying the diabetic foot according to its severity in order to allow a proper decision making regarding hospitalization, antimicrobial use and surgical behaviors. Can be considered as mild (superficial ulcers with minimal cellulitis), moderate (deeper and with more extensive cellulitis), and severe (with systemic signs of sepsis).

In case of deep ulcers it is useful the probe to bone test for diagnosing osteomyelitis. It consists of introducing a sterile metal probe into the ulcer. In the case of contact the bone is considered positive. This test has a sensitivity of 65% and

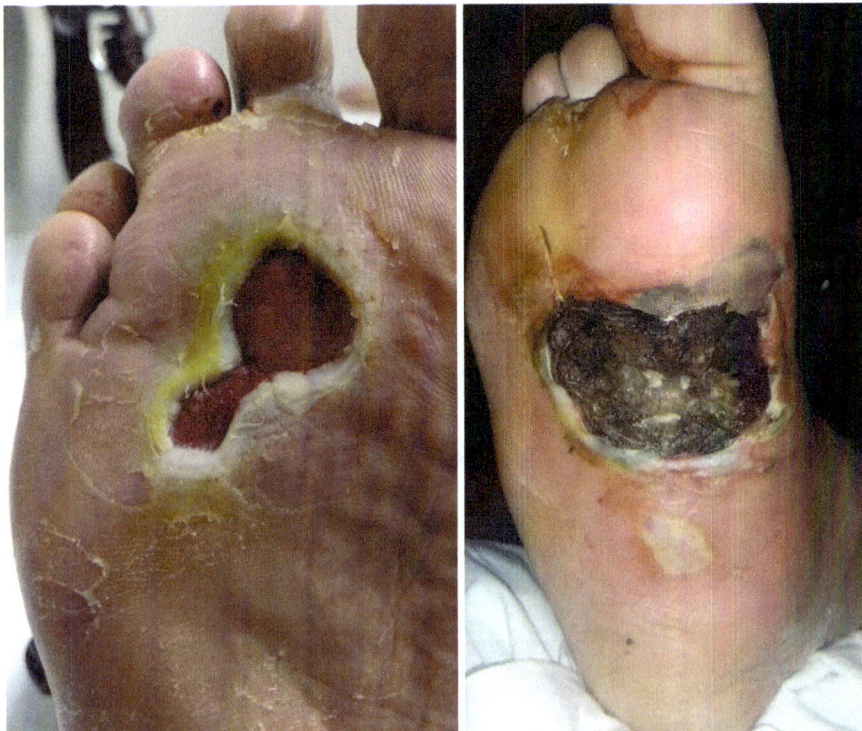

Fig. 10.1 Clinical characteristics of uninfected (*left*) and infected ulcers (*right*) (© D. Stecher)

specificity of 85% for osteomyelitis diagnosis, with positive predictive value of 89% and negative of 56% [7].

The examination should be supplemented with a vascular and neurological evaluation. For the vascular, the palpation of the pulses and the ankle-arm index must be performed. The latter consists of measuring the blood pressure in the ankle and brachial artery, if possible using a Doppler with the tensiometer). Values below 0.90 are interpreted as arterial obstruction being severe below 0.40 [3].

The neurological evaluation should contemplate the tactile sensitivity using a monofilament and the vibratory sensitivity with a diapason.

Complementary Studies

Laboratory

Leukocytosis with left-sided deviation, accelerated erythrocyte sedimentation rate (ESR), and an increased C-reactive protein (CRP) are markers suggestive of infection, of poor response to treatment, and can be used as a criterion for discontinuation of treatment [3, 4]. Some authors have demonstrated the utility of procalcitonin dosage as a predictor of severity [8]. Other studies that must be requested are glycemia, renal function tests and electrolytes.

Images

Imaging studies allow evaluation of bone involvement, which is of great importance due to the high frequency of osteomyelitis as a complication of the diabetic foot. The simple radiography may not show images compatible with infection until several weeks after it is produced, so it is suggested to repeat it between 15 and 30 days later if no findings are found (Fig. 10.2). Magnetic resonance imaging (MRI) is the most accurate study for the diagnosis of bone infection (Fig. 10.3) [3, 4]. Due to the costs and availability is recommended its use in case of doubtful diagnosis. In cases of evident radiological images or bone exposure evidenced by the clinic or the bone probe, MRI is not considered necessary.

As the studies by radioisotopes have low specificity, they are not usually used for the diagnosis of osteomyelitis in the diabetic foot.

Sampling for Microbiological Diagnosis

Due to the usual colonization of the skin, the sampling for microbiological diagnosis should be reserved for those cases with clinical diagnosis of infection, not to be sampled uninfected ulcers.

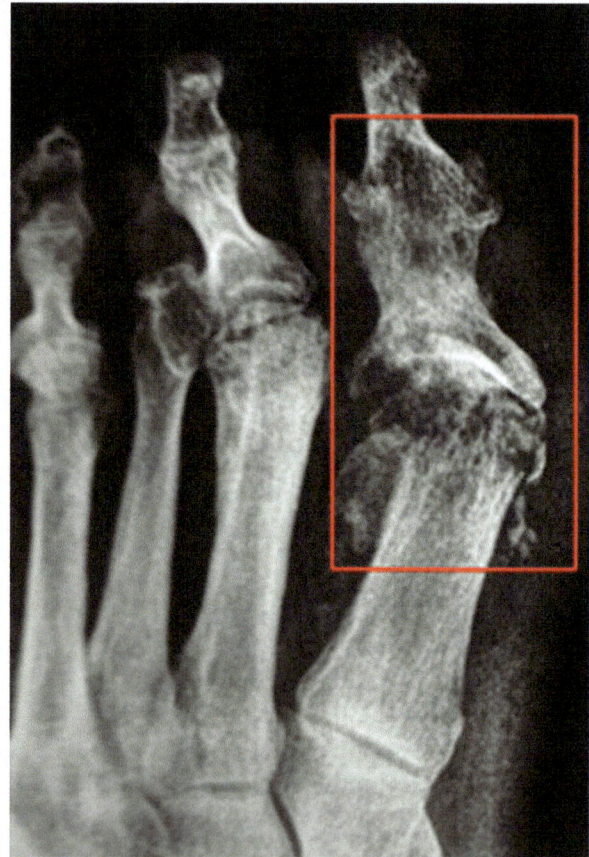

Fig. 10.2 Osteolytic lesions on plain radiography (© D. Stecher)

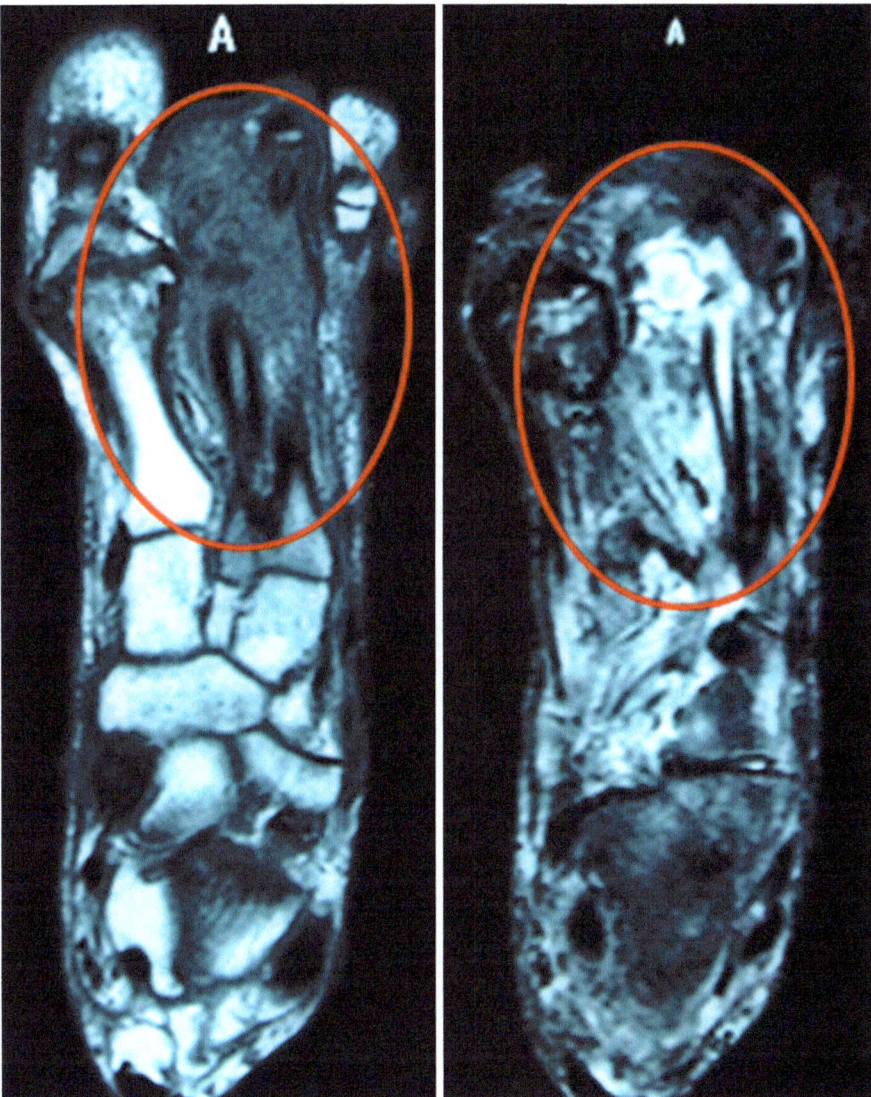

Fig. 10.3 Osteomyelitis in MRI: hypointense signal in T1 and hyperintense in T2 (© D. Stecher)

The recommended ulcers sample is the scraping of its bottom with an unsharpened curette [9, 10] (Fig. 10.4). A study carried out in our hospital by Bello and col. showed that the success of this methodology was 87.5%, being 93% in the cases which had previously received antibiotics [11].

For cases of collections or cellulitis, puncture or the study of surgical samples are suggested if any procedure is performed.

In all cases, direct examination, bacterial culture, germ identification and antibiotic sensitivity study, should be done.

Fig. 10.4 Sample
collection technique by
scraping the ulcer bottom
(© D. Stecher)

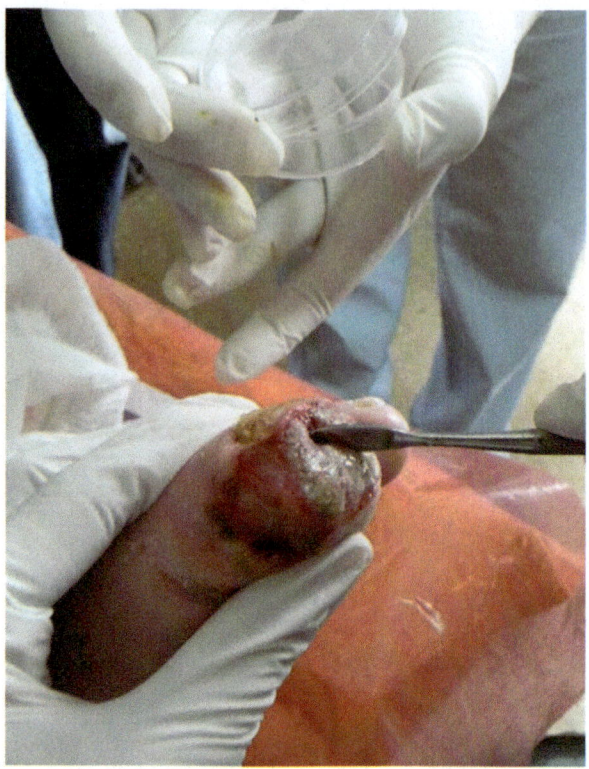

Osteomyelitis

Osteomyelitis occurs in the diabetic patient with a cutaneous infection that compromises the bone by contiguity. It is seen in 50% of severe infections and in 10–20% of apparently milder ones [4]. It should be suspected in patients with ulcers or other skin lesions, recurrent or multiple. Some elements that differentiate osteomyelitis from cellulitis are an ulcer of more than 3 mm deep, CRP (C-reactive protein) over 3.2 mg/dL and an ESR over 60 mm/h [4].

As discussed in the previous sections, exposure of the bone, positive probe bone test and the images, allow suspecting the osteomyelitis diagnosis. Bone biopsy allows its confirmation through the histological study and the identification of the etiological agent(s) by culture. Indications for its realization include the following:

1. Diagnosis not cleared by images
2. Necessity to confirm the diagnosis to define the duration of antibiotic treatment
3. Poor response to empirical treatment
4. Situations in which a metal implant is planned to be placed in an infection suspicion bone.

Referring the methodology, it can be performed by conventional surgery (especially in cases where surgical resection is required) or percutaneous puncture.

A differential diagnosis to consider with osteomyelitis is neuropathic osteoarthropathy or Charcot's disease that is shown as an important foot edema with radiological diffuse osseous lesions especially of the middle tarsal region [12].

Etiology

Several studies on the etiology of diabetic foot infections have shown that it is usually a polymicrobial infection [9–11]. In the study by Citron and col. in patients with moderate to severe infections, of 454 samples, the 94% of the cultures were positive with an average of 2.7 aerobic organism and 2.3 anaerobes per sample. In the previously cited study by Bello and col. which included 64 samples of mild, moderate and severe infections, the results were 87.5% positive and 1.8 organism per sample.

Among the most common findings in both studies are the following:

Gram positive cocci	*Staphylococcus aureus* (oxacillin sensitive and resistant), Coagulase-negative staphylococci, *Streptococci, Enterococcus spp*
Gram negative bacteria	*Enterobacteriaceae, Pseudomonas spp*
Anaerobes	*Bacteroides fragillis Fusobacterium spp., Prevotella spp., Clostridium spp.* Anaerobic cocci
Gram positive bacteria	*Corynebacterium spp*
Yeast	*Candida albicans*

Treatment

The treatment of diabetic foot infections involves the use of medical and surgical resources to which the improvement of perfusion, the local treatment of the lesions and the management of the foot discharge should be added. It is therefore a multidisciplinary work that requires the formation of a team that includes specialist in infectious diseases, diabetes, traumatology, vascular surgeons, wound care specialist, nurses and microbiologists among others [3, 4] (*See* Chap. 13).

Criteria for Hospitalization

The hospitalization is recommended for all patients with severe infections and those with moderate complication factors such as peripheral artery disease or difficulties to perform an outpatient treatment. Those who despite having been treated on an outpatient basis had a poor evolution or intolerance to treatment should be hospitalized as well.

Antibiotic Treatment

The use of antibiotics is essential in the treatment of diabetic foot infections. Although there are several studies that compare different schemes it should be taken into account for their interpretation that most of them are studies of non-inferiority and that they use different criteria to define severity of infections, so that their comparison is inappropriate [13]. On the other hand the polymicrobial nature of the infections and their varied etiology make difficult the selection of an effective empirical treatment. It is therefore recommended for an optimal selection of an antibiotic treatment to make a correct etiological diagnosis. The use of antibiotics is indicated only on suspicion or confirmation of infection. It should not be administered in the case of uninfected ulcers. The treatment can be administered orally in the case of mild infections, and should be parenteral in moderate forms requiring hospitalization and in the severe ones. The choice of the scheme will depend, as mentioned previously, on the germs involved. In cases of severe infections it is recommended to initiate an empirical treatment that should then be adjusted according to the microbiological findings. Parenteral treatments may be continued orally when the patient is stable and should be used those antibiotics with good bioavailability.

Table 10.1 summarizes the empirical antibiotic treatments recommended for the initial management of diabetic foot infections based on the most probable etiologies and level of severity.

The treatment duration depends on the clinical form. The IDSA guideline for the management of the diabetic foot infections recommends in soft tissue infections a duration of one to 4 weeks depending on severity and clinical response. For osteomyelitis it will depend on the type of surgical treatment and its outcome. In cases of total resection such as amputation will be 2–5 days whereas if the resection is partial will vary according to the viability of the remaining bone: 4–6 weeks if viable and more than 12 if there is necrotic bone. However, a study by Tone [14] demonstrated that a treatment duration of 6 weeks is equally effective but with less adverse events than 12 weeks in cases of osteomyelitis without surgical resection.

Surgical Treatment

Surgery is a common component in the management of these infections due to the most of the cutaneous lesions will require a debridement in order to evaluate its depth and perform a resection of the necrotic or devitalized material. In the case of severe forms, interventions will consist of drainage of collections, debridement of necrotizing fasciitis and bone resections or amputations in osteomyelitis. The objective of the surgery included reduce the bacterial load, removed necrotic tissues that cannot be reached by antibiotics and prevent bone deformity [15].

Another common surgical intervention is revascularization in cases where perfusion is compromised.

Table 10.1 Empiric antibiotics suggested treatments for diabetic foot infections

Severity	Etiologic agent	Antibiotics	Administration
Mild	MSSA	Cephalexin	Oral
	Streptococcus spp	Amoxicillin-clavulanate	Oral
		Clindamycin	Oral
	MRSA	Trimethoprim/sulfamethoxazole	Oral
Moderate or severe	MSSA *Streptococcus spp.*	Levofloxacin + clindamycin	Oral or parenteral
	Enterobacteriaceae Anaerobes	Ceftriaxone + clindamycin	Parenteral
		Sulbactam Ampicillin	Parenteral
		Carbapenem (imipenem, meropenem or ertapenem)	Parenteral
	MRSA	Vancomycin	Parenteral
		Daptomycin	Parenteral
	Pseudomonas aeruginosa	Piperacillin tazobactam	Parenteral
Severe	MRSA Anaerobes *Enterobacteriaceae* *Pseudomonas aeruginosa*	Vancomycin or daptomycin + Piperacillin tazobactam or carbapenem	Parenteral

MMSA methicillin susceptible *Staphylococcus aureus*, *MRSA* methicillin resistant *Staphylococcus aureus*

Signs that predict an infection that may compromise the limb and require surgery are as follows [3]:

1. Rapid progression of infection
2. Necrosis or extensive gangrene
3. Crepitation on the palpation or gas in the tissues on the radiograph
4. Ecchymosis or extended petechiae
5. Hemorrhagic bullae
6. New wound with anesthesia
7. Local pain disproportionate to clinical findings
8. Recent loss of neurological function
9. Critical limb ischemia
10. Extensive tissue loss
11. Extensive bone destruction
12. Failure to medical treatment response

Bone resection in osteomyelitis should include not only the need to remove compromised bone while retaining as much of the limb as possible, but also the patient's functionality in order to avoid surgeries that compromise support and generate new ulcers, the so called transfer syndrome [16]. Therefore these resections or amputations should be performed by surgeons with experience in this type of interventions. Amputations may be urgent or programmed according to the patient's clinical situation (life-threatening infection in the first case or recurrent ulcers, significant tissue loss that compromises support or prediction of prolonged hospitalization with more frequent complications in the second).

Revascularization either by surgical methods or by angioplasty is indicated in patients with critical ischemia (ankle arm index less than 0.40). It is recommended to be performed early to avoid ineffective antibiotic treatments because poor perfusion prevents their arrival in tissues. However, it is not acceptable to postpone surgical debridement if revascularization is delayed for some reason [3].

Other Therapeutic Interventions

Local Treatment of Ulcers
Local treatments using alginates or colloides have proven useful for accelerating ulcer healing.

Off-Loading Pressure
The use of total contact casts and removable walkers that redistribute the load and pressure on the ulcers contributes to its healing and prevents its recurrence.

Adjuvant Therapies
There is currently insufficient evidence to recommend the use of a hyperbaric chamber, colony stimulating factor or platelet-rich plasma in the treatment of diabetic foot ulcers.

Conclusion
Diabetic foot is a severe complication, the consequences of which involve, in some cases, the loss of the limb. The management of it requires a multidisciplinary team due to the different components that are required for a successful treatment.

References

1. Centers for Disease Control and Prevention. National Diabetes Statistics Report 2017. Estimates of Diabetes and its burden in the United States. https://www.cdc.gov/diabetes/pdfs/data/statistics/national-diabetes-statistics-report.pdf.
2. Diabetes. In Tercera Encuesta Nacional de Factores de Riesgo para Enfermedades No Transmisibles. Primera Edición. Buenos Aires. Ministerio de Salud de la Nación, Instituto Nacional de Estadísticas y Censos, 2015, p. 101–108. http://www.msal.gob.ar/images/stories/bes/graficos/0000000544cnt-2015_09_04_encuesta_nacional_factores_riesgo.pdf.
3. Lipsky BA, Berendt AR, Cornia PB, Pile JC, Peters EJ, Armstrong DG, Deery HG, Embil JM, Joseph WS, Karchmer AW, Pinzur MS, Senneville E, Infectious Diseases Society of America. 2012 Infectious Diseases Society of America clinical practice guideline for the diagnosis and treatment of diabetic foot infections. Clin Infect Dis. 2012;54(12):e132–e173. doi:https://doi.org/10.1093/cid/cis346.

4. Lipsky BA, Aragón-Sánchez J, Diggle M, Embil J, Kono S, Lavery L, Senneville É, Urbančič-Rovan V, Van Asten S, International Working Group on the Diabetic Foot, Peters EJ. IWGDF guidance on the diagnosis and management of foot infections in persons with diabetes. Diabetes Metab Res Rev. 2016;32(Suppl 1):45–74. https://doi.org/10.1002/dmrr.2699.

5. Mendelevich A, Kramer M, Maiarú M, Módica M, Ostolaza M, Peralta F, Amputations. A five-year epidemiological study in Buenos Aires City. Medicina (B Aires). 2015;75(6):384–6.

6. Ulbrecht JS, Cavanagh PR, Caputo GM. Foot problems in diabetes: an overview. Clin Infect Dis. 2004;39(Suppl 2):S73–82.

7. Grayson ML, Gibbons GW, Balogh K, Levin E, Karchmer AW. Probing to bone in infected pedal ulcers. A clinical sign of underlying osteomyelitis in diabetic patients. JAMA. 1995;273(9):721–3.

8. Jeandrot A, Richard JL, Combescure C, et al. Serum procalcitonin and C-reactive protein concentrations to distinguish mildly infected from non-infected diabetic foot ulcers: a pilot study. Diabetologia. 2008;51:347–52.

9. Citron DM, Goldstein EJ, Merriam CV, Lipsky BA, Abramson MA. Bacteriology of moderate-to-severe diabetic foot infections and in vitro activity of antimicrobialagents. J Clin Microbiol. 2007;45(9):2819–28; Epub 2007 Jul 3.

10. Sapico FL, Canawati HN, Witte JL, Montgomerie JZ, Wagner FW Jr, Bessman AN. Quantitative aerobic and anaerobic bacteriology of infected diabetic feet. J Clin Microbiol. 1980;12(3):413–20.

11. Bello N, Braver D, Ferreira M, Soto L, Echenique S, Barberis C, Stecher D, Paravano L, Finocchietto P. Implementation of a diagnostic methodology in the etiology of infected ulcers in the diabetic foot. XVI Congress of the Argentine Society of Infectology. Mendoza, R. Argentina, Mayo 2016.

12. Short DJ, Zgonis T. Medical imaging in differentiating the diabetic charcot foot from osteomyelitis. Clin Podiatr Med Surg. 2017;34(1):9–14. https://doi.org/10.1016/j.cpm.2016.07.002.

13. Lipsky BA, Berendt AR, Deery HG, Embil JM, Joseph WS, Karchmer AW, LeFrock JL, Lew DP, Mader JT, Norden C, Tan JS. Infectious diseases society of America. Diagnosis and treatment of diabetic foot infections. Clin Infect Dis. 2004;39(7):885–910.

14. Tone A, Nguyen S, Devemy F, Topolinski H, Valette M, Cazaubiel M, Fayard A, Beltrand É, Lemaire C, Senneville É. Six-week versus twelve-week antibiotic therapy for nonsurgically treated diabetic foot osteomyelitis: a multicenter open-label controlled randomized study. Diabetes Care. 2015;38:302–7.

15. Senneville E, Robineau O. Treatment options for diabetic foot osteomyelitis. Expert Opin Pharmacother. 2017;18(8):759–65. https://doi.org/10.1080/14656566.2017.1316375.

16. Aragón-Sánchez J. Treatment of diabetic foot osteomyelitis: a surgical critique. Int J Low Extrem Wounds. 2010;9(1):37–59. https://doi.org/10.1177/1534734610361949.

Dermatoses Most Frequently Related to Diabetes Mellitus

11

Emilia Noemí Cohen Sabban

Many dermatoses, some more common than others, have been historically linked to Diabetes. With the exception of glucagonoma syndrome, any of them can occur in non-diabetic patients.

Nowadays, the coexistence of Diabetes Mellitus (DM) with this heterogeneous group of diseases that affect the skin remains in the field of speculation, and many of them are not universally accepted.

However, over the course of our experience and based on clinical observation, we can state that many dermatoses are often undeniably linked.

Since our first publications on the subject in the nineties and thanks to the knowledge from the last decade, we have reformulated their classification according to their possible linkage mechanisms with DM (Table 11.1) [1].

When I started working in the Nutrition and Skin Division of the Dermatology Department of the Hospital de Clínicas, University of Buenos Aires, Argentina, we conducted a study in which we included diabetic patients with associated dermatoses to describe which ones occur more frequently (Table 11.2).

The results showed that psoriasis was the most common associated dermatosis and then, in descending order, eruptive xanthomas and vitiligo. Acrochordons and localized itching occurred with the same frequency and finally, generalized itching was the one with lower incidence [1, 2].

This chapter presents an overview of each pathology, especially focusing on the DM impact on such disease and its possible linkage with DM.

E.N. Cohen Sabban, M.D.
Dermatology Department, Instituto de Investigaciones Médicas A. Lanari,
University of Buenos Aires (UBA), Buenos Aires, Argentina
e-mail: emicohensabban@gmail.com

© Springer International Publishing AG 2018
E.N. Cohen Sabban et al. (eds.), *Dermatology and Diabetes*,
https://doi.org/10.1007/978-3-319-72475-1_11

Table 11.1 Diabetes and related dermatoses. Classification according to possible linkage mechanisms

Metabolic mechanism	Immunological mechanism	Unknown mechanism
Porphyria Cutanea Tarda	Vitiligo	Lichen planus
Eruptive xanthomas	Bullous pemphigoid	Kaposi's sarcoma
Necrolytic migratory erythema		Acquired perforating dermatoses
Itching		
Acrochordons or skin tags		

Dermatoses, diabetes mellitus, psoriasis

Table 11.2 Associated dermatoses in patients with DM

Dermatoses	N = 237	%
Psoriasis	9	3.79
Vitiligo	6	2.50
Alterations of the lipid metabolism	6	2.53
Skin tags	4	1.68
Localized itching	4	1.68
Generalized itching	3	1.26

Metabolic Mechanism

Porphyria Cutanea Tarda

The porphyria cutanea tarda (PCT) is probably the most common type of porphyria; it usually affects adults between 30 and 60 years of age and both sexes equally. It occurs due to the specific blockage of the uroporphyrinogen decarboxylase (UROD), a liver enzyme that participates in the heme synthesis. The enzymatic failure can be inherited (autosomal dominant), but the sporadic forms in genetically predisposed patients are more common. In both cases, there is an accumulation of uroporphyrins in the skin and liver.

The alteration of the liver function of the enzyme through an iron-dependent mechanism explains the increase of iron parameters such as serum ferritin levels in the analytical laboratory.

Cutaneous and extracutaneous manifestations are described. The cutaneous clinical picture is dominated by the photosensitivity caused by the accumulation of porphyrins, resulting in the onset of three manifestations: blisters, hyperpigmentation and ageing. *Tense blisters* have serous or serohematic content, appear on healthy skin in photo-exposed areas and cure leaving scars and *milium* cysts; the *cutaneous hyperpigmentation* can be the presentation sign of the disease; it's progressive and affects sun exposure areas; skin *premature ageing* gives that yellowish color and thickened aspect with comedones and cysts. Another characteristic sign is *skin fragility* in which minor injuries result in painful erosions.

Hypertrichosis is an early sign which could be the first manifestation of the disease and is observed in the frontotemporal and malar regions of the face. On the contrary, sclerodermiform changes are described in long-term PCT and affect exposed areas. Finally, this disease is one of the causes of *diffuse alopecia* that generally has a sudden onset, unlike the rest of the manifestations that have a gradual onset (Figs. 11.1, 11.2, 11.3, 11.4, and 11.5).

In the extracutaneous clinical manifestations, liver involvement is present in almost all patients and indicates prognosis. Eye, neurological, musculoskeletal and digestive involvement can also occur.

While in histopathology the presence of a subepidermal blister with slight inflammatory infiltrate and PAS-positive thickening of the vessel walls can be proved, the diagnosis is made based on the detection of porphyrins in blood and uroporphyrins, whose accumulation give the typical urine coral fluorescence with Wood's light. Plasma iron overload expressed by a high rate of saturation of transferrin and ferritin increase are additional laboratory parameters.

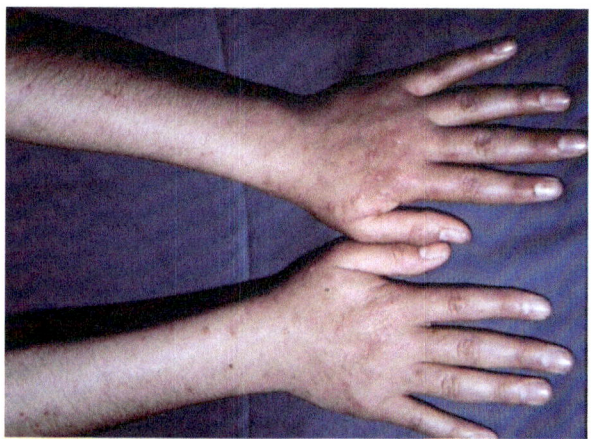

Fig. 11.1 Tense blisters in photo-exposed areas. Healing with milium cysts

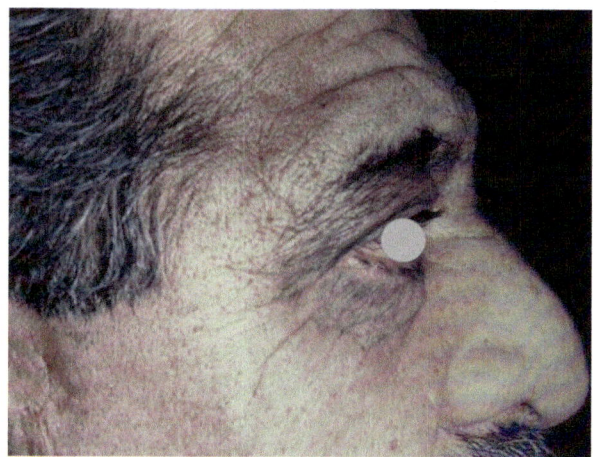

Fig. 11.2 Malar hypertrichosis, pigmentation, conjunctival injection, thickening of the skin

Fig. 11.3 Hypertrichosis, conjunctival injection, skin ageing

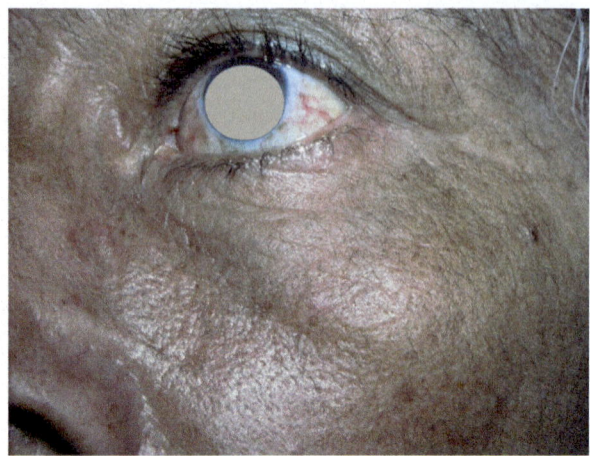

Fig. 11.4 Aging skin with residual lesions where blisters and milium cysts developed

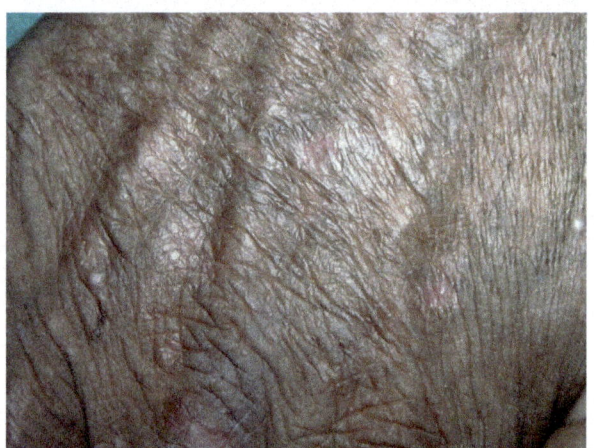

Fig. 11.5 Dried blisters covered with crusts in photo-exposed areas and residual lesions. Significant skin ageing

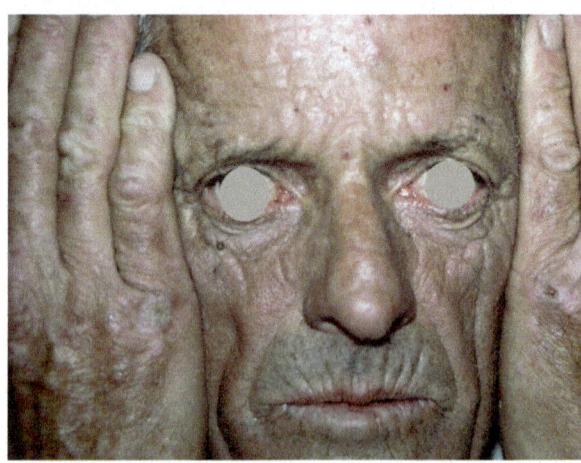

Only 1% of diabetic patients also suffer from PCT, which is included in the metabolic group since the chronic hyperglycemia of DM would be the responsible for the non-enzymatic glycation (NEG) of the heme group, with the resulting association. On the contrary, 25% of porphyric patients, more frequently men between 45 and 75 years of age, has DM [3]. It has been shown that the iron overload observed in patients with PCT has an impact on carbohydrate metabolism, revealing a statistically significant association between these parameters and blood glucose levels and glycated hemoglobin (HbA1c).

Eruptive Xanthomas

Eruptive xanthomas are lesions caused by localized lipid deposits in the skin. They are considered cutaneous markers from a wide range of primary diseases (caused by a genetic disorder) like some types of familial lipoproteinemias or secondary to other processes, including DM. They are observed in patients with a poor control of the disease, with hyperglycemia, hypertriglyceridemia and glycosuria. Both its onset and disappearance are useful to monitor the internal metabolism; on the one hand, metabolic control can result in a rapid disappearance that sometimes occurs in weeks, and on the other hand, contrary to the above, its sudden onset forces us to discard some underlying metabolic disease [4].

They are clinically described as little yellowish papules of one to two millimeters in diameter, or nodules, surrounded by an inflammatory erythematous halo with sudden onset. They are generally asymptomatic, but they can be pruritic. They appear on the buttocks, extensor areas of the limbs (knees and elbows) and the back. They can also result from the Köebner phenomenon in sites of friction or pressure points [5] (Figs. 11.6 and 11.7). The diagnosis is eminently clinical. If it was necessary to perform a biopsy of the lesion, we would observe that the presence of foamy macrophages with lipid content in a perivascular distribution in the superficial dermis and clear spaces that represent the lipid deposition in the dermis, are the histological key. Occasionally, Touton-type giant cells can be observed.

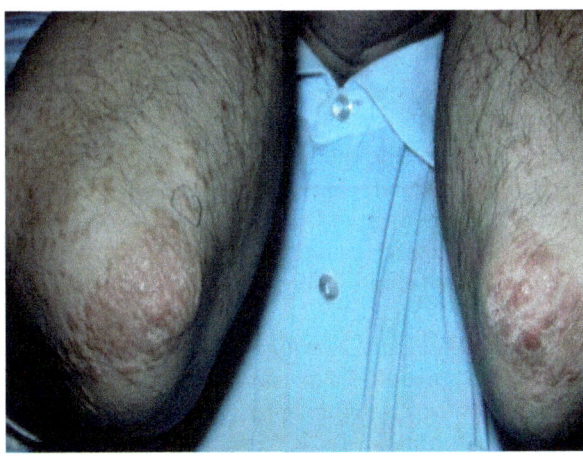

Fig. 11.6 Eruptive xanthomas. Yellowish papules that coalesce forming plaques on the extensor area of the upper limbs

Fig. 11.7 Multiple
eruptive xanthomas

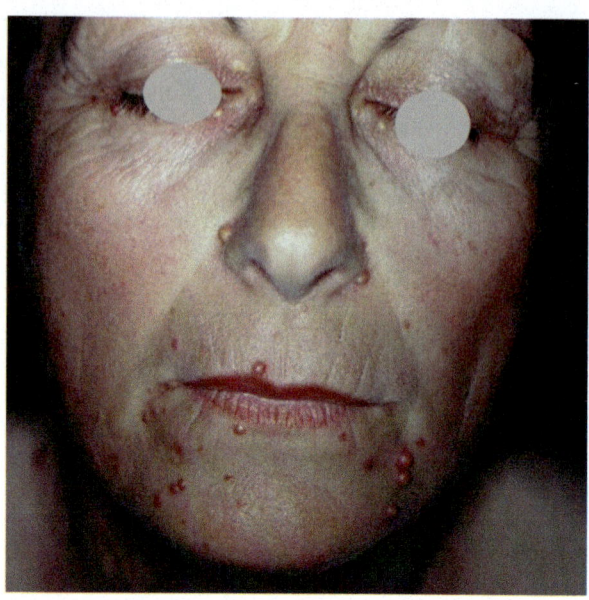

The metabolism of carbohydrates and lipids are closely related. Insulin activates the lipoprotein lipase enzyme (LpL) which produces a clearance of plasma triglycerides and lipoproteins rich in triglycerides. Due to insulin deficiency and therefore LpL inactivity, this is one of the reasons why DM is accompanied by hyperlipidemia, with hypertriglyceridemia and an increase of chylomicrons and very-low-density lipoproteins (VLDL) [6].

Carbohydrates normalization and insulin adjustments will have a direct impact on lipid regulation, for which we also have statins and fibrates [7].

Although the incidence of EX is less than 0.1% of diabetic patients, such association is well established.

Necrolytic Migratory Erythema

The necrolytic migratory erythema (NME) is a characteristic, but not pathognomonic, lesion of the glucagonoma, a rare pancreatic neuroendocrine tumor of the pancreatic α-cells.

Its clinical manifestations constitute the so-called glucagonoma syndrome which is based on a tripod: glucagon hypersecretion, mild to moderate DM or abnormal glucose tolerance test in 76–94% of patients (due to glucagon action on the glycogen stored in muscle and adipose tissues) and mucocutaneous manifestations that the dermatologist must know: [8]

- *Necrolytic migratory erythema*: It is the presentation sign in 50–70% of the cases and it can precede the diagnosis of glucagonoma in 1–6 years; therefore, its presence must be a warning sign. Its pathogenesis has not been clarified yet. Clinically,

they are annular erythematous plaques or vesicobullous and pustules that tend to coalesce. They show central regression and centrifugal growth forming large geographical areas of circinate well-defined limits, leaving or not residual hyperpigmentation when healing. They predominantly appear in intertriginous and periorificial areas (perinasal, peribucal, perineal and perianal areas), as well as buttocks and limbs. Histological findings are not NME-specific as they are also found in other conditions such as pellagra, necrolytic acral erythema, among others. Immunohistochemistry can be positive for glucagon, synaptophysin and chromogranin. Its progression follows a chronic and cyclical course characterized by spontaneous remissions and new lesions outbreaks.
- Painful *atrophic and red tongue* (glossitis).
- *Angular cheilitis.*
- *Blepharitis* [9].

Moreover, there are debilitating signs (weight loss, anemia, diarrhea, etc.), high incidence of thromboembolic phenomena that can cause death in 50% of the cases and neuropsychiatric symptoms in 20% of the patients.

The diagnosis of glucagonoma is based on the clinical recognition of skin rash and DM, associated with increased glucagon serum levels. Imaging studies, such as computed tomography (CT) and magnetic resonance imaging (MRI), are very useful, as well as selective (celiac and hepatic) angiography, though invasive, are considered the gold standard, since it is a hypervascularized tumor.

The treatment of choice is surgery as the glucagonoma is resistant to chemotherapy. It is a slow-growing tumor with a global 5-year survival rate of 70%. The surgical removal of the primary tumor will result in the skin lesions regression. The prognosis and survival depend on the tumor stage, which is already in metastatic disease in almost 50% of the cases at the time of diagnosis.

As metastases are surgically difficult to resect, although there is no consensus on its effectiveness, long-acting somatostatin analogues, such as octreotide and lanreotide, are being used as palliative treatment, which inhibit tumor secretion of glucagon, significantly reducing its concentration and actions [10].

The relationship between DM and glucagonoma differs from other associations described in this chapter. In this case, DM is an example of a disease secondary to other pathological process. The early recognition by the dermatologist, who can be the first physician to suspect the underlying tumor in early stages of the disease, is vitally important [11].

Itching

Itching, the most common skin symptom, is an unpleasant feeling that causes the desire to scratch. If it is intense, it has a direct impact on the quality of life of patients, being the sleep disorders, one of the most frequent consequences.

It is divided into generalized or localized depending on its extension and it could be acute or chronic if it lasts less or more than 6 weeks and it is refractory to the conventional treatments, respectively. According to its origin, it has been related to skin, systemic, neurological or psychogenic diseases (Figs. 11.8, 11.9, 11.10, 11.11, and 11.12). Systemic diseases include endocrine diseases such as DM, like other hepatic, renal and hematological diseases. From patients with generalized itching with no apparent skin cause, 14–24% are from systemic cause and DM is one of them. Obviously, it is not pathognomonic of DM, but it is very common, and most importantly, it can be the presentation symptom.

Regarding localized itching, the most common occurs in anal/genital areas, scalp and lower limbs. Generalized itching is less common than the foregoing and a positive correlation with postprandial glucose levels was found, suggesting that their control could result in symptom relief. On the contrary, these authors could not demonstrate an interrelation between generalized itching and HbA1c levels [12].

Itching etiology in diabetic patients is attributed to several physiotopathogenic mechanisms, in which different pathways and mediators are involved, probably

Fig. 11.8 Pruritus. Lesions due to scratching on the trunk

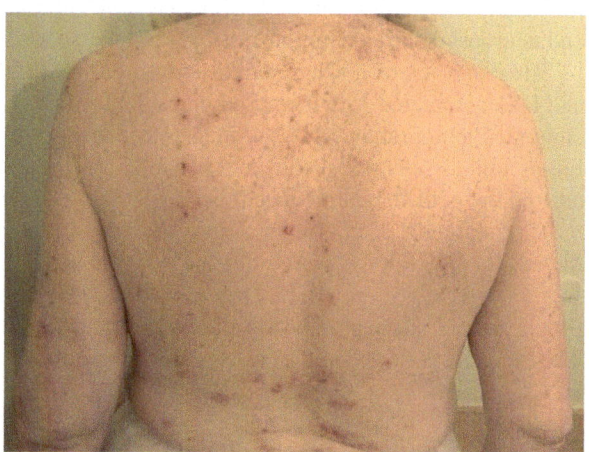

Fig. 11.9 Pruritus. Lesions are predominantly affecting the upper part of the body

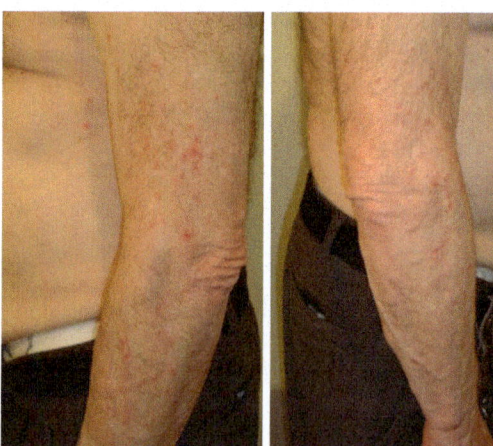

Fig. 11.10 Pruritus.
Typical linear distribution
of lesions due to scratching

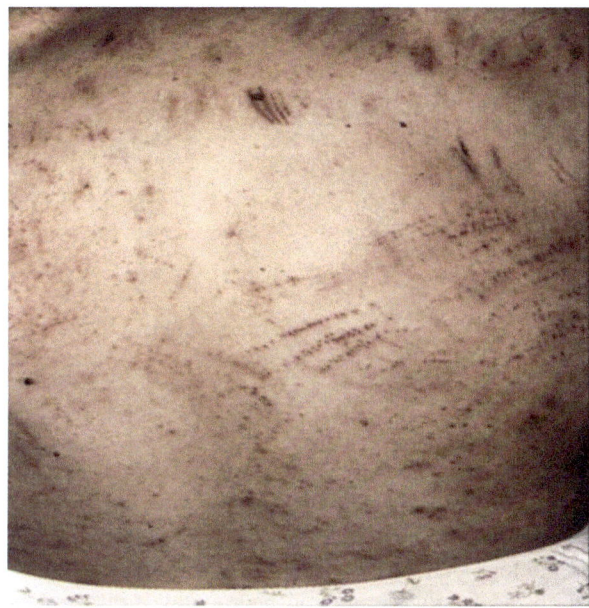

Fig. 11.11 Generalized
itching

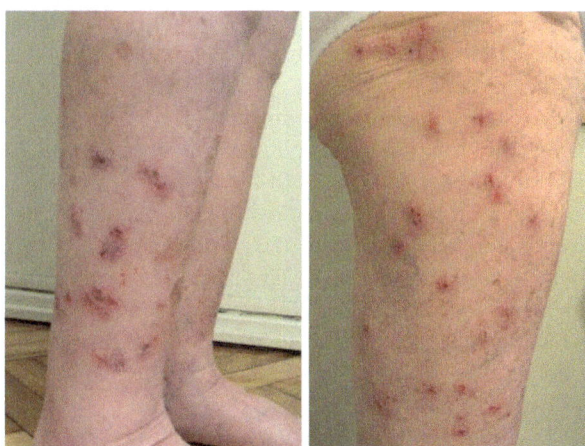

related to metabolic changes of the disease. And that's how different causes are recognized, existing in some cases a superposition among them: [13]

- Skin conditions of diabetic patients.
- Linked to DM complications.
- Consequences of drug reactions to antidiabetic treatment (see Chap. 12).
- Skin conditions of diabetic patients

The association of itching with xerosis, fungal infections such as dermatophytosis and candidiasis is well known.

Fig. 11.12 Excoriations
due to scratching. Linear
lesions in a hemodialyzed
diabetic patient with
chronic kidney failure

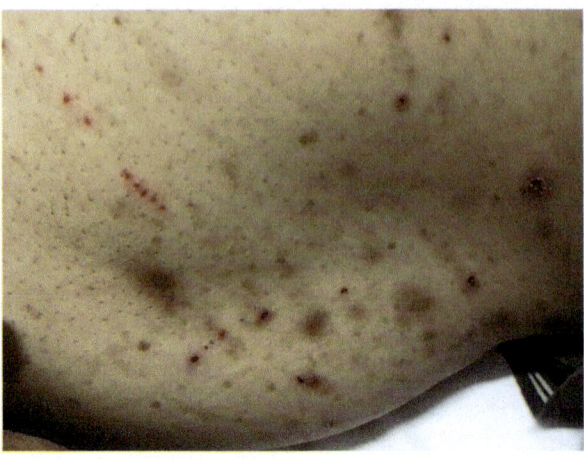

Xerosis, a very common manifestation of DM related to itching, is observed in 25% of diabetic patients, especially in lower limbs. It is caused in part by skin barrier defects that generate dryness. But in its onset, it overlaps sudomotor alterations produced by the autonomic neuropathy with the resulting hypo/anhidrosis (See Chap. 5). If we consider the most distal parts of the limbs, we must not forget *tinea pedis*, another cause of itching resulting from a dermatophyte infection, complicating even more the whole situation (See Chap. 9).

The presence of xerosis is a warning sign, since itching can cause superinfections and erosions/ulcers that we must prevent with a proper skin hygiene using moisturizing soft soap and hydration immediately after the daily bath that should be brief and with not too hot water [14].

Itching in anal or genital regions is observed in up to 20% of diabetic women; candidiasis must be discarded (C. Albicans, C. Glabrata) and it reveals a poor metabolic control (See Chap. 9). They require a longer antifungal oral treatment, supplemented by local treatment, for instance, with boric acid suppositories [15].

Localized itching in scalp is closely related to peaks of hyperglycemia and it improves significantly with DM control.

– Linked to more serious DM complications

For some authors, itching is a polyneuropathy marker. Sensitive peripheral neuropathy of small unmyelinated nerve fibers or C fibers occurs with a type of itching, the truncal pruritus of unknown origin (TPUO); it was related to other neuropathy parameters such as Achilles tendon areflexia or sensitive neuropathy signs in palms and soles such as pins and needles, among others [16].

– Consequences of drug reactions to antidiabetic treatment

It can be a consequence of drug reactions to antidiabetic treatment. Itchy rashes had already been described due to therapies that have now fallen into disuse, such as first-generation sulfonylureas. Recently and with pharmacological advances, the same adverse event has been reported with the latest class of diabetes drugs, SGLT2 inhibitors (sodium glucose transporter 2) and in particular canagliflozin [17].

Itching treatment is beyond the scope of this chapter and it must consider its possible etiological factors to choose the most appropriate topical or topical and systemic therapy in each case. We must not forget the general measures to implement in skin care, whatever the underlying causes may be. We must also highlight the importance of an interdisciplinary approach for the itching in general and the diabetic patient in particular.

There is a close interrelation between itching and systemic diseases. Every patient with itching but no skin lesions must be studied in depth, facing the possibility of an underlying DM. Itching is related to DM mainly through a metabolic mechanism; greater hyperglycemia, greater itching.

Acrochordons or Skin Tags

Acrochordons, also known as skin tags (ST), are the most common benign fibro-epithelial tumors. They are small exophytic pedunculated proliferations, predominantly appearing in neck, eyelids and folds (axillary, inframammary and inguinal folds). They are most common in obese women and its prevalence increases with age. They are considered multiple when there are at least eight (Figs. 11.13, 11.14, 11.15, 11.16, 11.17, 11.18, and 11.19). ST frequency in diabetic patients with signs of IR reaches 26.2%, its association is widely reported in the literature and it is also related to acanthosis nigricans (AN) and metabolic syndrome [18].

Shah et al. demonstrated the correlation between acrochordons and an atherogenic profile (increase in total cholesterol, triglycerides, LDL cholesterol, low HDL cholesterol) and high blood pressure [19].

The association with DM is well established especially if they are numerous, bilateral and voluminous [20].

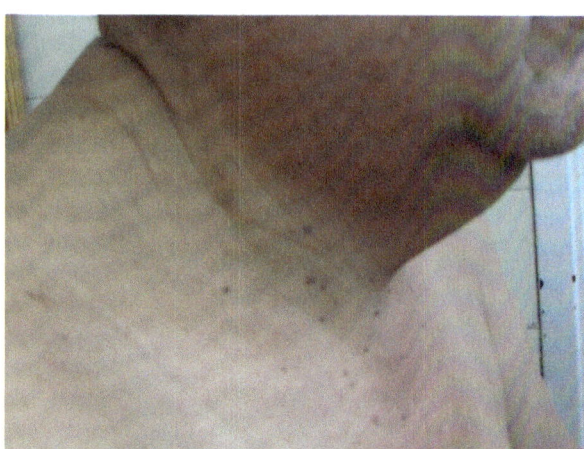

Fig. 11.13 Skin Tags or acrochordons

Fig. 11.14 Skin Tags

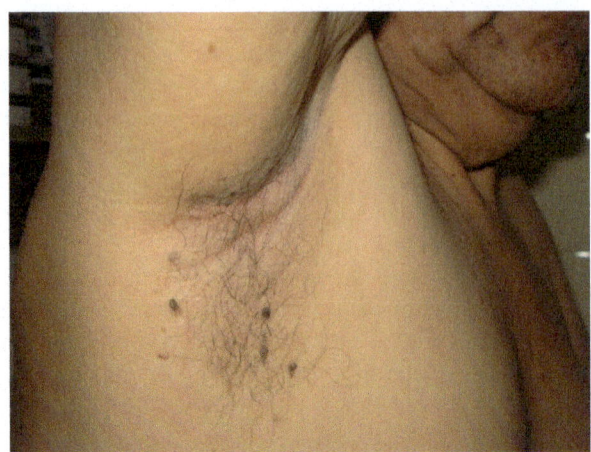

Fig. 11.15 Skin Tags

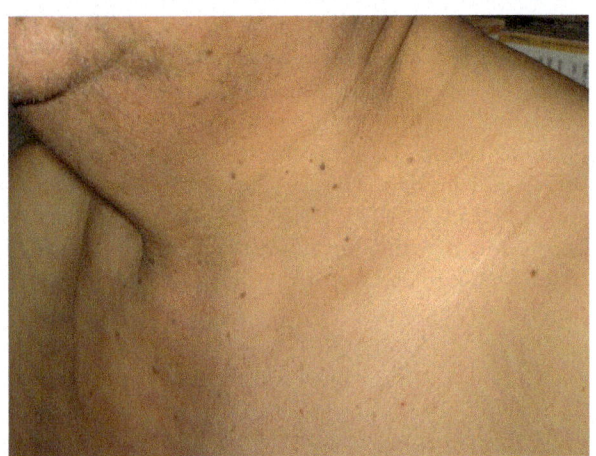

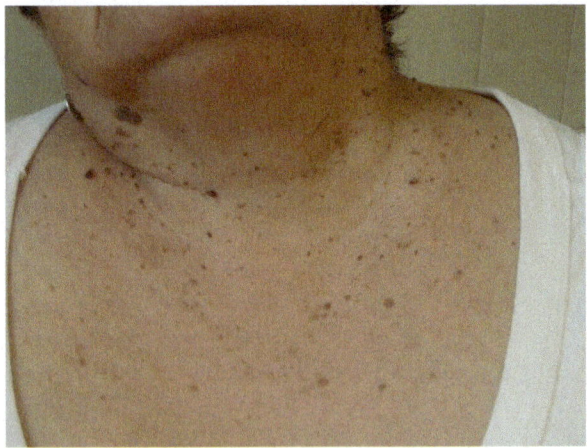

Fig. 11.16 Skin Tags

Fig. 11.17 Skin Tags

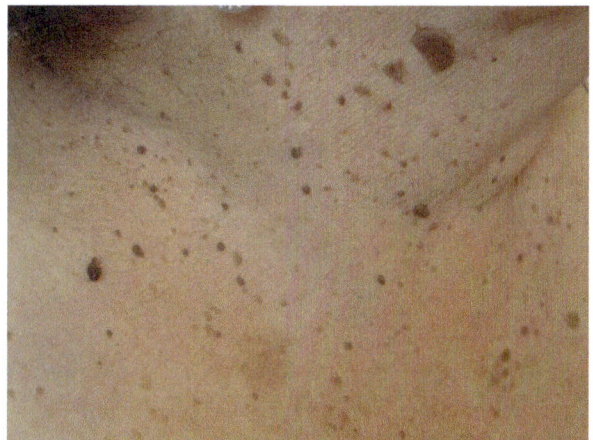

Fig. 11.18 Skin Tags

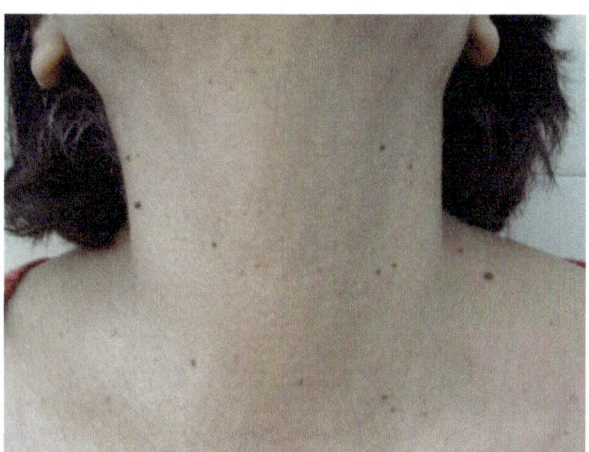

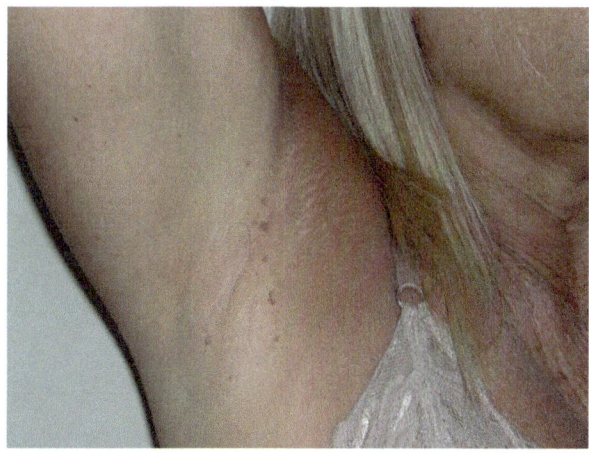

Fig. 11.19 Skin Tags

Immunological Mechanism

Vitiligo

It is a chronic pigmentation disorder characterized by the loss of melanocytes. Finding serum anti-melanin antibodies explains the clinical and subclinical association of vitiligo with other organ-specific autoimmune diseases. Among these diseases, we highlight thyroid autoimmune disorders, DM or the autoimmune polyglandular syndrome (APS).

The autoimmune and inflammatory hypothesis of its pathogenesis is the most solid one, in which the lack or dysfunction of melanocytes is explained as a result of a melanocyte-specific cytotoxic immune response in a prone skin due to a defect in the adherence of melanocytes. Apparently, the melanocytes of patients with vitiligo have an intrinsic defect of the adhesion molecules and that's why they lose cohesion under stress conditions [21].

Clinically, it presents as symmetrical and bilateral asymptomatic hypo/achromic macules with well-defined limits, located in periorificial areas (eyes, nose, mouth, ears, navel, genitals), acral regions, torso and abdomen, affecting hair in the zone concerned (Figs. 11.20, 11.21, and 11.22). The lack of melanin in the affected skin

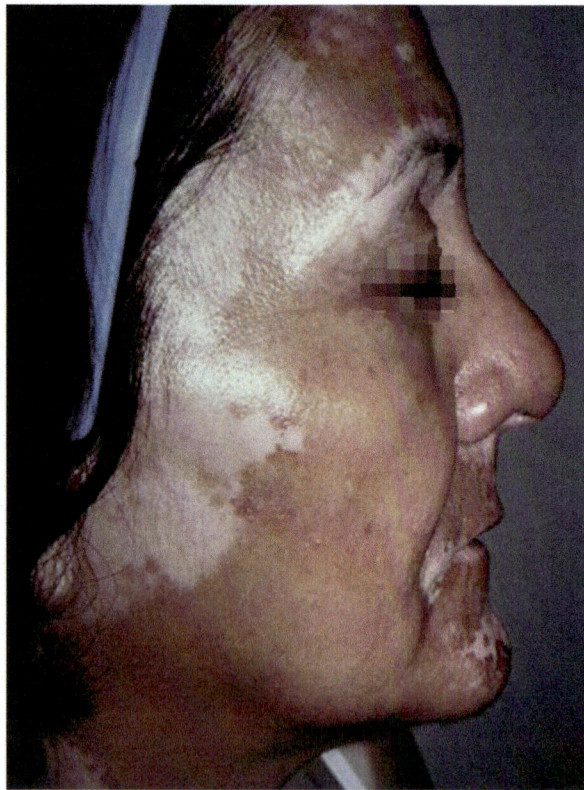

Fig. 11.20 Vitiligo. Achromic macules in the periorificial areas of the face

Fig. 11.21 Periocular vitiligo. Hypo/achromic macules with well-defined limits

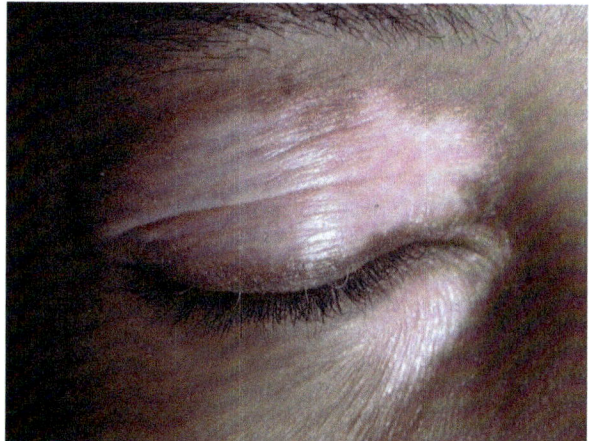

Fig. 11.22 Vitiligo on acral areas in a patient who also had granuloma annulare plaques

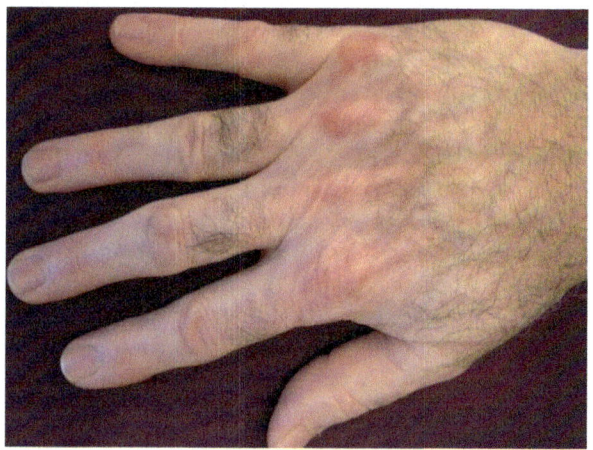

makes it more sensitive to sunburns. Between 10 and 30% of patients with vitiligo have ocular alterations.

In most cases, its course is chronic and only a few resolve spontaneously. Unfortunately, its treatment until now has been unsuccessful. It will depend on the (localized or generalized) extension if we use a local therapy or if we also add a systemic therapy with immunosuppressive drugs, phototherapy, lasers, etc. Photoprotection must be strict due to the lack of melanin in the affected areas. Although it is asymptomatic, it has a great impact on the quality of life, that's why covering makeup is a cosmetic solution to consider [22].

The association between both diseases is unquestionable. Vitiligo is more frequent in diabetic patients than in general population, reaching up to 7%. As a result, it is important to discard the presence of other diseases such as DM in patients with vitiligo. 30% of cases have a family history of vitiligo [23].

Bullous Pemphigoid

The bullous pemphigoid (BP) is an autoimmune disease that affects more women over 60 years old. Blisters develop through detachment at the lamina lucida level of the basement membrane zone (BMZ) in the dermoepidermal junction, due to antibodies (Ab) directed against proteins of hemidesmosomes. There are two antigenic fractions: 230 kD (BPAG1) and the other one with lower molecular weight, 180 kD (BPAG2) [24].

It is clinically characterized by tense blisters that appear on normal or erythematous skin, urticarial plaques and eczema-like lesions that mainly affect limbs (especially lower limbs), abdomen, trunk, groins and armpits. It can affect mucous membranes of the digestive, respiratory and genital systems. It is generally pruritic with a varying level of intensity. It is classified into localized or generalized, depending on how many anatomical regions are involved (Figs. 11.23, 11.24, 11.25, 11.26, 11.27, and 11.28).

Under clinical suspicion, the confirmation will come with the skin blister biopsy and the direct immunofluorescence of the perilesional skin in which the linear deposit of immunoglobulin G (IgG) and/or complement C3 and C4 fractions along the BMZ will be found, and as result of salt-split technique, they are attached to the epidermal side of the blister. Serological studies will detect circulating IgG autoantibodies in 70% of patients. They have a diagnostic value but not a prognostic value, as they are not related to the activity of the disease.

Among the list of comorbidities, arterial hypertension, DM and neurological diseases are the most reported ones. For this reason, despite the large evidence that systemic corticosteroids (CST) are the first-choice drugs, their adverse effects resulted in the incorporation of CST-sparing drugs, such as immunosuppressant, to the therapeutic arsenal of BP [25–27]. Another approach could be tetracyclines and nicotinamide or plasmapheresis in order to remove autoantibodies. Unfortunately, DM has a negative impact on the course, response to treatment and higher mortality incidence on BP, where heart diseases and infections are the most frequent causes of death [28].

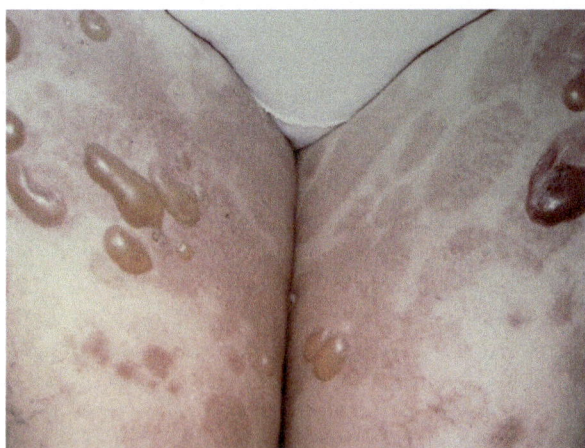

Fig. 11.23 Bullous pemphigoid. Skin erythematous plaques on which blisters develop

Fig. 11.24 Bullous pemphigoid. Tense blisters with serous content

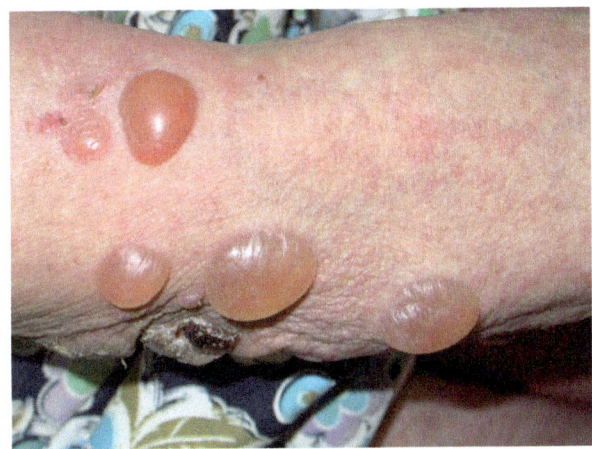

Fig. 11.25 Bullous pemphigoid. Some blisters do not have liquid content and they are covered with crusts

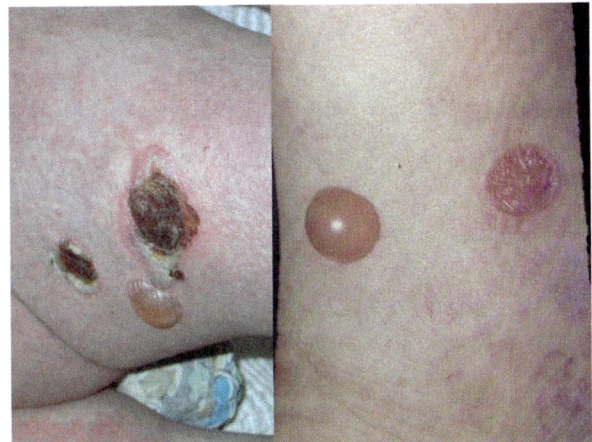

Fig. 11.26 Bullous pemphigoid. The disease is still active and there are new small blisters near the ones that were already present

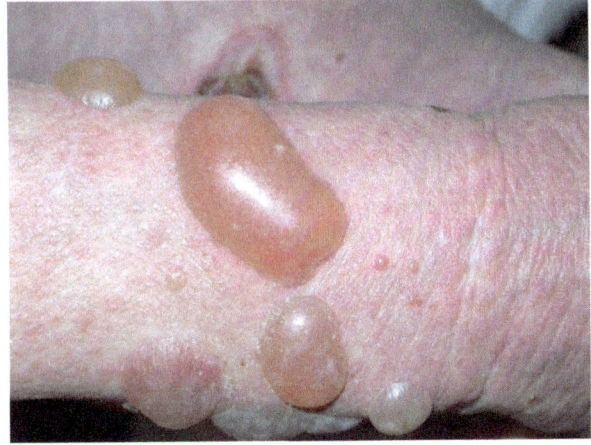

Fig. 11.27 Bullous pemphigoid can be very pruritic; clinically, we observe erythematous edematous plaques and lesions due to scratching, which complicate the diagnosis

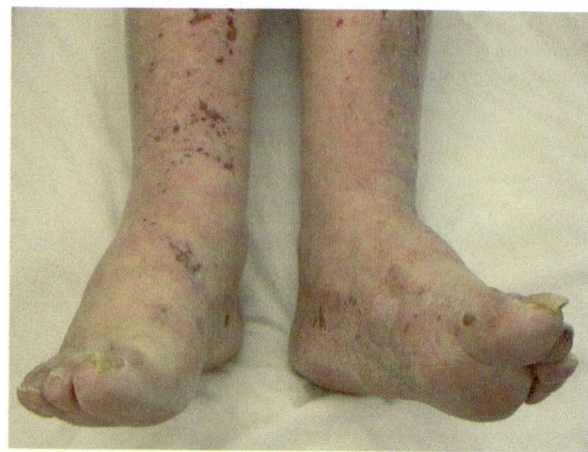

Fig. 11.28 Bullous pemphigoid. Oral mucosal involvement

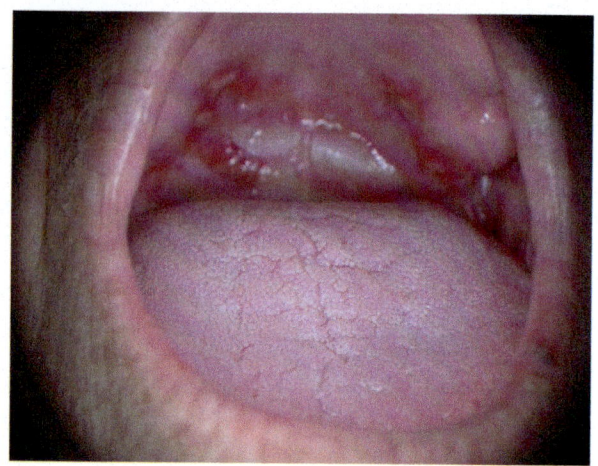

The association between DM and BP is frequent and it reaches an incidence of 20–41%. Its linkage is classified according to an immunological mechanism that could be related to the antigenicity conferred by the NEG of the proteins of the dermoepidermal junction, resulting in the formation of Ab that will cause the detachment and the arising of blisters clinically.

Metabolic and Immunological Mixed Mechanism

Psoriasis

Psoriasis (Ps) is an immune-mediated chronic inflammatory dermatosis. It is currently considered a systemic disease with high risk of developing cardiometabolic comorbidities such as DM, obesity, insulin resistance (IR) and metabolic syndrome

(MetS). Up to 73% of patients present at least one comorbidity, related to a higher risk of global morbimortality, especially young patients with severe psoriasis.

The main disorder is focused on the acceleration of the cell cycle of keratinocytes, shortened to 4 days. Hyperproliferation is accompanied with angiogenesis and inflammation that clinically appear as erythematous papules and plaques, covered by whitish scales. They are bilateral and symmetrical, generally located in extensor surfaces of the body like elbows and knees, scalp, lumbosacral region, etc [29] (Figs. 11.29, 11.30, 11.31, 11.32, and 11.33). When facing a minor trauma, as it is described in the isomorphic Köebner phenomenon, new psoriasis lesions arise in the affected site. Itch is present in variable intensity and also depends on location. While most of the cases improve with exposure to ultraviolet radiation (UVR), there is a small percentage of patients who have photosensitivity.

In the association between Ps and its comorbidities, there would be genetic links, environmental factors and common underlying inflammatory pathways. Systemic inflammation status with an increase of non-specific markers such as C-reactive

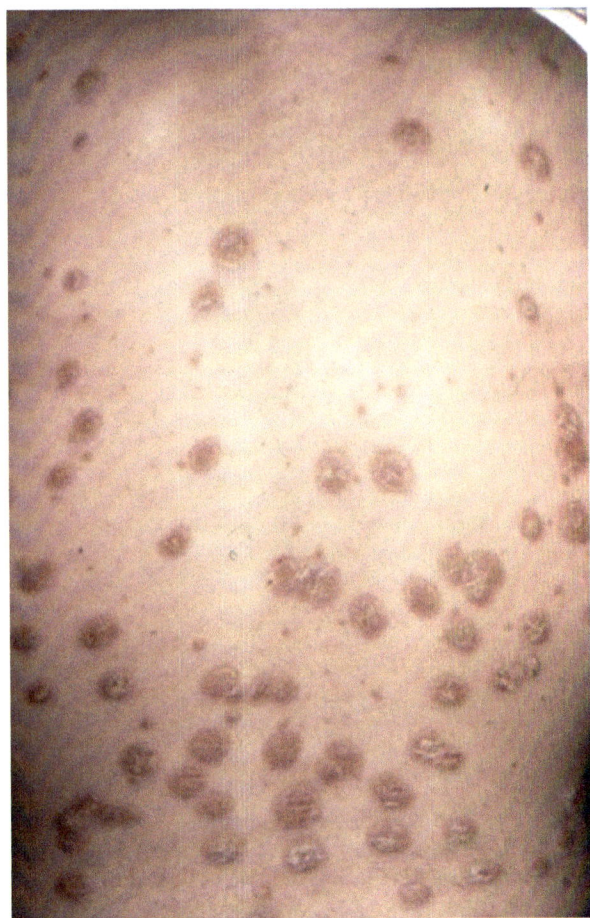

Fig. 11.29 Psoriasis. Multiple Psoriasis plaques in the trunk

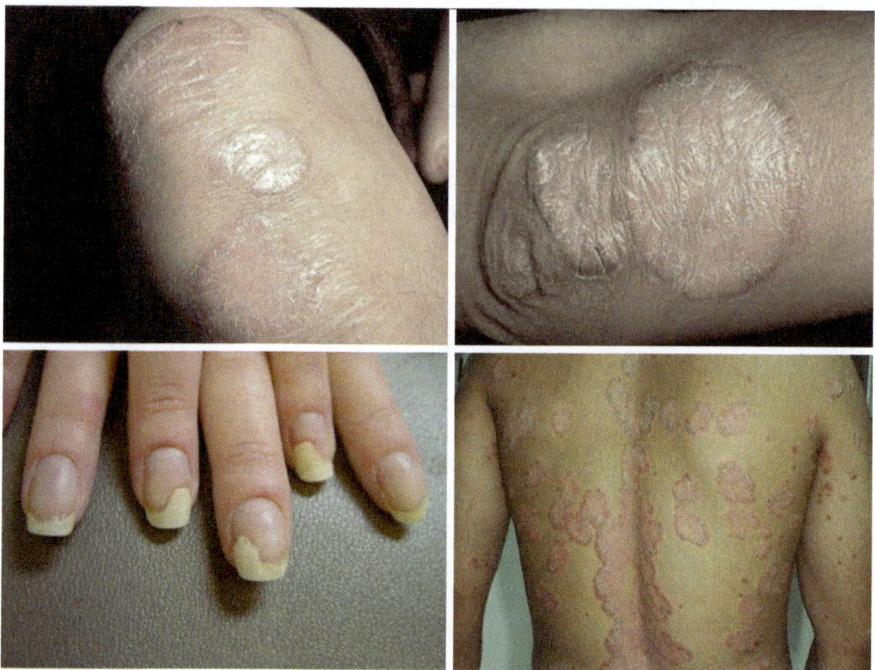

Fig. 11.30 Psoriasis in plaques and nail involvement

Fig. 11.31 Psoriasis.
Plaques in lower limbs

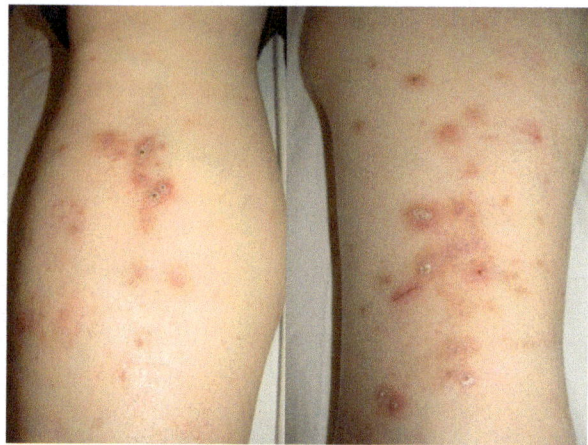

protein (CRP) and proinflammatory cytokines such as tumor necrosis factor-alpha
(TNF- α) and interleukins (IL) (IL-6, IL-17, IL-20, IL-22 and IL-23) would seem to
be the common denominator of all these associations. Cytokines produced by the
adipocyte adiponectin, leptin and resistin, are also involved in the pathogenesis of
Ps as well as MetS, DM, obesity, IR, etc. These adipokines have metabolic and

Fig. 11.32 Psoriasis in plaques

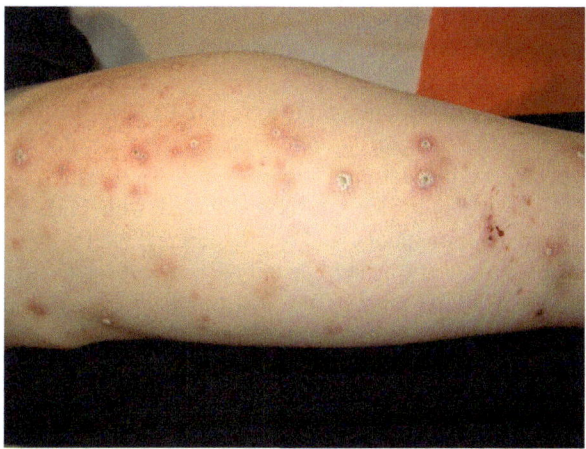

Fig. 11.33 Psoriasis. Plantar involvement

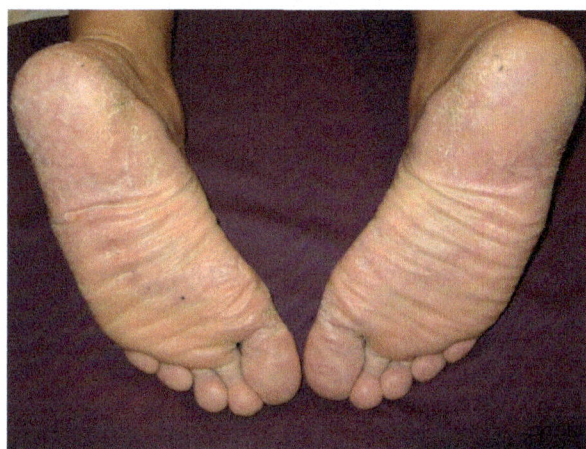

immunological functions like inducing the release of cytokines and the differentiation of T lymphocytes [30].

Adiponectin, which stimulates insulin sensitivity, participating in the metabolism of glucose and lipids, is anti-inflammatory and antiatherogenic and it is diminished at a plasma level in Ps, DM, MetS, etc. Leptin and resistin are proinflammatory; the first one stimulates the formation of TNF- α and IL-6, while the second one favors IR and both are present in Ps and chronic diseases such as DM and obesity. Insulin participates in the normal proliferation and differentiation of keratinocytes; therefore, it is expected that IR status has an impact on cutaneous homeostasis and hence in Ps. TNF- α, one of the main actors in the pathogenesis of Ps, alters the insulin signaling pathway, acting on adipocytes and muscle cells and reducing adiponectin secretion from fat cells [31].

At the same time, when trying to understand even more the connection between Ps and its metabolic alterations that increase cardiovascular risk, patients with Ps have a higher body mass index (BMI) than controls, resulting in the accumulation of fat tissue and the release of adipokines [32].

Treatment is beyond the aim of this book, but it is important to highlight that those patients with moderate to severe Ps must be treated rapidly and effectively, as well as emphasizing on addressing cardiovascular risk factors and, in particular, obesity and the smoking habit.

It is the only dermatosis associated with DM, whose linkage mechanism is mixed, both metabolic and immunological, and is widely evidenced [33].

Psoriasis is the most frequently dermatosis related to DM. DM prevalence found in different studies ranges from 2.35 to 37.4% in psoriasis in general and from 7.5 to 41.9% in patients with severe psoriasis [34].

In a recent study, DM incidence in patients with psoriasis was 8.44% and DM appeared to develop several years after the diagnosis of Ps. Undoubtedly, this association is completely supported by evidence [35].

Unknown Mechanism

Lichen Planus

Lichen planus (LP) is a disease of unknown etiology, whose chronicity ranges from periods of exacerbations and remissions. It is more frequent in women between 30 and 60 years of age and it involves the mucous membranes (oral and genital), skin, nails and scalp. Oral lichen planus (OLP), the mucosal counterpart of cutaneous LP, is the most affected.

Clinically, it is characterized by the appearance of small, itchy, shiny, violaceous flat papules of polygonal shape. They are located in the skin of the flexor surface of wrists and forearms, anterior surface of the legs and the trunk, but it can be spread. In the mucosa, it adopts different clinical patterns among which the erosive variant is part of the triad described by Dr. Grinspan: erosive oral Lichen planus, Diabetes and arterial hypertension. This association was observed in poorly controlled patients with T1DM and smokers or with the habit of chewing tobacco [36] (Figs. 11.34, 11.35, 11.36, 11.37, 11.38, 11.39, 11.40, 11.41, 11.42, and 11.43).

While its etiopathogenesis is not totally clarified, the expression of auto-antigen (Ags) by basal keratinocytes (Kc) would be an initial step. These Ags are presented by Langerhans cells (LC) to the T lymphocytes, stimulating their epidermotropism (CD8+), resulting in cytotoxicity of Kc by apoptosis, mediated by cytokines, TNF-α, FasL, etc [37].

The diagnosis is confirmed with the skin or mucosal biopsy. There are not specific laboratory studies that contribute to its accurate identification.

This disease has been described in association with different systemic conditions such as high blood pressure, DM, hepatitis C, primary biliary cirrhosis, etc. There are reports about the relationship among chronic inflammatory conditions, such as LP, MetS and cardiovascular risk factors, especially in patients with oral LP [38].

Fig. 11.34 Lichen Planus. Generalized involvement

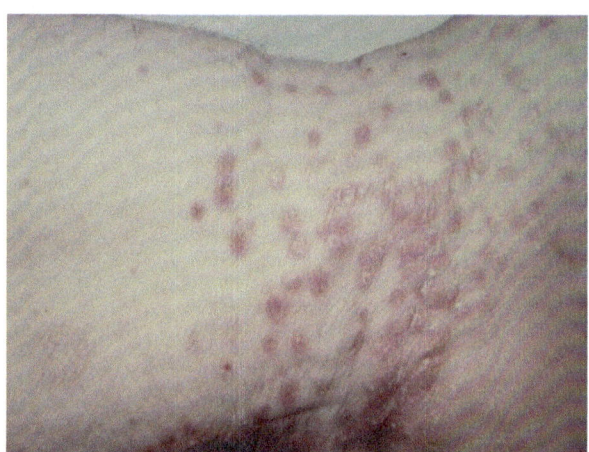

Fig. 11.35 Lichen planus

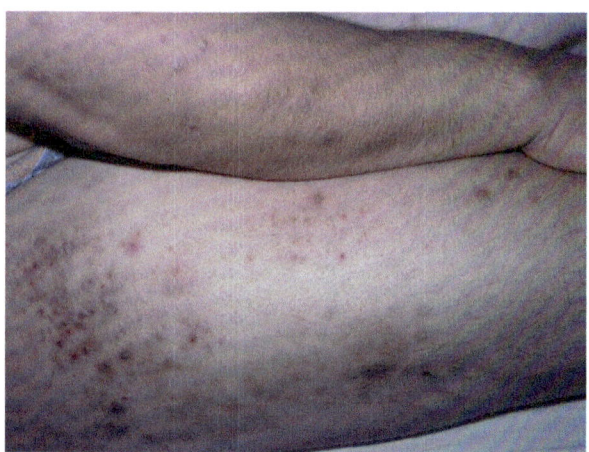

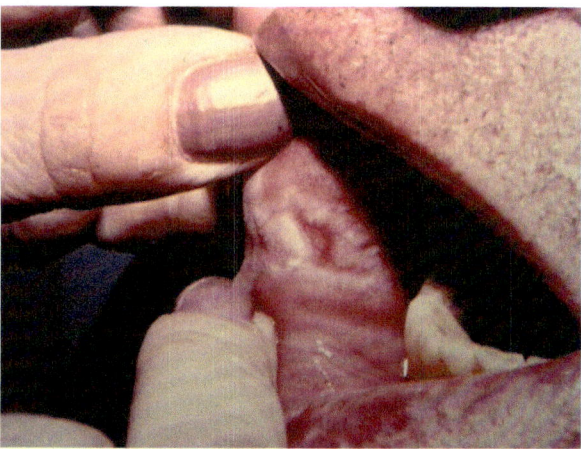

Fig. 11.36 Erosive oral lichen planus

Fig. 11.37 Lichen planus. Multiple, erythematous violaceous, polygonal papules with fine white lines, called Wickham striae

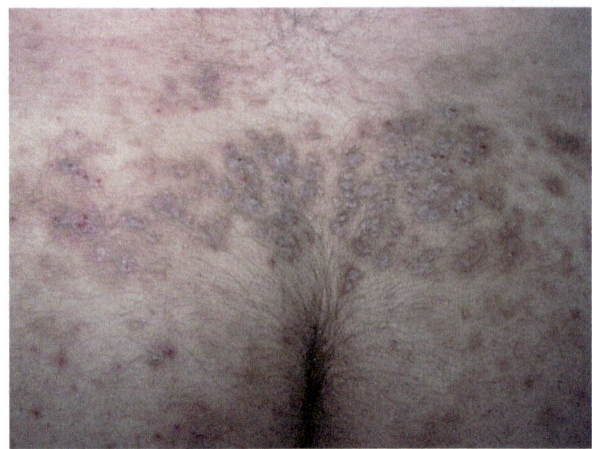

Fig. 11.38 Erosive lichen on the edge of the tongue

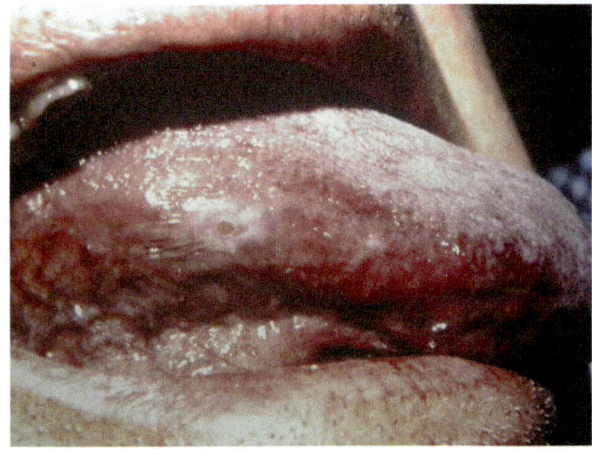

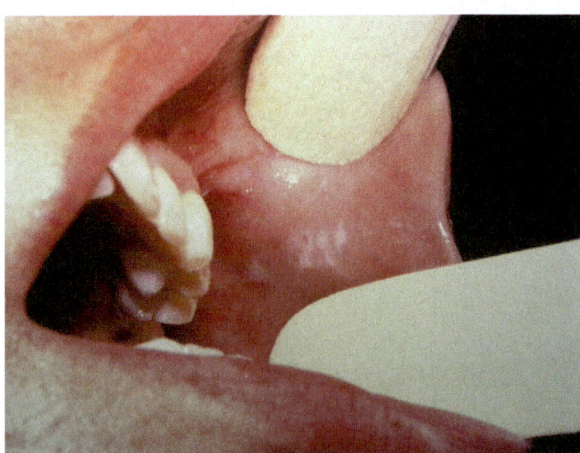

Fig. 11.39 Lichen planus on the buccal mucosa in the form of a whitish plaque

Fig. 11.40 Lichen planus. Papules coalesce forming plaques

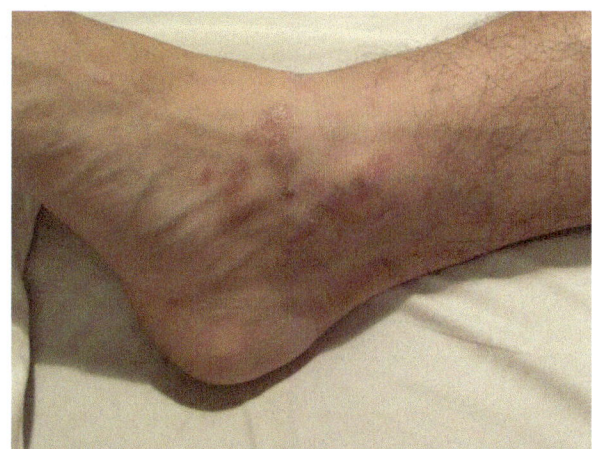

Fig. 11.41 Lichen planus. Typical erythematous violaceous lesions in the lower limb

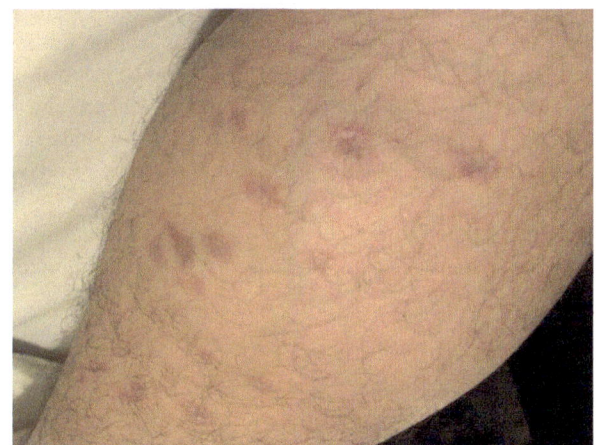

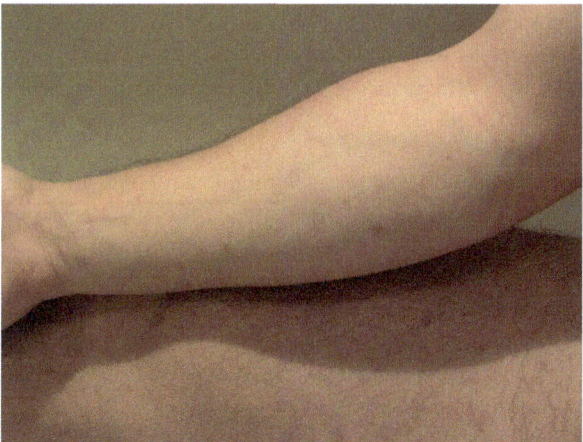

Fig. 11.42 Lichen planus. Lesions in upper limbs

Fig. 11.43 Lichen planus

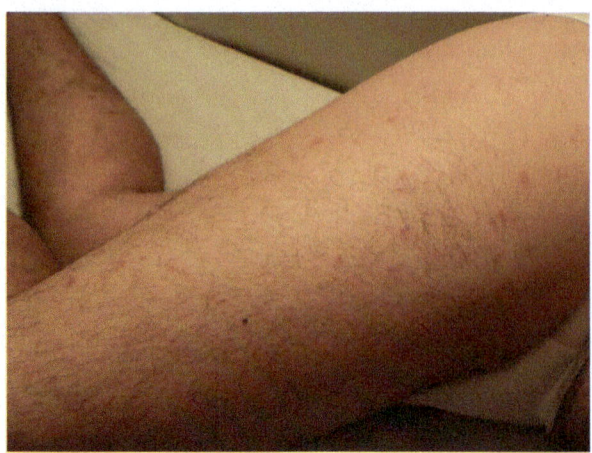

In a study carried out in India, 60 from 200 diabetic patients presented cutaneous manifestations from which lichen planus was observed in 3.33% and it was related to high levels of HbA1c, a fact that should be confirmed in the future [39].

The relationship between OLP and DM is endorsed by numerous publications. Although previous studies were not conclusive, a meta-analysis confirmed the association between DM and OLP with a prevalence range from 0.5 to 9.3% in diabetic patients [40].

The association between DM and LP, although it exists, is not yet clear under which mechanism occurs. Apparently, both could be related to a chronic inflammation state.

Kaposi's Sarcoma

Classic Kaposi's sarcoma (KS) is a slow-growing neoplasm that affects skin, nodes and internal organs, affecting more elderly men of Mediterranean and Eastern European origin or their descendants. Its etiological agent is the Kaposi sarcoma-associated virus or human herpesvirus-8 (HHV-8), whose infection induces the release of different cytokines that stimulate the proliferation of endothelial cells [41].

Nowadays, there is no doubt about the participation of the virus in the KS onset. Antibodies (Abs) against the virus have been detected, but there are epidemiological differences between one geographical region and the other and also between different ethnic groups from the same region. The areas where KS incidence is higher correspond to different HHV-8 infection rates [42].

Lesions consist of macules, plaques or asymptomatic reddish-violaceous tumors, that can ulcerate causing bleeding and pain (Figs. 11.44, 11.45, 11.46, and 11.47). They generally appear in feet and lower third of the legs; even though the dissemination is rare, it can be spread to other regions such as the trunk or the face. It also affects the mucous membranes, especially the oral. It has a good prognosis.

Fig. 11.44 Classic Kaposi's sarcoma in lower limbs

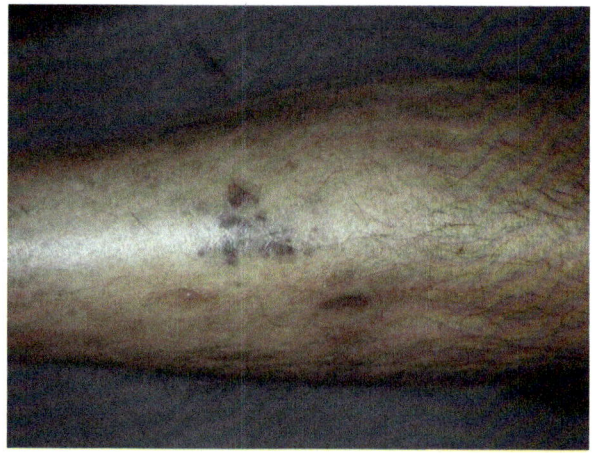

Fig. 11.45 Classic Kaposi's sarcoma in early macule stage

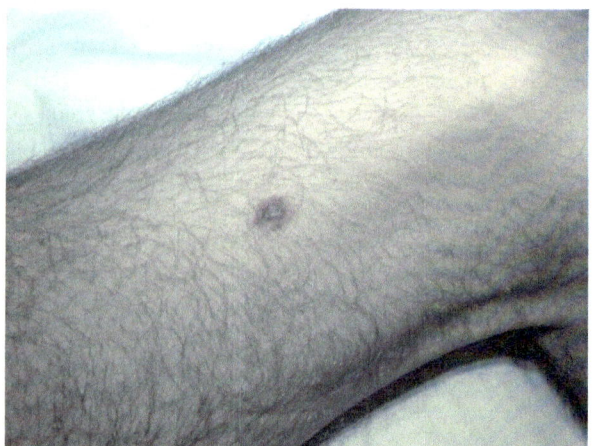

Fig. 11.46 Classic Kaposi's sarcoma

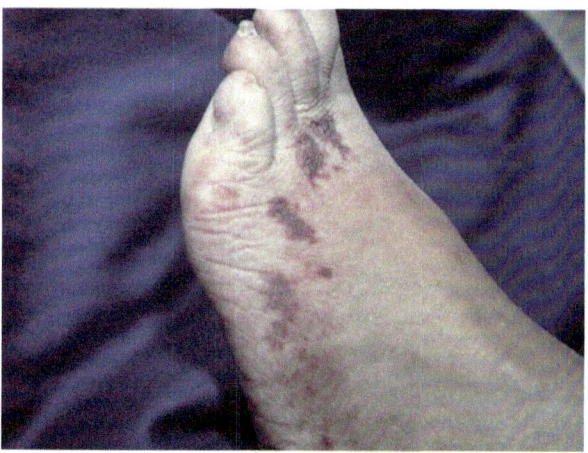

Fig. 11.47 Classic
Kaposi's sarcoma in tumor/
plaque stage

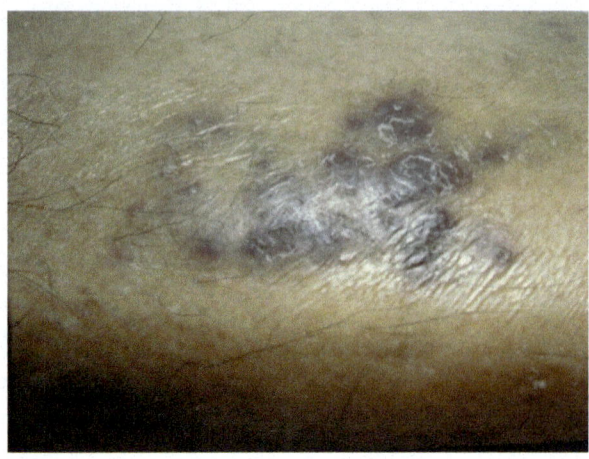

The histological study confirms the diagnosis, which could be complemented by immunohistochemical techniques (CD31, CD34, factor VIII, positive D2-40) and the detection of Abs against HHV-8.

KS treatments such as radiotherapy, surgery and chemotherapy produce severe side effects, even more in diabetic patients. In order to avoid systemic effects, local treatments with intralesional injection of vinblastine have been tried [43].

The association between Kaposi's sarcoma and DM is controversial. For some authors, both pathologies together are more frequent than expected. It is an unanswered question how DM would increase the risk of suffering from classic KS, but there is a relationship with insulin-dependent pathways (insulin-like growth factor-I, insulin receptor expression), and with the alteration of microcirculation which in turn results in hypoxia that allows viral replication, and, as a consequence, there is no doubt that one is facilitating the other [44].

Acquired Perforating Dermatoses

Acquired perforating dermatoses (APD) are a group of diseases whose common denominator is the transepidermal elimination of dermal components. According to the eliminated material, they are classified into four classic variants: [45] (Table 11.3).

They generally appear in adulthood and they are related to systemic diseases such as advanced chronic kidney failure and under treatment with hemodialysis, high blood pressure and DM that sometimes is the cause of kidney failure at the beginning of adulthood, among others.

Its pathogenesis is unknown and it is probably multifactorial because one cause, like microdeposits of substances difficult to remove with hemodialysis such as calcium salts, would not explain the presence of APD in patients that are not under such treatment. The same happens if we refer to diabetic microangiopathy as the underlying cause of collagen deterioration and we do not know what happens in non-diabetic patients. Chronic itching has a more comprehensive explanation, since

Table 11.3 Classification of acquired perforating dermatoses according to the eliminated material

Perforating dermatosis	Eliminated material
Reactive perforating collagenosis (RPC)	Collagen fibers detected by Masson's trichrome stain
Perforating folliculitis (PF)	Follicular necrotic tissue. There can be collagen and/or elastic fibers in the eliminated material
Elastosis perforans serpiginosa (EPS)	Thickened elastic fibers detected by Verhoeff van Gieson stain
Kyrle disease (KD)	Keratotic material but no fibers

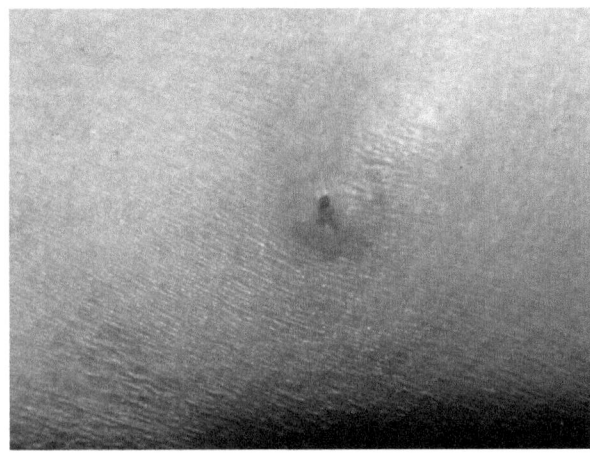

Fig. 11.48 Acquired perforating dermatoses. Typical dome-shaped lesion

it is the predominant symptom and is present in most patients. It has been suggested that trauma from scratching in a poor irrigated tissue due to vasculopathy could cause its necrosis and subsequent elimination through the epidermis. Inflammatory cells release mediators such as interleukin-1 (IL-1) that stimulates metalloproteinase synthesis which degrades the extracellular matrix [46, 47].

Its clinical aspect is characteristic and it has a major diagnostic value. Lesions are erythematous papules with a central umbilication in which we find the eliminated material (keratotic plug) or itchy nodules (Figs. 11.48, 11.49, 11.50, and 11.51). It can adopt a linear distribution in response to a trauma (Köebner phenomenon). They are preferably located in lower limbs, the trunk and the dorsum of the hands, and less frequently, in the face.

From the clinical and histological point of view, the separation among these four classic variants is not always so clear and findings overlap.

Dermoscopy, a diagnostic tool over the last years, can be useful. There are shiny white areas in the center of the lesion that belongs to the dilated hair follicle infundibulum, full of keratin and cellular detritus, surrounded by a non-structure grayish area from the combination of epidermal and dermal changes [48].

First line dermatological treatment includes antihistamines to relieve itching and corticosteroids and/or topical keratolytic drugs (retinoids, salicylic acid, urea) with

Fig. 11.49 Acquired perforating dermatoses. Raised lesion in which the typical central crater with transepidermally eliminated material can be observed

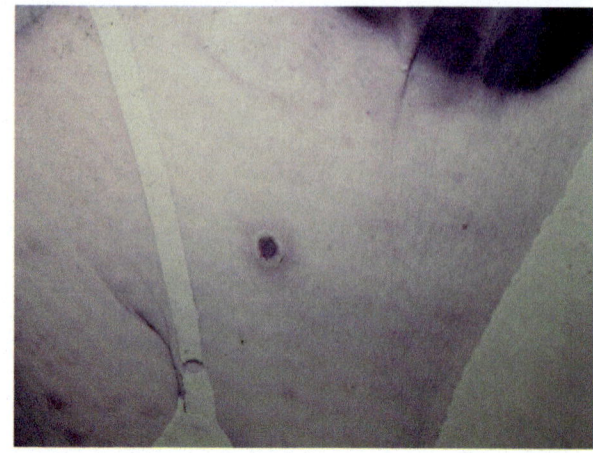

Fig. 11.50 Acquired perforating dermatoses. Lesions in different progression stages and residual pigmented lesions

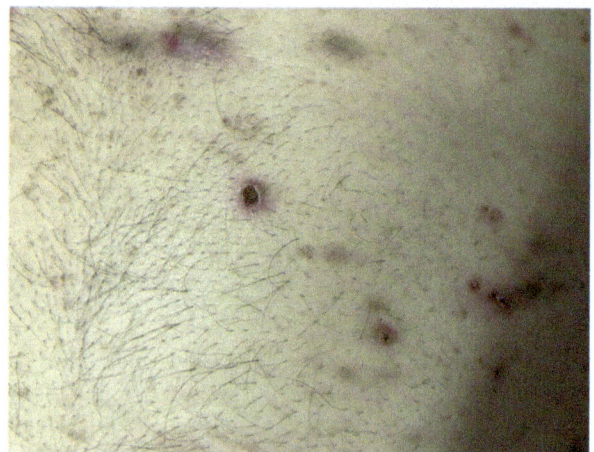

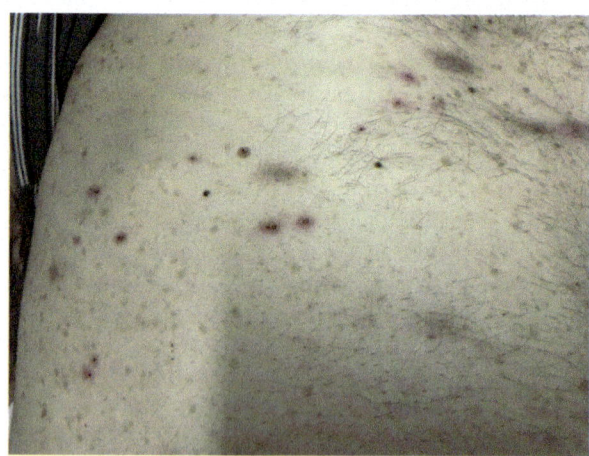

Fig. 11.51 Acquired perforating dermatoses. Lesions in different stages and residual pigmented lesions

emollients. If necessary, oral retinoids, phototherapy and allopurinol are also indicated. The discontinuation of the treatment generally causes relapse. But we must not ignore the context in which these dermatoses appear and the control of the disease or underlying diseases which is fundamentally important.

Finally, acquired perforating dermatoses or transepidermal elimination diseases in adulthood are related to diabetic patients and especially to those with nephropathy in chronic kidney failure status. In some cases, 70% of APD were found in patients with chronic kidney failure and 50% of them were diabetics. While its linkage mechanism is not yet clarified, the association between DM and the subsequent onset of APD is widely described in the literature [49].

Conclusions

Knowing the long list of dermatoses most frequently related to DM has a triple importance:

From the diagnostic point of view, it allows us to suspect and make an early diagnosis of an unknown DM.

From the prognostic point of view, these dermatoses in diabetic patients progresses more torpidly than in general population.

Finally, and related to the previous concept, treatment must be more aggressive and prolonged.

References

1. Cohen Sabban E. Enfermedades que se asocian con frecuencia a la Diabetes. En: Prof. Dr. Horacio Cabo (ed). Manifestaciones Cutáneas de la Diabetes Mellitus. Bueno Aires: Ed A. Macchi; 1996. p. 139–163.
2. Cohen Sabban E, Cabo H. Dermatoses most frequently related to diabetes. J Clin Dermatol. 1999;2:15–22.
3. Muñoz-Santos C, Guilabert A, Moreno N, Gimenez M, Darwich E, To-Figueras J, Herrero C. The association between porphyria cutanea tarda and diabetes mellitus: analysis of a long-term follow-up cohort. Br J Dermatol. 2011;165:486–91.
4. Kashif M, Kumar H, Khaja M. An unusual presentation of eruptive xanthoma: a case report and literature review. Medicine (Baltimore). 2016;95(37):e4866.
5. Wani AM, Hussain WM, Fatani MI, et al. Eruptive xanthomas with Koebner phenomenon, type 1 diabetes mellitus, hypertriglyceridaemia and hypertension in a 41-year-old man. BMJ Case Rep. 2009;2009. https://doi.org/10.1136/bcr.05.2009.1871.
6. Kala J, Mostow EN. Images in clinical medicine. Eruptive xanthoma. N Engl J Med. 2012;366:835.
7. Abdelghany M, Massoud S. Eruptive xanthoma. Cleve Clin J Med. 2015;82(4):209–10. https://doi.org/10.3949/ccjm.82a.14081.
8. Guerrero Vázquez R, Oliva Rodríguez R, Cuenca Cuenca JI, Sánchez Alberdi F, Navarro González E. Malignant glucagonoma: an uncommon cause of new onset diabetes. Endocrinol Nutr. 2011;58:199–201.
9. Halvorson SAC, Gilbert E, Hopkins RS, Liu H, Lopez C, Chu M, Martin M, Sheppard B. Putting the pieces together: necrolytic migratory erythema and the glucagonoma syndrome. J Gen Intern Med. 2013;28(11):1525–9.
10. John AM, Schwartz RA. Glucagonoma syndrome: a review and update on treatment. J Eur Acad Dermatol Venereol. 2016;30(12):2016–22.

11. Granero Castro P, Miyar de León A, Granero Trancón J, Álvarez Martínez P, Álvarez Pérez JA, Fernández Fernández JC, García Bernardo CM, Barneo Serra L, González González JJ. Glucagonoma syndrome: a case report. J Med Case Rep. 2011;5:402.
12. Ko MJ, Chiu HC, Jee SH, et al. Postprandial blood glucose is associated with generalized pruritus in patients with type 2 diabetes. Eur J Dermatol. 2013;23(5):688–93.
13. Vinik A. Barely scratching the surface. Diabetes Care. 2010;33(1):210–2.
14. Horton WB, Boler PL, Subauste AR. Diabetes mellitus and the skin: recognition and management of cutaneous manifestations. South Med J. 2016;109(10):636–46.
15. Atabek ME, Akyürek N, Eklioglu BS. Frequency of vaginal candida colonization and relationship between metabolic parameters in children with type 1 diabetes mellitus. J Pediatr Adolesc Gynecol. 2013;26(5):257–60.
16. Yamaoka H, Sasaki H, Yamasaki H, Ogawa K, Ohta T, Furuta H, Nishi M, Nanjo K. Truncal pruritus of unknown origin may be a symptom of diabetic polyneuropathy. Diabetes Care. 2010;33(1):150–5.
17. Vasapollo P, Cione E, Luciani F, Gallelli L. Generalized intense pruritus during canaglifozina treatment: Is it an adverse drug reaction? Curr Drug Saf. 2016.
18. Baselga Torres E, Torres-Pradilla M. Manifestaciones cutáneas en niños con diabetes mellitus y obesidad. Actas Dermosifiliogr. 2014;105:546–57.
19. Shah R, Jindal A, Patel N. Acrochordons as a cutaneous sign of metabolic syndrome: a case-control study. Ann Med Health Sci Res. 2014;4(2):202–5.
20. Barbato MT, Criado PR, Silva AK, Averbeck E, Guerine MB, Sá NB. Association of acanthosis nigricans and skin tags with insulin resistance. An Bras Dermatol. 2012;87(1):97–104.
21. Boniface K, Taïeb A, Seneschal J. New insights into immune mechanisms of vitiligo. G Ital Dermatol Venereol. 2016;151(1):44–54.
22. Mendes AL, Miot HA, Junior HV. Diabetes mellitus and the skin. An Bras Dermatol. 2017;92(1):8–20.
23. Sheth VM, Guo Y, Qureshi AA. Comorbidities associated with vitiligo: a ten-year retrospective study. Dermatology. 2013;227(4):311–5.
24. Furue M, Kadono T. Bullous pemphigoid: What's ahead? J Dermatol. 2015;43(3):237–40. https://doi.org/10.1111/1346-8138.13207.
25. Jedlickova H, Jana Racovska J, Niedermeier A, Feit J, Hertl M. Anti-basement membrane zone antibodies in elderly patients with pruritic disorders and diabetes mellitus. Eur J Dermatol. 2008;18(5):534–8.
26. Kibsgaard L, Bay B, Deleuran M, Vestergaard C. A retrospective consecutive case-series study on the effect of systemic treatment, length of admission time, and co-morbidities in 98 bullous pemphigoid patients admitted to a tertiary centre. Acta Derm Venereol. 2015;95(3):307–11.
27. Sakanoue M, Kawai K, Kanekura T. Bullous pemphigoid associated with type 1 diabetes mellitus responsive to mycophenolate mofetil. J Dermatol. 2012;39(10):884–5.
28. Lee JH, Kim SC. Mortality of patients with bullous pemphigoid in Korea. J Am Acad Dermatol. 2014;71:676–83.
29. Cabo H, Cohen Sabban E. Psoriasis y Diabetes. Texto para libro con formato de Disco Compacto 2002. Autores: E. Chouela; A.Bessone; N. Poggio.
30. Napolitano M, Megna M, Monfrecola G. Insulin resistance and skin diseases. Sci World J. 2015;2015:479354.
31. Vachatova S, Andrys C, Krejsek J, Salavec M, Ettler K, Rehacek V, Cermakova E, Malkova A, Fiala Z, Borska L. Metabolic syndrome and selective inflammatory markers in psoriatic patients. J Immunol Res. 2016;2016:5380792. https://doi.org/10.1155/2016/5380792.
32. Balci A, Balci DD, Yonden Z, Korkmaz I, Yenin JZ, Celik E, Okumus N, Egilmez E. Increased amount of visceral fat in patients with psoriasis contributes to metabolic syndrome. Dermatology. 2010;220(1):32–7.
33. Carvalho AV, Romiti R, Souza CD, Paschoal RS, Milman LM, Meneghello LP. Psoriasis comorbidities: complications and benefits of immunobiological treatment. An Bras Dermatol. 2016;91(6):781–9.

34. Daudén E, Castañeda S, Suárez C, García-Campayo J, Blasco AJ, Aguilar MD, Ferrándiz C, Puig L, Sánchez-Carazo JL. Abordaje integral de la comorbilidad del paciente con psoriasis. Actas Dermosifiliogr. 2012;103(Suppl 1):1–64.
35. Shah K, Mellars L, Changolkar A, Feldman SR. Real-world burden of comorbidities in US patients with psoriasis. J Am Acad Dermatol. 2017;77:287–92.
36. Gupta S, Jawanda MK. Oral lichen planus: an update on etiology, pathogenesis, clinical presentation, diagnosis and management. Indian J Dermatol. 2015;60(3):222–9.
37. Krupaa RJ, Sankari SL, Masthan KM, Rajesh E. Oral lichen planus: an overview. J Pharm Bioallied Sci. 2015;7(Suppl 1):S158–61.
38. Baykal L, Arıca DA, Yaylı S, Örem A, Bahadır S, Altun E, Yaman H. Prevalence of metabolic syndrome in patients with mucosal lichen planus: a case-control study. Am J Clin Dermatol. 2015;16(5):439–45.
39. Ghosh K, Das K, Ghosh S, Chakraborty S, Jatua SK, Bhattacharya A, Ghosh M. Prevalence of skin changes in diabetes mellitus and its correlation with internal diseases: a single center observational study. Indian J Dermatol. 2015;60(5):465–9.
40. Mozaffari HR, Roohollah Sharifi R, Sadeghi M. Prevalence of oral lichen planus in diabetes mellitus: a meta-analysis study. Acta Inform Med. 2016;24(6):390–3.
41. de la Puente Martín M, Pallardo Rodil B, Valverde Moyar MV, Fernández Guarino M, Barrio Garde J, Gómez-Pavón J. Classic Kaposi sarcoma. Rev Esp Geriatr Gerontol. 2015;50(4):200–5.
42. Mohanna S, Maco V, Bravo F, Gotuzzo E. Epidemiology and clinical characteristics of classic Kaposi's sarcoma, seroprevalence, and variants of human herpesvirus 8 in South America: a critical review of an old disease. Int J Infect Dis. 2005;9:239–50.
43. Vassallo C, Carugno A, Derlino F, Ciocca O, Brazzelli V, Borroni G. Intralesional vinblastine injections for treatment of classic Kaposi sarcoma in diabetic patients. Cutis. 2015;95(5):E28–34.
44. Anderson LA, Lauria C, Romano N, Brown EE, Whitby D, Graubard BI, Li Y, Messina A, Gafà L, Vitale F, Goedert JJ. Risk factors for classical Kaposi sarcoma in a population-based case-control study in Sicily. Cancer Epidemiol Biomark Prev. 2008;17(12):3435–43.
45. Nair PA, Jivani NB, Diwan NG. Kyrle's disease in a patient of diabetes mellitus and chronic renal failure on dialysis. J Family Med Prim Care. 2015;4(2):284–6.
46. Wieczorek A, Matusiak L, Szepietowski JC. Acquired peforating dermatosis associated with end-stage diabetic kidney failure in a hemodialysis patient. Iran J Kidney Dis. 2016;10(3):164–7.
47. Fernandes KA, Lima LA, Guedes JC, Lima RB, D'Acri AM, Martins CJ. Acquired perforating dermatosis in a patient with chronic renal failure. An Bras Dermatol. 2016;91(5 suppl 1):10–3.
48. Ramirez-Fort MK, Khan F, Rosendahl CO, Mercer SE, Shim-Chang H, Levitt JO. Acquired perforating dermatosis: a clinical and dermatoscopic correlation. Dermatol Online J. 2013;19(7):18958.
49. Saray D, Seçkin B, Bilezikçi B. Acquired perforating dermatosis: clinicopathological features in twenty-two cases. J Eur Acad Dermatol Venereol. 2006;20:679–88.

Cutaneous Manifestations Induced by Antidiabetic Treatment

12

Marina Luz Margossian and Emilia Noemí Cohen Sabban

The increased prevalence of diabetes mellitus (DM) as a global pandemic positions it among the most important non-transmissible chronic diseases in recent years. Currently, we have multiple groups of hypoglycemic drugs, which are associated with various adverse events, including dermatological effects. Although the advent of new technologies in drugs and supplies could diminish the appearance of some of them, it is important to know the most common drug reactions seen in this group of patients. In turn, we must consider that any of these effects would negatively impact on the therapeutic patient adherence. A review of the different pharmacological groups used in DM (oral, insulin and injectable non-insulin) and their cutaneous side effects will be performed.

The cutaneous manifestations induced by antidiabetic treatment, which according to the general classification belong to group 4, are divided based on the therapeutic modality instituted by oral hypoglycemic agents, non-insulin subcutaneous hypoglycemic agents and insulins (Table 12.1).

M.L. Margossian (✉)
Diabetes Division, Hospital de Clínicas José de San Martín, University of Buenos Aires (UBA), Buenos Aires, Argentina
e-mail: marinamargossian@yahoo.com.ar

E.N. Cohen Sabban
Dermatology Department, Instituto de Investigaciones Médicas A. Lanari, University of Buenos Aires (UBA), Buenos Aires, Argentina
e-mail: emicohensabban@gmail.com

© Springer International Publishing AG 2018
E.N. Cohen Sabban et al. (eds.), *Dermatology and Diabetes*,
https://doi.org/10.1007/978-3-319-72475-1_12

Table 12.1 Hypoglycemic agents

ORAL HYPOGLYCEMIC AGENTS	
Sulfonylureas	First generation: Chlorpropamide, Tolbutamide
	Second generation: Glibenclamide, Gliclazide, Glipizide
	Third generation: Glimepiride
Meglitinides	Repaglinide, Nateglinide
Biguanides	Metformin
Thiazolidinediones	Rosiglitazone, Pioglitazone
Dipeptidyl peptidase-4 inhibitor (Gliptins)	Sitagliptin, Saxagliptin, Vildagliptin, Linagliptin, Alogliptin, Teneligliptin
SGLT2-inhibitors (Gliflozins)	Dapagliflozin, Canagliflozin, Empagliflozin
Alpha-glucosidase inhibitors	Acarbose
NON-INSULIN SUBCUTANEOUS HYPOGLYCEMIC AGENTS	
GLP-1 agonists	Exenatide, Liraglutide, Lixisenatide
	Albiglutide
INSULINS	
Animal-source	Bovine, Porcine
Human	Rapid-acting insulin: Regular
	Intermediate-acting insulin: NPH
Analogues (modified human insulins)	Ultra short-acting insulins: Aspart, Lispro, Glulisine
	Long-acting insulins: Levemir, Glargine, Degludec
	Pre-mixed insulins: (short and long- acting insulins) Lispro protamine + Lispro 75/25, Lispro protamine + Lispro 50/50, Aspart Protamine + Aspart 70/30

Oral Hypoglycemic Agents

Sulfonylureas

Sulfonylureas stimulate insulin release by blocking ATP sensitive potassium channels in the Beta cells, reducing potassium permeability. This causes depolarization of the cell and increases calcium intake, increasing insulin secretion.

First-Generation Sulfonylureas (Chlorpropamide, Tolbutamide)

Between 1 and 5% of patients under treatment with first-generation sulfonylureas develop skin reactions within the first 2 months of treatment. The most frequent form of manifestation consists of a maculopapular exanthema that disappears with the discontinuation of the drug. Between 10 and 30% of patients taking chlorpropamide develop alcohol induced flushing, acute vasomotor syndrome manifested by erythema and heat, nauseas, vomiting, headaches, tachycardia and, occasionally, dyspnea beginning 15 min after alcohol consumption. In fact, it may cause a flushing skin reaction after alcohol ingestion by inhibiting the metabolism of acetaldehyde. The symptoms usually disappear after an hour. This pattern of reaction appears to be of an autosomal dominant inheritance.

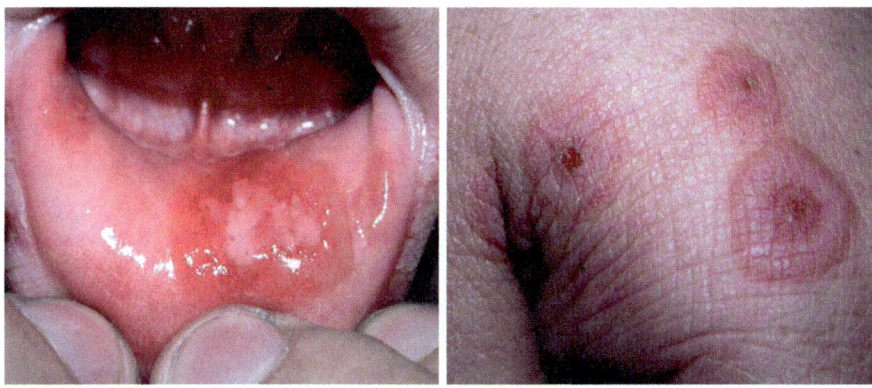

Fig. 12.1   First-generation Sulfonylureas adverse event. Erythema multiforme

Fig. 12.2   First-generation
Sulfonylureas adverse
event. Erythema nodosum

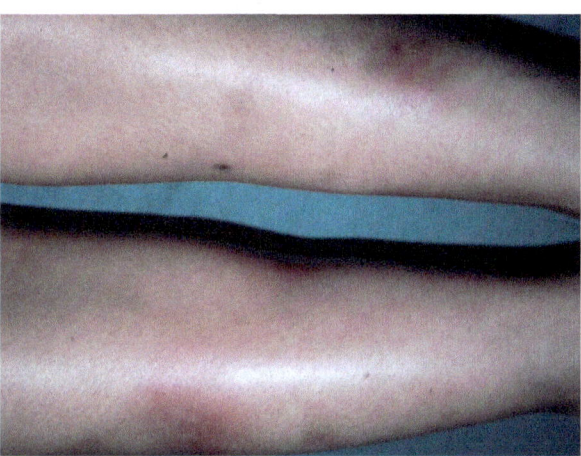

Fig. 12.3   Erythema
nodosum

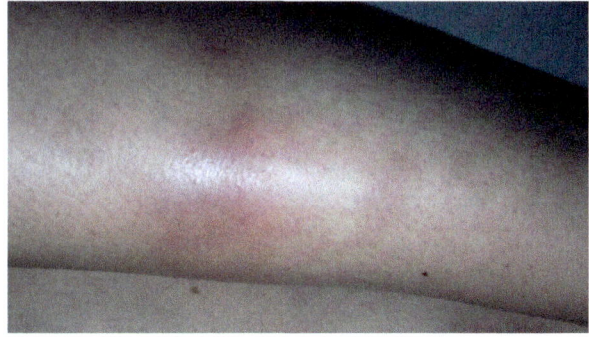

Both phototoxic and photoallergic reactions may occur. Other skin reactions, including urticaria, pruritus, fixed erythema, erythema multiforme (Fig. 12.1) erythema nodosum (Figs. 12.2, 12.3 and 12.4), Lyell's syndrome and toxic epidermal necrolysis, have also been observed. This group of drugs is not currently used.

Fig. 12.4 Erythema nodosum

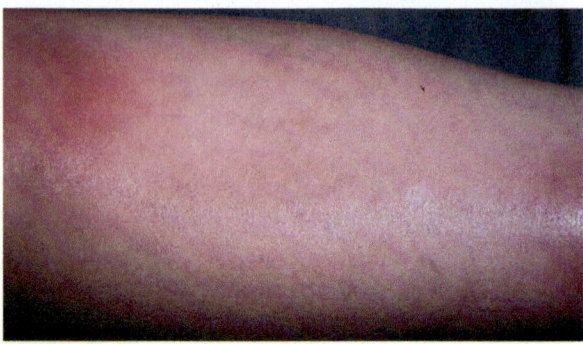

Fig. 12.5 Photosensitive drug reaction to Glipizide

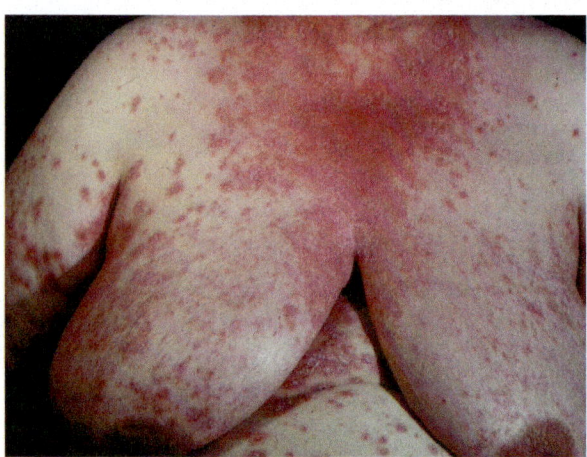

Second-Generation Sulfonylureas (Glibenclamide, Glipizide, Gliclazide)

This group also produces skin reactions. Of those associated with glipizide, photosensitivity (Fig. 12.5), urticaria and pruritus were mentioned, which are less frequent with glimepiride (third-generation) [1, 2].

Biguanides

Metformin has a widespread use and it is the only available of its group. It is a biguanide with insulin sensitivity effect and it is considered the first-line oral treatment for DM2 patients. Its main action is to inhibit the hepatic production of glucose and increase peripheral tissue sensitivity to insulin. Cutaneous adverse events include psoriasiform reactions, leukocytoclastic vasculitis (Fig. 12.6) and erythema multiforme. Erythema, rash, pruritus, urticaria, photosensitivity and lichenoid eruption (Fig. 12.7) have also been reported [2].

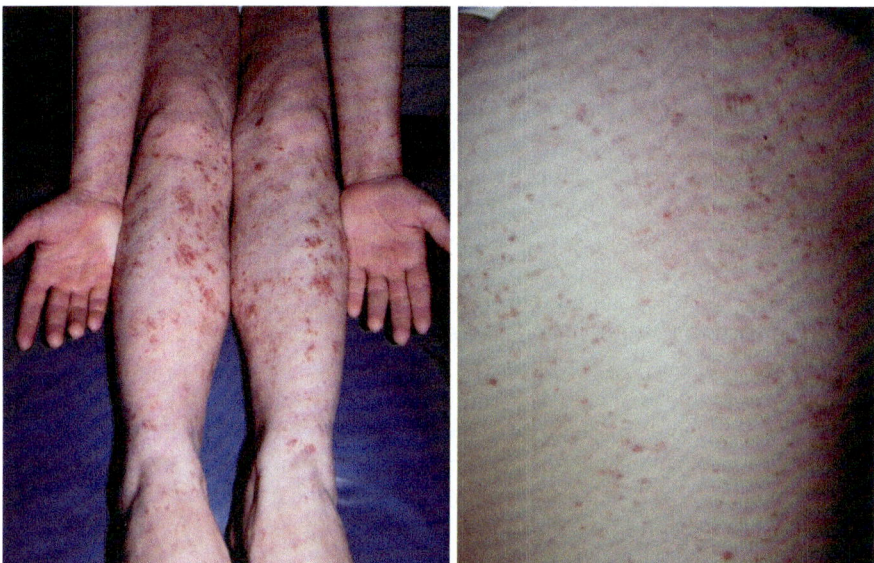

Fig. 12.6 Leucocitoclastic vasculitis due to Metformin

Fig. 12.7 Lichenoid eruption induced by Metformin

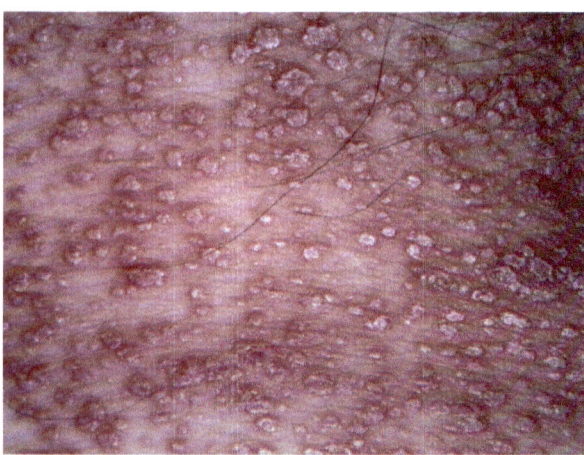

Leukocytoclastic vasculitis (LV) is a cutaneous vasculitis characterized by small vessel inflammation and necrosis. Lesions are often localized in the skin, but other organs may be involved. Drugs are implicated in 20% of reported cases of LV. The pathogenesis of drug-induced LV is little known. It is suggested that it could be an immune-mediated reaction to a triggering antigen. There is no clinical or biochemical form to differentiate drug-induced LV from other types of vasculitis. The diagnosis is based on medical history including patient's medication, exclusion of other known causes of LV, improvement of symptoms when the drug is discontinued and the recurrence of lesions when treatment restarts [3].

Drug rash with eosinophilia and systemic symptoms (DRESS syndrome) is a severe, idiosyncratic reaction to a drug characterized by a prolonged latency period, 2–8 weeks after initiating the offending drug. It is manifested as fever, rash, lymphadenopathy, eosinophilia and mild to severe systemic presentations like abnormal liver function tests, which can mimic viral hepatitis.

The cutaneous manifestations typically consist of an urticarial, maculopapular eruption and, in some instances, vesicles, bullae, pustules, purpura, target lesions, facial edema, cheilitis and erythroderma. Visceral involvement (hepatitis, pneumonitis, myocarditis, pericarditis, nephritis and colitis) is the major cause of morbidity and mortality in this syndrome. Many cases are associated with leukocytosis with eosinophilia (90%) and/or mononucleosis (40%).

DRESS syndrome is a life-threatening reaction with a mortality rate around 10% according to multiple studies. It should be distinguished from other processes that cause similar symptoms, including Stevens-Johnson syndrome and toxic epidermal necrolysis. Once the diagnosis is made, administration of the causative drug should be discontinued. The treatments of choice are systemic corticosteroids (CST) (oral or parenteral) if internal organs are involved and topical treatment with CST and emollients [4].

The first report linking metformin to the DRESS syndrome was published by Voore P et al., in a 40-year-old man with pruritus, lymphadenopathy, rash and eosinophilia after metformin treatment. The lesions disappeared when the drug was stopped [5].

Thiazolidinediones

The thiazolidinediones (TZDs) or 'glitazones' are a class of oral antidiabetic drugs, which act through the improvement of insulin sensitivity. TZDs exert their antidiabetic effects through a mechanism that involves activation of the gamma isoform of a nuclear receptor, the peroxisome proliferator-activated receptor (PPARγ). PPARγ are transcription factors belonging to the superfamily of nuclear receptors and, as such, they regulate the expression of numerous genes that affect glycemic control, lipid metabolism, vascular tone and inflammation [6].

TZDs decrease insulin resistance in adipose tissue, muscle and the liver. They reduce the levels of free fatty acids in insulin-resistant patients and change the distribution of body fat. These drugs not only improve the control of blood glucose and diminish insulin resistance, but also improve many abnormalities that are part of the insulin resistance syndrome, such as dyslipidemia, hypertension, glucose intolerance, hypercoagulability, obesity, hyperinsulinemia and mild inflammation, all cardiovascular risk factors [7, 8]. It is known that through the peroxisome proliferator-activated receptor (PPARγ), which is expressed in endothelial cells, endothelial function is modified and vascular complications of DM are prevented or decreased [9].

In a randomized, open-label, parallel-group study, TZDs were compared with sulfonylureas, and the authors found that, in 6 months, glycosylated hemoglobin

(HbA1c) decreased, but only TZDs had modulation effects on circulating RAGE levels. Edema has been reported as a cutaneous side effect of rosiglitazone and pioglitazone [10].

Rosiglitazone was put under selling restrictions in the United States and withdrawn from the market in Europe due to some studies suggesting an increased risk of cardiovascular events. Upon re-evaluation of new data in 2013, the FDA lifted the restrictions. Other TZDs cutaneous reactions, such as blistering, peeling or red skin, rash and swelling in hands, ankles or feet have been described.

Alpha Glycosidase Inhibitor

Acarbose inhibits the absorption of glucose at the intestinal level. It rarely causes adverse events since it is minimally absorbed in the digestive tract. Erythema multiforme and generalized acute exanthematous pustulosis induced by the drug have been reported [11].

Incretins

The "incretin effect" is known as the insulin release after glucose administration and is equivalent to 60% of the total insulin release after ingestion. Faced with the observation that this phenomenon is diminished in DM2, a new pharmacological target appears to counteract this deficit.

Incretins are a group of hormones produced in the gut in response to food intake. There are two main peptides and they are generated at the duodenal level: Glucose-dependent insulinotropic polypeptide (GIP) and glucagon-like peptide-1 (GLP-1). When nutrients are ingested, these peptides are secreted causing increased glucose-dependent pancreatic secretion of insulin, suppression of postprandial glucagon secretion and slow down gastric emptying [12, 13].

Incretins in turn are divided into two pharmacological subgroups to treat DM2:

- *Inhibitors of dipeptidyl-peptidase 4 (DPP-4)* inhibit the enzyme dipeptidyl peptidase 4 (DPP-4) that degrades incretins. Therefore, they increase endogenous levels of GIP and GLP-1, prolonging their half-life, stimulating the production and their hypoglycemic effect. As monotherapy, they do not produce hypoglycemia because they have a glucose dependent mode of action, which means that they do not act with glycemias inferior to 77 mg%. This subgroup includes sitagliptin, saxagliptin, vildagliptin, alogliptin, linagliptin and teneligliptin. They are indicated orally, alone or in combination with other drugs. Among their general adverse events, we can mention headache, nasopharyngitis, urinary tract infections and hypoglycemia (in a combined therapeutic regimen). At the cutaneous level, blister and blistering diseases produced by all but teneligliptin. The others are described as follows:

- – Hypersensitivity reactions (sitagliptin, saxagliptin, teneligliptin).
- – Skin rash (sitagliptin, linagliptin, teneligliptin).
- – Angioedema (sitagliptin, linagliptin).
- – Steven-Johnson syndrome (sitagliptin).
- – Anaphylaxis (sitagliptin).
- – Facial edema (saxagliptin).
- – Eczematous reactions (tenegliptin) (Fig. 12.8).
- – Pruritus (tenegliptin).
- – Hyperhidrosis by vildagliptin when it is associated with sulfonylureas.

Several cases of Bullous Pemphigoid (BP) associated with DPP-4 inhibitors, and more specifically with vildagliptin and sitagliptin, have recently been reported. Bullous pemphigoid is the most common autoimmune blistering disease in which autoantibodies against hemidesmosomes, components of the basement membrane zone (BMZ) of the skin, are produced. In the cases described, although in most of them gliptin was associated with metformin, there are no cases of BP reported in patients treated with metformin alone. On the other hand, the association between DM and BP is well-known, but the participation of the drug was clear when, despite oral or topical treatment with CST such as clobetasol dipropionate 0.05% with which a transient improvement was achieved after 3 months, the final remission was only obtained by gliptin discontinuation. The exact underlying mechanism is still unknown, but it is believed that gliptins could modify the immune response in genetically predisposed patients or could alter the antigenicity of membrane proteins of the BMZ. However, prospective confirmatory studies should be performed to see if the effect of these drugs could trigger a subclinical disease or its exacerbation in the group of elderly diabetic patients with pruritic dermatosis [14–21].

Mendonça FM et al. have reported one case of bullous pemphigoid in an 82-year-old man, under linagliptin therapy, who developed the reaction after 45 days of treatment. He had an itchy cutaneous eruption in the head and neck. He was first medicated with dexamethasone and antihistamines for 3 weeks, and the lesions

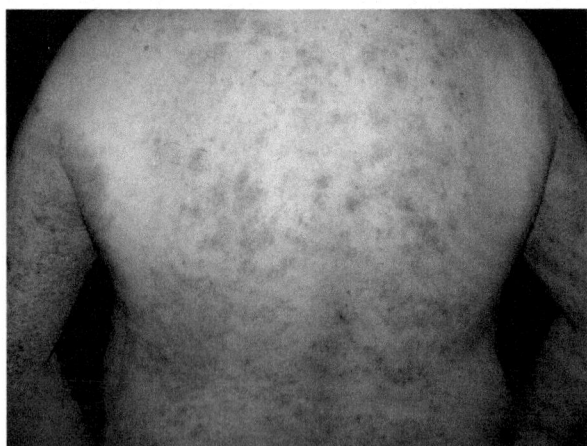

Fig. 12.8 Eczematous reaction (tenegliptin)

healed without scarring. Skin biopsy was performed and the diagnosis of BP was confirmed. Linear IgG and granular C3 deposition were found on the epidermal side of perilesional skin direct immunofluorescence with salt split technique. Treatment with oral prednisolone and local antibiotic was enough to control the symptoms, but the lesions reappeared when CST were discontinued. Finally, linagliptin was discontinued after the second skin reaction and there were no recurrences [22].

From: Skin disorders associated with gliptins published by pharmacovigilance of the European Medicines Agency until August 2014 in the European Economic Area (Tables 12.2 and 12.3) [19].

- *Glucagon-like peptide-1 agonists* maintain an incretin-mimetic effect. This group belongs to the non-insulin subcutaneous hypoglycemic agents. These drugs are molecularly analogous to the GLP-1 peptide, binding to its receptor with an affinity similar to incretins. They act as the native peptide, but they are not degraded by the enzyme DPP-4. Among their pharmacological effects, we can mention the stimulation of insulin secretion by the pancreatic β-cells and the inhibition of glucagon secretion. Unlike DPP-4 inhibitors, they slow down gastric emptying and act on the hypothalamic center of satiety, giving a sensation of postprandial fullness, decreased appetite and, consequently, helping in weight loss. They are administered subcutaneously daily or weekly, according to their formulation. Among the drugs of this subgroup, we can mention exenatide, liraglutide, lixisenatide and albiglutide. Adverse events include nauseas, vomiting, diarrhea, dyspepsia, asthenia, pancreatitis, renal failure and hypoglycemia (in association with sulfonylureas). Several cutaneous manifestations were described; we highlight pruritus, urticaria, anaphylactic and allergic reaction at the injection site. In addition, post-marketing reports of exenatide include hyperhidrosis, alopecia, maculopapular exanthema and angioneurotic edema, while with lixisenatide, reactions to the excipient metacresol were reported in the literature.

Table 12.2 Cases of blistering diseases associated with gliptines according to reaction [high-level terms (HLT) of the MedDRA Terminology Classification] [19]

	Vildagliptin	Sitagliptin	Saxagliptin	Linagliptin
Blistering diseases	121	70	6	6

Table 12.3 Description of the different blistering diseases associated with gliptines according to reaction [preferred terms (PT) of the MedDRA Terminology Classification] [19]

Injury	Vildagliptin	Sitagliptin	Saxagliptin	Linagliptin
Blister	40	23	3	4
Blistering dermatitis	32	8	1	1
Pemphigoid blister	72	28	2	1
Pemphigus	8	2	–	–
Erythema multiforme	1	6	–	–
Toxic epidermal necrolysis	2	–	–	–
Stevens Johnson syndrome	–	4	–	–

Injection site reactions were reported in 3.9% of patients receiving the drug over a 24-week period, versus 1.4% of the placebo group. As the intensity of these was mild, no treatment was required. Allergic reactions were observed in 0.4% of patients versus 0.1% of the placebo group, and they were mild in intensity and included anaphylactic reaction, angioedema and urticaria [12–14].

Sodium-Glucose Cotransporter 2 Inhibitors (SGLT-2)

This is the newest group of oral hypoglycemic agents. Sodium-glucose cotransporter 2 (SGLT-2) is a protein that is expressed at the proximal renal tubule level and acts as a sodium-glucose cotransporter with low affinity and high capacity, reabsorbing more than 90% of the filtered glucose. Inhibitors of this transporter inhibit glucose reabsorption, resulting in glycosuria, a β-cell non-dependent mechanism. The glycosuria of approximately 70 g/day produces a transient increase of natriuresis and excretion of uric acid, in addition to helping in weight loss. It also promotes an improvement in blood pressure. Dapagliflozin, canagliflozin and empagliflozin belong to this group. The adverse events of these drugs are genitourinary infections, symptoms of volume depletion (dizziness, hypotension and dehydration), increased creatinine and hypoglycemia. Some skin adverse events include hyperhidrosis, stomatitis and herpes zoster, but they are very rare. In the genital area, erythema, itching, balanoposthitis and vaginitis can be seen [23–25].

Vasapollo P et al. reported a 61-year-old woman who developed an intense and severe pruritus during the treatment with canagliflozin. Clinical and laboratory findings excluded the presence of systemic or skin diseases able to induce pruritus. The discontinuation of canagliflozin and the treatment with pioglitazone and metformin induced a remission of the symptom [26].

Insulin Therapy

Insulin therapy is associated with significant adverse events on the skin, which may interfere with kinetic of insulin absorption and cause hypo or hyperglycemia [27]. Fortunately, these complications have been decreasing since the advent of the new generations of insulin. However, we should mention them:

• Administration failures: Intraepidermal injection.
• Idiosyncrasy.
• Insulin allergy.
• Lipodystrophies.

Other complications such as keloids, keratotic papules, purpura, infectious abscesses and circumscribed pigmentation may appear from the injection of insulin [27–29].

Insulin Allergy

Impurities in the preparation, presence of animal-origin proteins (bovine, porcine), insulin molecule in itself, preservatives or additives can cause allergic reactions to insulin [30]. They can be localized or generalized and they are classified as follows:

- Immediate-localized.
- Immediate-generalized.
- Delayed hypersensitivity reaction.
- Biphasic.

Local allergic reactions to insulin clinically manifest with erythema, papules and nodules with pruritus and induration at the injection site. These reactions are usually transient and resolve spontaneously within weeks. The immediate-localized form appears after the application, reaches their maximum intensity in 15–30 min and usually disappears within the first hour. Under clinical examination, the presence of erythema, which may evolve into urticarial wheals probably mediated by immunoglobulin E (IgE), is observed. The immediate localized form may progress to a generalized form similar to an accelerated urticarial reaction or, less frequently, to an Arthus reaction [27, 30]. The delayed hypersensitivity reaction is the most common, it appears around 2 weeks after the initiation of insulin therapy, as an itchy nodule at the application site, 4–24 h after the injection. The biphasic or dual reaction is extremely rare and it consists of a delayed local reaction and general malaise similar to serum sickness. They are considered to be immune-mediated reactions of Arthus type [30]. The treatment of choice for the immediate localized allergic reaction is to rotate to a more purified insulin. Other options include antihistamines, the addition of CST to insulin, discontinuing insulin and desensitization, or changes in the delivery system. The most important immunological problem is the IgE-mediated anaphylaxis, which can be controlled by decreasing the dose or by desensitization to insulin [27].

Lipodystrophies

The lipodystrophy is a complication of subcutaneous insulin injection and it includes lipoatrophy and lipohypertrophy, which can coexist in the same patient. They are more common in obese children and women.

Lipoatrophy can be caused by lipolytic components of the preparation or by an inflammatory process mediated by immune complexes. Other theories refer to cryotrauma of refrigerated insulin, mechanical trauma due to injection angle, surface contamination with alcohol or local hyperproduction of tumor necrosis factor-alpha (TNF-α) by macrophages induced by insulin injection. Insulin deposits have also been implicated, and that is the reason why some authors suggest its replacement with rapid-acting insulin.

Since the introduction of highly purified recombinant human insulin, lipoatrophy (Fig. 12.9) is quite unusual. It occurs clinically as a depressed and circumscribed area of the skin at the site of application, 6–24 months after therapy initiation. Histologically, there is a decrease or absence of subcutaneous fat without inflammatory signs. Repeated use of the injection at the same site increases the risk of lipoatrophy; over time, patients learn that these areas are relatively painless and continue to use them. However, insulin absorption in the lipoatrophic areas is erratic and frequently leads to the difficulty of achieving optimal blood glucose control [31].

With the increasing use of rapidly absorbed modified insulin analogues, the frequency of lipoatrophy has declined in recent years. The probability of its appearance can be reduced through the regular rotation of the injection site or by changing the insulin's brand [27, 32].

Lipohypertrophy (Figs. 12.10, 12.11 and 12.12) is the most common cutaneous complication of insulin therapy, regardless of its origin or mode of administration [33]. Clinically, it resembles a lipoma and presents as a soft consistency tumor in the dermis, at the injection site. It is considered as a local response to the anabolic action of insulin over the fat metabolism. It may present along with hypoalgesia. Histologically, an increase of groups of local adipocytes separated by fibrous tracts is observed.

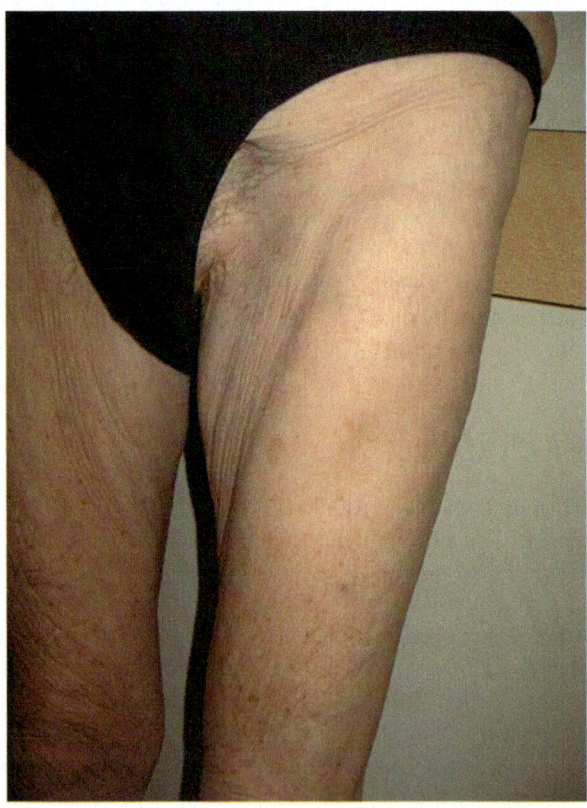

Fig. 12.9 Lipoatrophy

Fig. 12.10
Lipohypertrophy

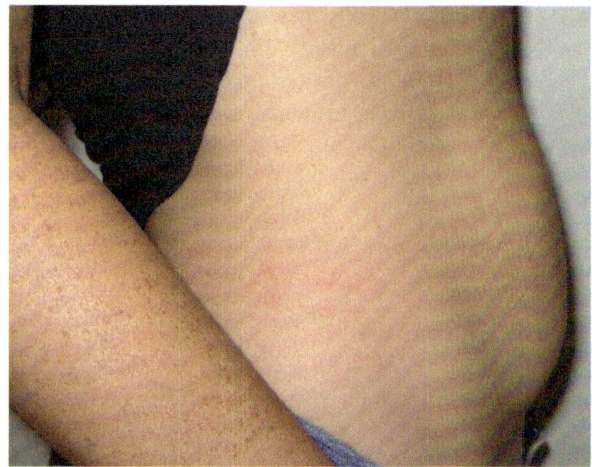

Fig. 12.11
Lipohypertrophy

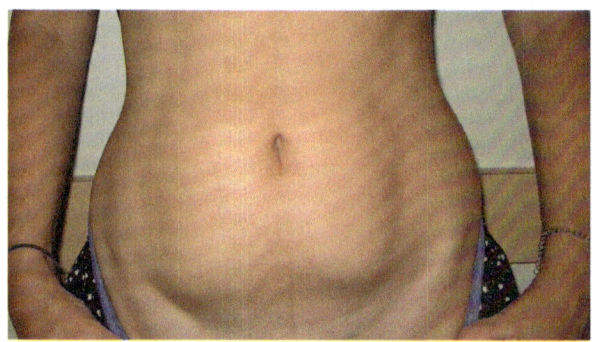

Fig. 12.12
Lipohypertrophy

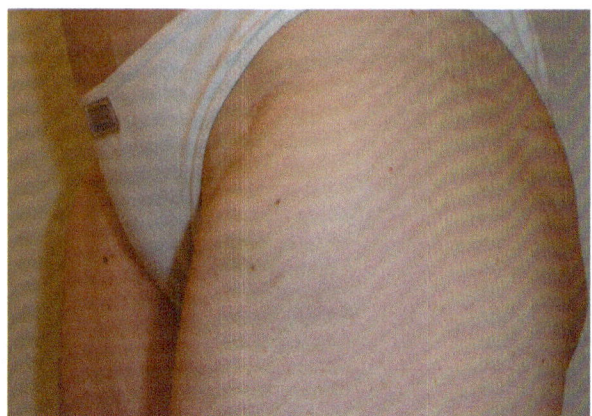

Like with lipoatrophy, new insulins have also reduced their prevalence significantly, although their adverse effects on DM control are similar due to worsening of insulin absorption into the systemic circulation [27]. The introduction of new therapies and new delivery systems (continuous subcutaneous insulin infusion) would seem to reduce skin manifestations associated with long-term insulin use, although many of the cutaneous reactions are decreasing with the use of new insulins. However, it could influence glycemic control and increase the risk of hypoglycemia, as well as cause some cosmetic impact (Table 12.4).

Insulin Analogues

They are modified human insulins that have allowed a more stable control, that is, with less intraindividual variability in the patient's glycemic profile. Lipoatrophy was commonly seen with old animal insulins (bovine and porcine), but at present it is rarely observed since the introduction of insulin analogues.

Although not common, some cases of IgE-mediated anaphylaxis, a case of vitiligo (insulin lispro), allergy (insulin glargine) and local reactions at the application site (insulin detemir) have been reported. At present and since the introduction of insulin analogues (altered amino acid sequence compared to natural insulin), cases of lipoatrophy have decreased, although there are reported cases [34]. The exposure to insulin analogues (lispro, aspart, glargine and detemir) prior to the development of lipoatrophy varies significantly between 4 weeks and 2 years [35]. The treatment include desensitization, changes in insulin type, rotation of the injection site, changes in the delivery system (continuous subcutaneous insulin infusion [CSII] through a portable pump) or a combination of the above [30].

Babiker A. et al. have reported 4 patients with DM 1, under treatment with insulin detemir, aspart or biphasic aspart, who developed lipoatrophy 2–3 years after the onset of insulin therapy. Two of the patients resolved by rotating the application site, suggesting that the cause was local factors. However, the lipoatrophy developed in the other two patients required a change in the insulin type that was being used. The lesion resolved after 1–2 years in all patients and did not recur after 4 years of follow-up. Therefore, poor insulin absorption at the site of lipoatrophy could contribute to worsening the patient's glycemic control, increasing glycated hemoglobin levels. Many studies have demonstrated an association between high insulin antibodies and lipoatrophy [34].

Andrade P. et al. have published one case of IgE-mediated allergy to insulin analogue lispro and Mix 25 in a DM2 patient. An itchy urticarial lesion has raised at the injection site and disappeared by rotating the insulin to an oral hypoglycemic agent. Due to the risk of anaphylactic shock, angioedema and hyperglycemia, suspicion of insulin hypersensitivity should lead to change the treatment to an oral agent. Then, it is important to perform a diagnosis confirmation by complete immunologic work up. It would also have to consider other substances of the insulin molecule that could also act as allergens: protamine, zinc and metacresol, although they are more infrequent [36].

Table 12.4 Skin manifestations induced by the pharmacological treatment of diabetes mellitus [40]

Type of drug	Incidence	Skin manifestation	Pathogenesis	Treatment
Non-insulin				
Sulfonylureas	1–5%	• Maculopapular rash	• Unknown	Change treatment
	1–5%		• Mediated by cells	Suspend drug
	1–5%	• Photoallergy		
	10–30%	• Phototoxicity	• Toxic	
		• Flushing (Chlorpropamide)	• Opioids IV	
		• Acute vasomotor		
DPP-4 inhibitors	Infrequent	• Pemphigoid blister	• Alteration of immune response	Suspend drug
			• Antigenic modification in BMZ	
GLP-1 analogs	Infrequent	• Urticaria	IgE-mediated reaction	Rotate application site
		• Pruritus		
		• Allergic reaction at injection site		
SGLT-2 inhibitors	Infrequent	Hyperhidrosis stomatitis and herpes zoster	Not known	Suspend drug
Insulin				
Animal origin	10–50%	• Lipoatrophy	• IgE cell mediation; IgG	Rotate the IHR
		• Erythema		
		• Papules and pruriginous nodules (urticarial reaction)	• Changes in tertiary structure	
Human recombinant	Rare <3%	Lipoatrophy	Lipolytic components of insulin and immune complexes	Highly purified IHR injection in the periphery

DPP-4 dipeptidyl-peptidase 4, *IV* intravenous, *GLP-1* glucagon-like peptide, *IgE* immunoglobulin E, *IgG* immunoglobulin G, *IHR* recombinant human insulin, *SGLT-2* sodium-glucose contransporter-2, *BMZ* basement membrane zone

Continuous Subcutaneous Insulin Infusion (CSII)

Insulin pump users worldwide depend on insulin infusion set for predictable delivery of insulin to the subcutaneous tissue. The insulin infusions sets are associated with many pump-related adverse events, like skin manifestations, and may contribute to potentially life-threatening problem of hyperglycemia.

The infusion set of patients using a CSII consists of four parts: the pump itself, the reservoir, the needle cannula and the inserter. The set is composed of a subcutaneous catheter connected by a tube to the insulin reservoir. In this way, continuous infusion of insulin is performed. The infusion set and the reservoir are disposable and must be replaced every 2 days for steel and 3 days for teflon. Patients who have difficulty inserting their infusion set manually may prefer a mechanical insertion device. Auto inserters are generally recommended when the cannula is made of teflon [37].

For reasons that are still unknown, some patients can exceed advised wear-time without developing skin reactions or worsening of glycemic control, whereas other must change their sets more frequently than recommended to prevent adverse events. More researches, including skin biopsies, will be needed to distinguish the mechanism behind these individual differences. Patients should be educated on the importance of inserting the cannula into healthy subcutaneous tissue, avoiding underlying muscle as well as areas of skin irritation, infection, scarring and lipohypertrophy. Therefore, it was hypothesized that teflon cannulae used in the pump system may have induced the local immune reaction (Figs. 12.13 and 12.14).

Fig. 12.13 Local immune reaction induced by insulin analogues, delivered by CSII

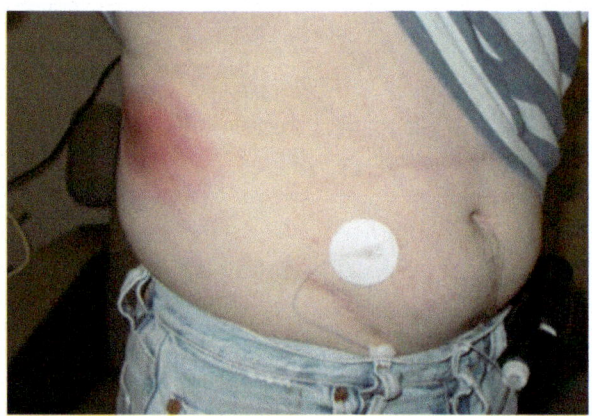

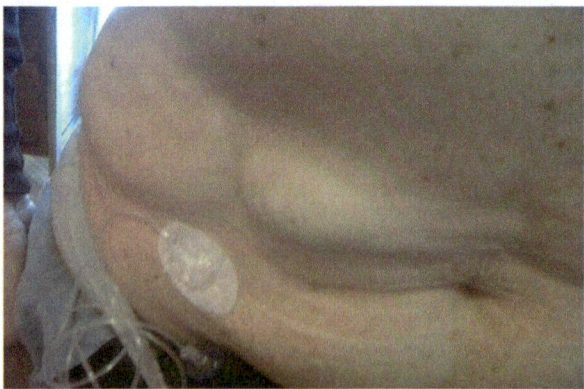

Fig. 12.14 Lipohypertrophy induced by insulin analogues, delivered by CSII

Patients should be encouraged to self-inspect sites, to identify healthy tissue for set insertion. It is recommended to perform glycemic self-monitoring in case of rotating from injured to healthy tissue, since by improving the absorption of insulin, the dose should be reduced.

The correct handling of the adhesive is essential to prevent site irritation and cannula movement, and the patient should perform the change of the infusion set in a sterile manner. It is advisable to change the infusion set every 3 days to prevent it from being clogged, and the onset of infections such as Staphylococcus Aureus abscesses. Occasionally, irritation can be caused by adhesive tape, which is recommended to be hypoallergenic. It is important to avoid stretching the tape over the skin, which can make the removal very difficult. If the irritation is caused by the use of soap or alcohol, antibacterial soap is recommended. Antimicrobial body washes may be helpful in patients prone to skin infections. Hands should be washed thoroughly before cannula insertion, and the top of the insulin vial should be cleaned with alcohol [37].

Glycemic Self-Monitoring

The glycemic self-monitoring is an essential tool in the self-care of a patient with DM. The results of this procedure are used to determine the metabolic state of the disease, assess the efficiency of the treatment and make the necessary adjustments to achieve therapeutic goals. The frequency of monitoring will depend on the metabolic control and the type of treatment, as it will be greater in those patients that use insulin. For this procedure, the patient must prick his/her fingers with specific lancets for each sensor. As this can be painful, the technique tends to be resisted due to the discomfort that can cause, generally to those who perform delicate manual tasks.

It is recommended to wash hands thoroughly before the puncture and use the lateral part of the middle, ring and little fingers. It is not recommended to prick the thumb and index finger, as those are the fingers involved in the gripping action, nor the fingertips to avoid losing sensitivity. It is common to see post-traumatic lesions caused by lancets in the fingers of patients with long-standing DM (Fig. 12.15). In order to reduce these lesions, it is convenient to use new lancets in each control and rotate the

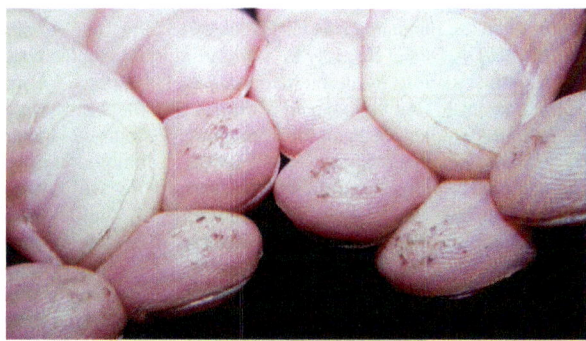

Fig. 12.15 Residual lesions at hemoglucotest sites

puncture site. Currently, there are continuous glucose monitoring systems. In this device, the sensor is inside a needle that is inserted in the subcutaneous adipose tissue, which uses the glucose oxidase enzyme for the dosage of interstitial glucose and it performs 288 daily determinations. This modality prevents the patient to prick him/her, but it represents a higher cost and it is used in particular cases [38, 39].

References

1. Sola D, Rossi L, Schianca G, et al. Sulfonylureas and their use in clinical practice. Arch Med Sci. 2015;11(4):840–8.
2. Santamaría VG, Barrios EG. Educación médica continua—manifestaciones cutáneas de la diabetes mellitus. Rev Cent Dermatol pascua. 2001;10(1).
3. Salem CB, Hmouda H, Slim R, et al. Rare case of metformin-induced leukocytoclastic vasculitis. Ann Pharmacother. 2006;40(9):1685–7.
4. Choudhary S, McLeod M, Torchia D, et al. Drug reaction with eosinophilia and systemic symptoms (DRESS) syndrome. J Clin Aesthet Dermatol. 2013;6(6):31.
5. Voore P, Odigwe C, Mirrakhimov AE, et al. DRESS syndrome following metformin administration: a case report and review of the literature. Am J Ther. 2016;23(6):e1970–3.
6. Ruiz M, Lombardo F. Hipoglucemiantes Orales. In: Ruiz M (Ed). Diabetes Mellitus, Cuarta edición. Akadia; 2011. p. 259–72.
7. Lebovitz HE, Banerji MA. Insulin resistance and its treatment by thiazolidinediones. Recent Prog Horm Res. 2001;56:265–94.
8. Martens FM, Visseren FL, Lemay J, et al. Metabolic and additional vascular effects of thiazolidinediones. Drugs. 2002;62:1463–80.
9. Caballero AE, Saouaf R, Lim SC, et al. The effects of troglitazone, an insulinsensitizing agent, on the endothelial function in early and late type 2 diabetes: a placebo-controlled randomized clinical trial. Metabolism. 2003;52:173–80.
10. Tan KC, Chow WS, Tso AW, et al. Thiazolidinedione increases serum soluble receptor for advanced glycation end-products in type 2 diabetes. Diabetologia. 2007;50:1819–25.
11. Hollander P. Safety profile of acarbose, an α-glucosidase inhibitor. Drugs. 1992;44(3):47–53.
12. Ruiz M, Lombardo F. Nuevos fármacos: incretinas. In: Ruiz M (Ed). Diabetes Mellitus, Cuarta edición. Akadia; 2011. p. 273–86.
13. Meier J, Gethmann A, Nauck M, et al. The glucagon–like–peptide–1 metabolite GLP–1 amide reduces postprandial glycemia independently of gastric emptying and insulin secretions in humans. Am J Physiol Endocrinol Metab. 2006;290:e1118–23.
14. European Medicines Agency. 2017. http://www.ema. europa.eu. Accessed Feb 2017.
15. Bastuji Garin S, Joly P, Lemordant P, et al. Risk factors for bullous pemphigoid in the elderly: a prospective case–control study. J Invest Dermatol. 2011;131(3):637–43.
16. Béné J, Jacobsoone A, Coupe P, et al. Bullous pemphigoid induced by vildagliptin: a report of three cases. Fundam Clin Pharmacol. 2014;29(1):112–4.
17. Murrel DF, Daniel BS, Joly P, et al. Definitions an outcome measures for bullous pemphigoid: recommendations by an international panel of experts. J Am Acad Dermatol. 2012;66:479–85.
18. Sundaram M, Adikrishnan S, Murugan S. Co-existence of rheumatoid arthritis, vitiligo and bullous pemphigoid as multiple autoinmune sindrome. Indian J Dermatol. 2014;59(3):306–7.
19. Unidad de fármacovigilancia del País Vasco. Inhibidores de la dipeptidil peptidasa 4 (gliptinas) y penfigoide ampollar. Boletín n°38, septiembre 2014.
20. Attaway A, Mersfelder T, Vaishnav S, et al. Bullous pemphigoid associated with dipeptidyl peptidase IV inhibitors. A case report and review of literature. J Dermatol Case Rep. 2014;8(1):24–8.
21. Skandalis K, Spirova M, Gaitanis G, et al. Drug-induced bullous pemphigoid in diabetes mellitus patients receiving dipeptidyl peptidase–IV inhibitors plus metformin. J Eur Acad Dermatol Venereol. 2012;26(2):249–53.

22. Mendonça FM, Martín-Gutierrez FJ, Ríos-Martín JJ, Camacho-Martinez F. Three cases of bullous pemphigoid associated with dipeptidyl peptidase-4 inhibitors-one due to linagliptin. Dermatology. 2016;232(2):249–53.
23. Taharani AA, Barnett AH, Bailey CJ. SGLT inhibitors in management of diabetes. Lancet Diabetes Endocrinol. 2013;1:140–51.
24. Leiter L. Symposium of safety and adverse effects. The role of SGLT2 inhibitors in the treatment of type 2 diabetes. 74th Congress American Diabetes Association. San Francisco, California; 2014.
25. De Fronzo RA, Davidson J, Del Prato S. The role of the kidneys in glucose homeostasis: a new path towards normalizing glycaemia. Diabetes Obes Metab. 2012;141(1):5–14.
26. Vasapollo P, Cione E, Luciani F, Gallelli L. Generalized intense pruritus during canagliflozin treatment: Is it an adverse drug reaction? Curr Drug Saf. 2016.
27. Richardson T, Kerr D. Skin-related complications of insulin therapy: epidemiology and emerging management strategies. Am J Clin Dermatol. 2003;4:661–7.
28. Perez MI, Kohn SR. Cutaneous manifestations of diabetes mellitus. J Am Acad Dermatol. 1994;30:519–31.
29. Piérard-Franchimont C, Hermanns-Lê T, Scheen AJ, Piérard GE. Cutaneous complications of insulin therapy. A drug-induced condition on the decline. Rev Med Liege. 2005;60:564–5.
30. Van Hattem S, Bootsma A, Bing Thio H. Skin manifestations of diabetes. Cleve Clin J Med. 2008;75:772–87.
31. Del Olmo MI, Campos V, Abellán P, et al. A case of lipoatrophy with insulin detemir. Diabetes Res Clin Pract. 2008;80:20–1.
32. Saraceno EF. Manifestaciones Cutáneas del tratamiento Antidiabético. In: Cabo H, editor. Manifestaciones Cutáneas de la Diabetes Mellitus. Buenos Aires: Ed A. Macchi; 1996. p. 165–78.
33. Radermecker RP, Piérard GE, Scheen AJ. Lipodystrophy reactions to insulin: effects of continuous insulin infusion and new insulin analogs. Am J Clin Dermatol. 2007;8:21–8.
34. Babiker A, Datta V. Lipoatrophy with insulin analogues in type I diabetes. Arch Dis Child. 2011;96:101–2.
35. Holstein A, Stege H, Kovacs P. Lipoatrophy associated with the use of insulin analogues: a new case associated with the use of insulin glargine and review of the literature. Expert Opin Drug Saf. 2010;9:225–31.
36. Andrade P, Barros L, Gonçalo M. Type 1 Ig-E mediated allergy to human insulin, insulin analogues and beta-lactam antibiotics. An Bras Dermatol. 2012;87(6):917–9.
37. Deiss D, Adolfsson P, Alkemade-van Zomeren M, et al. Insulin infusion set use: European perspectives and recommendations. Diabetes Technol Ther. 2016;18(9):517–24.
38. Commendatore, Víctor F, Linari M, Dieuzeide G, et al. Automonitoreo y Monitoreo de Glucosa y Cetonas en la persona con diabetes. *Monografía en Internet*. Buenos Aires: Sociedad Argentina de Diabetes; 2014.
39. American Diabetes Association. 6. Glycemic targets. Diabetes Care. 2017;40(Suppl.1):S48–56.
40. Miracle López S, Barreda BF. Manifestaciones cutáneas de la diabetes mellitus, una manera clínica de identificar la enfermedad. Rev Endocrinol Nutr. 2005;13(2):75–87.

José Contreras-Ruiz and Ana Carolina Manzotti-Rodriguez

Wound Healing in Diabetics

To understand how Diabetes causes impaired repair of injured tissue, one must first understand how wounds are repaired under normal conditions. Therefore, a brief overview of this process is included in the following paragraphs.

Regardless of the mechanism of injury, wound healing represents a complex and dynamic process involving multiple cell types, growth factors and chemical signals that mediate tissue repair. This process has traditionally been divided into 4 phases: hemostasis, inflammation, proliferation and remodeling. These phases represent a continuum and overlap usually exists at some point in the process, including interactions between different cells and the matrix—an interaction known as dynamic reciprocity [1].

When tissue injury occurs, collagen is exposed to circulating platelets, which causes them to aggregate and adhere to sites of damage, thus initiating the coagulation cascade. Fibrinogen is eventually converted to fibrin forming a fibrin plug, which induces hemostasis. This process also causes a massive release of growth factors and cytokines that initiate cell migration to the wound. As cells arrive at the site of injury, the inflammatory phase of wound repair begins. Neutrophils are usually the first cells present at wound sites where they ingest and destroy bacteria and debris through phagocytosis and the production of toxic substances such as proteases and cathepsin. Neutrophil influx lasts for 48 h and is then followed by migration of macrophages to the wound site, which produce growth factors that promote

J. Contreras-Ruiz, M.D. (✉)
Division of Dermatology, Wound and Ostomy Care Center, Hospital General "Dr. Manuel Gea González", Mexico City, CDMX, Mexico
e-mail: dermayheridas@gmail.com

A.C. Manzotti-Rodriguez, M.D.
Dermatología Integral de Monterrey, Monterrey, Nuevo Leon, Mexico
e-mail: ana.cmanzotti@gmail.com

© Springer International Publishing AG 2018
E.N. Cohen Sabban et al. (eds.), *Dermatology and Diabetes*,
https://doi.org/10.1007/978-3-319-72475-1_13

angiogenesis and granulation in the wound bed, and lymphocytes which help regulate the production of new tissue, like collagen and extracellular matrix, needed for wound repair [2]. Once the site of injury is clear of debris new tissue must be formed to repair the wound; this complex process is known as the proliferative phase of wound repair. From the onset of injury, multiple chemical mediators such as platelet-derived growth factor and transforming growth factor-β induce angiogenesis in the wound bed. The same mediators also attract fibroblasts that produce collagen and extracellular matrix proteins laying down what is known as granulation tissue. Fibroblasts then transform to myofibroblasts and form a complex net capable of contracting to reduce the surface area of the wound. This is important because epithelial cells must migrate from the edges of the wound to replace the lost epithelium; a process known as reepithelization. As the wound contracts, the area that must be covered by new epithelium becomes progressively smaller. Finally, the remodeling phase takes place when type 1 collagen that was laid down during the proliferative phase is replaced by stronger, more organized type 3 collagen [3, 4].

Several factors contribute to delayed wound healing in diabetic patients. Ischemia, trauma, and neuropathy, the three main abnormalities responsible for diabetic foot, are also to blame for the disruption in the healing process [5]. Additionally, other factors such as infection and chronic inflammation can also have a negative impact on wound repair. The result is a failure of the wound to successfully progress through the normal healing process [3].

Multiple microvascular abnormalities are present in patients with Diabetes such as a reduction in capillary size, thickening of the basement membrane and arteriolar hyalinosis. Furthermore, peripheral arterial disease is a common comorbidity in these patients. The resulting reduction in blood flow produces altered migration of leukocytes, misdistribution of blood flow, altered physiological exchanges, and an increased susceptibility to pressure forces in the foot. Hypoxia also produces free oxygen radicals that further delay wound repair [5].

Neuropathy in patients with Diabetes affects motor, sensory and autonomic fibers. Motor dysfunction causes abnormal gait and anatomical deformities while the absence of pain associated with sensory dysfunction is to blame for a loss of protective symptoms. Both abnormalities combined lead to constant pressure on the affected limb that is responsible for the initiation and perpetuation of the wound. Damage to autonomic nerves causes misdistribution of blood flow and altered neurovascular response leading to decrease vasodilation which, combined with micro and macrocirculatory abnormalities, lead to decreased perfusion [5].

While inflammation is necessary for wound repair, the inflammatory response in patients with Diabetes is often protracted and ineffective due mainly to altered cell function. Macrophages and neutrophils have decreased phagocytic activity, fibroblasts show decreased proliferation, and keratinocytes show decreased differentiation. At the same time, high levels of metalloproteinases in the wound lead to increased extracellular matrix destruction causing further delay in the healing process [3].

Infections are a common complication in patients with Diabetes; at least half of all diabetic foot ulcers are infected at the time the patient presents to consult. More importantly, infected foot wounds precede two-thirds of lower extremity amputations

[6]. As previously mentioned, immune cells of patients with Diabetes have decreased phagocytic ability that is further affected by varying degrees of hypoxia caused by damage to blood vessels and an impaired macro and microcirculatory system [5]. Diabetics also have impaired chemotaxis and inhibition of the complement-mediated cascade that render them susceptible to more frequent and more severe infections [7].

These factors interact to make diabetic wounds particularly difficult to treat. Given that Diabetes is a multisystem disease it seems logical that a multidisciplinary team would be best suited to elaborate a treatment plan. When faced with one of these patients it is wise to think of the patient as a whole, and not just focus on their wound so that each of these factors can be taken into account and, if possible, properly addressed. In the following sections, specific treatment recommendations for each of these factors will be discussed (see below).

Common Wounds in Diabetics

By far, the most common form of cutaneous ulceration in the diabetic is the diabetic foot ulcer (see below). However, other forms of ulceration can occur in the diabetic and the clinician must know how to properly identify them and understand their pathophysiology to be able to effectively manage the wound.

Diabetic Foot Ulcers

Any loss of continuity of the stratum corneum (SC) below the malleoli of a person with Diabetes Mellitus (DM) should be considered a diabetic foot until proven otherwise (Fig. 13.1). The reason is that, as stated above, diabetic patients are prone to complications due to a severe decrease in the ability to heal and fight-off infection.

Multiple factors should be considered when assessing a diabetic foot. As circulation is determinant on prognosis, adequate vascular examination is of the outmost importance. Evaluating the circulation can be as simple as searching for pulses or

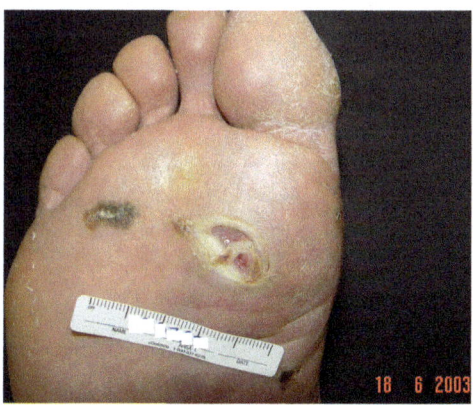

Fig. 13.1 Diabetic foot ulcer (UTex IIA)

obtaining an ankle-brachial index, or as complex as vascular laboratory testing such as angiotomography or arteriography.

The presence of infection may be obscured by delayed manifestations of inflammation caused by elevated glucose levels and leukocyte abnormalities. Infection in the diabetic foot ulcer needs to be classified into absent, mild, moderate or severe according to the criteria established by the Infectious Disease Society of America (IDSA) [8]. Increased pain, or the presence of pain in an ulcer that was anesthetic, should always be considered a sign of infection [9] and a positive probe to bone test or abnormalities in plain X-rays as signs of osteomyelitis [10].

Loss of protective sensation caused by peripheral neuropathy places diabetic patients at risk for the development of ulcers [11]. To assess for neuropathy the gold standard is the use of a biothesiometer, but this test is expensive and not readily available. To test the at-risk foot, one may use the nylon monofilament test [12] or even the simple Ipswich touch test [13]. These tests are simple methods to assess for loss of sensation in different areas of the foot and correlates with the presence of foot injuries (Fig. 13.2).

Related to the loss of protective sensation and neuropathy, patients commonly develop ulcers in pressure points such as the metatarsal heads and toes. Evaluating this continuous pressure and gait disturbances may lead to identifying areas of increased weight bearing or trauma. Since continued pressure or trauma to the ulcer leads to delayed healing, it must be addressed.

Finally, when an ulcer or skin rupture is evident, evaluation of the depth of the tissues involved is necessary since involvement of the subcutaneous fat and deeper tissues is associated with a worse prognosis [14].

Once the patient has been properly evaluated, the cutaneous ulceration must be classified. The authors prefer the University of Texas classification, provided in Table 13.1, since it has been validated and provides a logical treatment algorithm [15, 16].

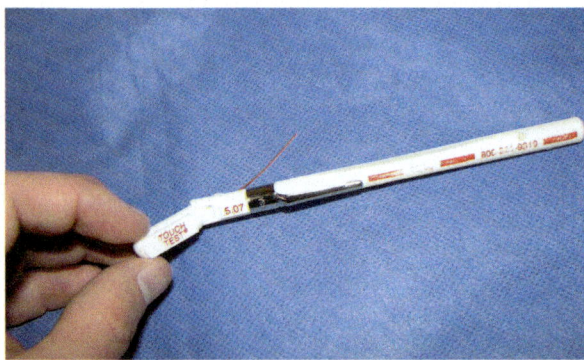

Fig. 13.2 10 g nylon monofilament test

Table 13.1 University of Texas diabetic foot classification

		Grade			
		0	I	II	III
		Pre- or post-ulcerative lesion completely epithelialized	Superficial wound down to the fascia	Wound penetrating to tendon or reaching the joint capsule	Wound penetrating to bone or joint
Stage	A	No infection or ischemia	No infection or ischemia	No infection or ischemia	No infection or ischemia
	B	Infected	Infected	Infected	Infected
	C	Ischemic	Ischemic	Ischemic	Ischemic
	D	Infected and ischemic	Infected and ischemic	Infected and ischemic	Infected and ischemic

Fig. 13.3 "Diabetic hand" with severe destruction due to infection. Note active infection and the presence of slough covering the wound

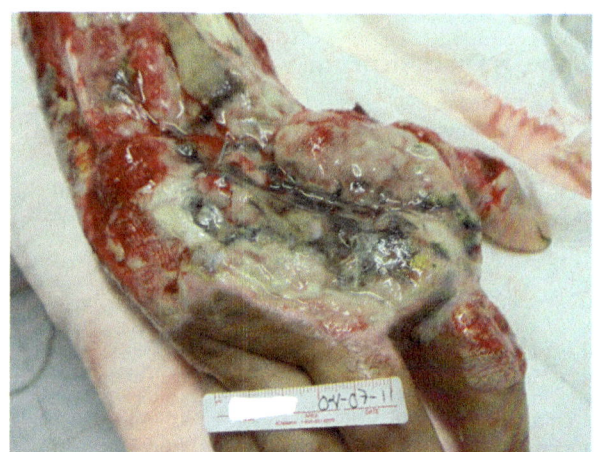

"Diabetic Hand" Ulcers

Similar to the diabetic foot, hand ulcers, although much less frequent, can have devastating consequences on the patient with Diabetes (Fig. 13.3). Also known as the "Tropical Diabetic Hand Syndrome", infectious complications of wounds on the hands may lead to aggressive debridement and even amputations. In the latter, associated factors leading to it are end stage renal disease, elevated hemoglobin A1c (more than 10%) and severe peripheral neuropathy [17]. Management of these ulcers is also multidisciplinary and hyperbaric oxygen therapy has been shown to be useful [18].

Fig. 13.4 Bullosis
diabeticorum on the hand
of a patient with type 2
diabetes

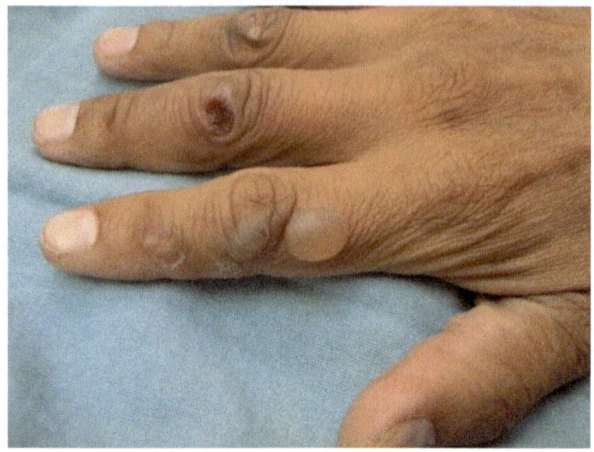

Bullosis Diabeticorum

This rare cutaneous marker of DM is characterized by the formation of spontaneous bullae that usually affect the skin of the lower extremities. These bullae are not associated with inflammation [19]. The etiology of this entity is still unknown but the treatment follows the basic wound care principles depicted below [20] (Fig. 13.4).

Leg Ulcers

Leg ulcers are not characteristic of the diabetic patient only, but given the co-morbidities associated with the metabolic syndrome, such as obesity and accelerated atherosclerosis, persons with Diabetes may develop chronic leg ulcers. Leg ulcers in the diabetic may be secondary to diverse conditions such as venous or arterial disease as well as more uncommon causes of leg ulceration.

Venous Leg Ulcers

Venous leg ulcers (VLU) are caused by increased resting venous pressure that may be due to valvular insufficiency, post-thrombotic syndrome or simply by affection of the ankle joint that in turn affects the "calf-muscle pump". This increased pressure leads to continuous inflammation and leakage of proteins and cells at the venous capillaries that eventually causes ulceration.

Even though venous leg ulcers are not characteristic of patients with Diabetes, they are highly prevalent in the ageing population. Furthermore, up to 20% of patients with a venous leg ulcer will have Diabetes as a co-morbid condition [21] (Fig. 13.5a).

VLU are usually located around the malleoli with cutaneous changes secondary to venous hypertension such as ochre pigmentation and the presence of varicosities.

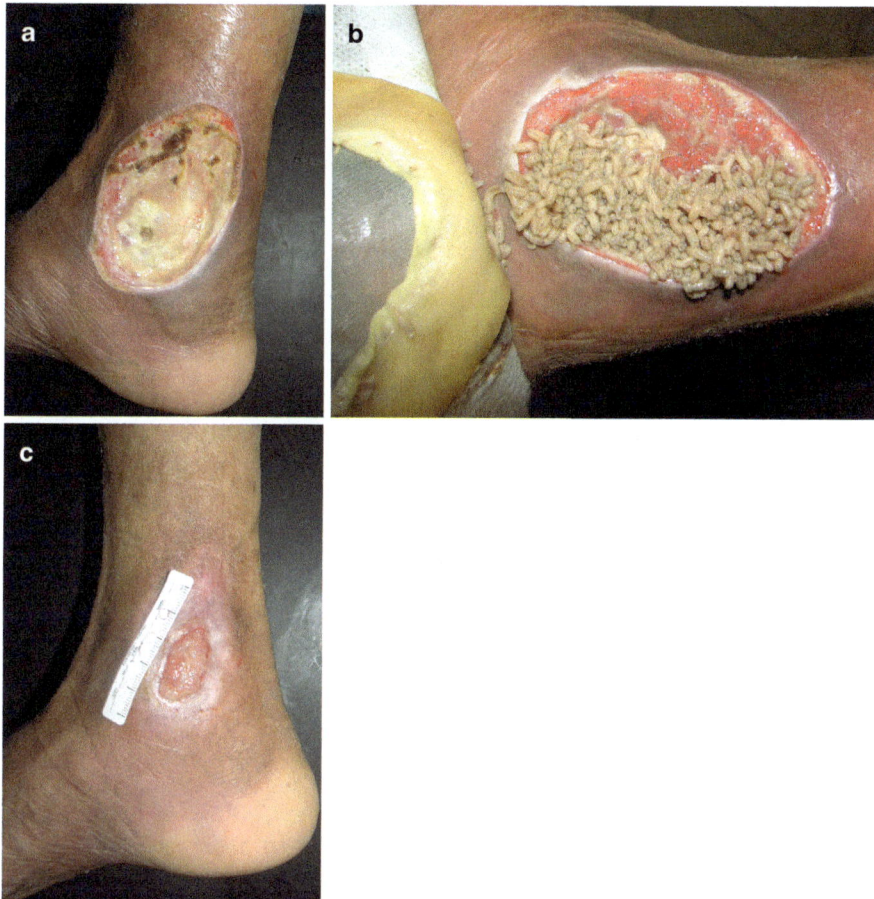

Fig. 13.5 Venous leg ulcer with necrotic tissue on the leg of a diabetic patient. (**a**) At presentation, (**b**) debridement with maggot therapy, (**c**) after moist interactive healing

The ulcer itself has a congestive wound bed, is irregularly shaped and highly exudative [22].

Arterial (Ischemic) Ulcers

Arterial or ischemic ulcers are the result of poor perfusion of the skin secondary to arterial vasocclusive disease. As Diabetes and the metabolic syndrome are associated with accelerated atherosclerosis, it is common for this type of ulcers to develop.

Arterial ulcers are characteristically covered with either necrotic eschar or pale slough. Their shape will depend on the size of the affected blood vessel. When the disease is due to the occlusion of a large vessel, very destructive deep ulcers develop while more discrete arterial disease will lead to round or wedge-shaped wounds [23] (Fig. 13.6).

Fig. 13.6 Arterial ulcer on
the ankle. Note the lack of
granulation tissue and depth

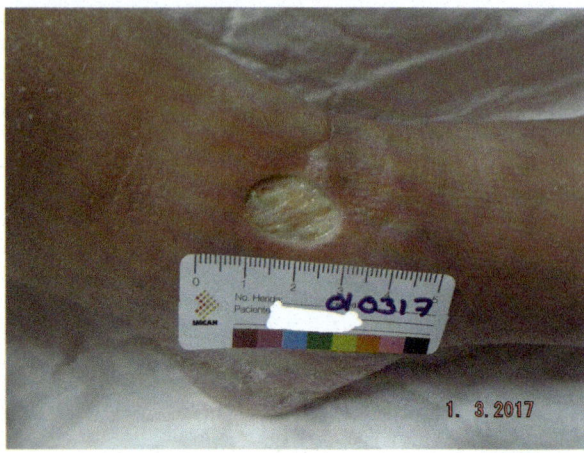

Other Causes of Leg Ulceration

Necrobiosis lipoidica diabeticorum may occasionally become ulcerated. These
ulcers are always located on the lower extremities and the diagnosis is relatively
simple once the typical associated findings are evident. The ulcerated plaques usually have a yellowish waxy and atrophic surface with one or multiple ulcers [24].
Ulcerated necrobiosis lipoidica may even precede diabetes in as much as 30% of the
cases. The cause of this cutaneous marker of DM is unknown, but it has been associated with microangiopathy, antibody-mediated vasculitis and disorders of neutrophil function (Fig. 13.7).

Other causes of leg ulceration in the diabetic are less frequent and must be ruled
out whenever the clinical picture suggest them, especially the presence of atypical
mycobacteria, fungi or complications of bacterial disease such as necrotizing
infections.

Pressure Injuries

Pressure-related injuries or pressure ulcers are related to increased pressure between
bony prominences and a surface (commonly the patient's bed) over a period of time.
Pressure injury may present in any patient with decreased mobility or lack of sensitivity, both of which occur commonly in hospitalizations due to other complications
of diabetes and because of neuropathy. The resulting injuries may range from small
blisters or abrasions to full thickness ulcerations reaching down to the bone. As their
name implies, the treatment is absolute removal of the causative factor (i.e. Pressure)
and proper wound care [25] (Fig. 13.8).

Fig. 13.7 Ulcerated
necrobiosis lipoidica
diabeticorum

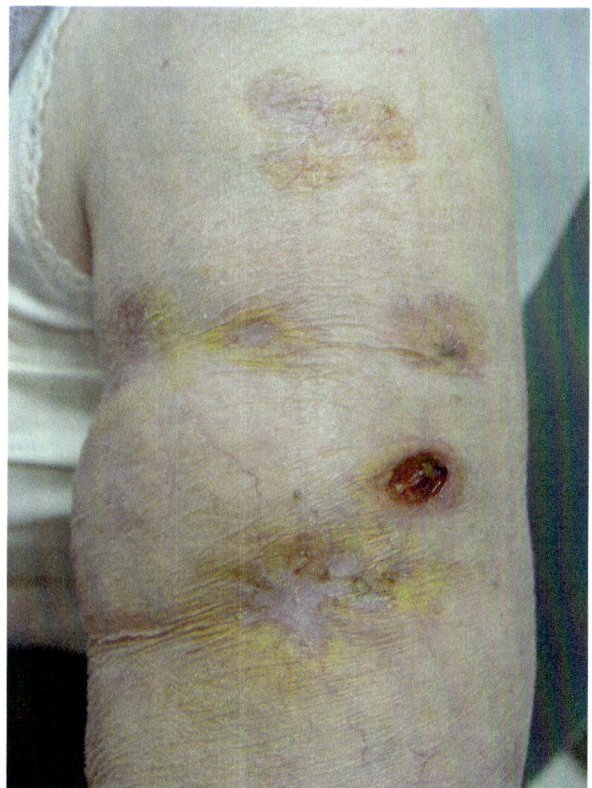

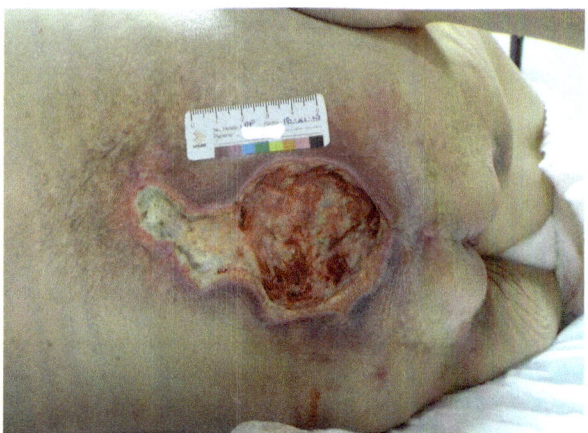

Fig. 13.8 Pressure-induced
injury (pressure ulcer) on the
sacral area of a diabetic
patient after hospitalization

Wound Care in Diabetic Patients

Advances in the understanding of wound healing in the past century have led to new treatment paradigms and technological improvements. Since 1962, when Winter showed [26] that allowing a wound to dry is definitely not beneficial to the healing process, and the later work by Hinman in 1963 [27] confirming this conclusion in humans, wound care has become almost a new specialty where scientific evidence and new exciting research has led to better outcomes. In the following sections, we will analyze some of these developments. A general approach to wound care in the diabetic is depicted in Fig. 13.9.

Wound Evaluation, Diagnosis and Treatment Goals

Whenever a patient presents to the clinic with a wound, the first step in their care is to perform an adequate evaluation. The dermatologist is able not only to properly diagnose an ulcer based on its location and morphology, but also to assess the condition of the surrounding skin, the associated possible complications (e.g. contact dermatitis) and any additional cutaneous signs that the patient may have (e.g. necrobiosis lipoidica). Full evaluation of a cutaneous ulcer includes wound measurement, assessment of the wound bed, borders, exudate, and the skin [28].

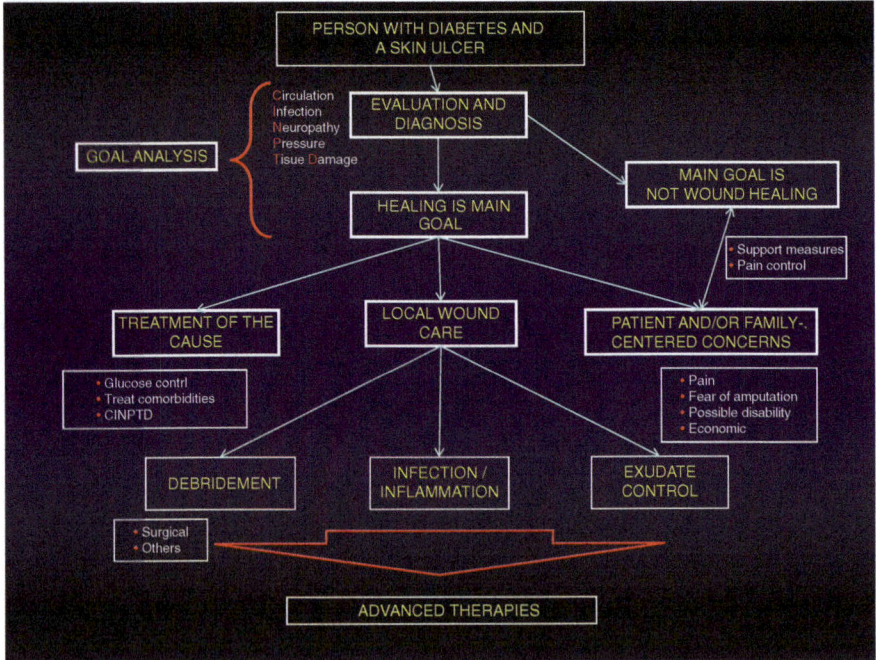

Fig. 13.9 General treatment algorithm for a person with diabetes and a cutaneous ulcer

Once the ulcer has been examined, a history of the present illness must be obtained. This includes asking when was the last time the patient had healthy skin on the area, how the ulcer began, past treatments, symptoms associated with the ulcer and relevant past medical history.

Proper assessment is key in obtaining an adequate diagnosis of the cause of the ulcer. Without an adequate diagnosis, one may not provide an ideal treatment plan, which should always, ideally, be driven by the patient's needs and desires and not solely on the clinician's.

The goals of treatment must take into consideration whether healing an ulcer is likely (e.g. critical ischemia), whether the patient is beyond treatment or if delaying a radical treatment (e.g. an amputation) may endanger his life or increase the risk of a higher amputation. Also, the physician must understand what the patient's main concern is (e.g. sometimes pain relief or odor control becomes more important than treating the wound itself).

Severe or Critical Ischemia Recommendations

One of the main factors affecting wound healing in the diabetic is cutaneous perfusion [29]. Ischemia leads to shortage of oxygen and nutrients necessary for wound healing, it affects the ability of the host to establish a proper immune response, and when severe enough, it will not allow for medications and antibiotics to reach the affected area. Therefore, reestablishing circulation is of paramount importance.

Unfortunately, sometimes this is not possible due to very advanced atherosclerosis or to a lack of human and economic resources to achieve successful revascularization, which is common in developing countries. When a cutaneous ulcer in a diabetic patient falls into this group, quality of life and avoiding further deterioration of the patient is the most important goal. To achieve the former, one must establish a close relationship with the patient, and take any possible measures to control the patient's pain; always taking into consideration that kidney function may be impaired. Pain may be due to associated ischemia, infection, or a combination of both. Therefore, the cause of the pain and any aggravating factors should be addressed.

Further deterioration of the wound, and of the patient's health, must be avoided. Although progressive ischemia may lead to deterioration, it is usually infection the main reason why these wounds become unstable. To avoid it, aggressive debridement is contraindicated (i.e. avoid removing necrotic tissue that is strongly adhered to the wound bed) since it will lead to a larger wound that will not heal anyway. In this scenario, moist healing (see below) is contraindicated for increasing humidity will also increase bacterial proliferation. The wound must be dried to allow for eschar formation and in some cases "mummification". Systemic antibiotics will be necessary in some cases to drive infection back while getting the patient in control [30, 31] (Fig. 13.10).

Finally, as stated before, if the pain becomes unbearable, the patient becomes unstable and there is risk of sepsis or the need for a higher level of amputation, or whenever the patient requests it, radical surgery by means of an amputation may be indicated.

Fig. 13.10 Crtilical limb
ischemia

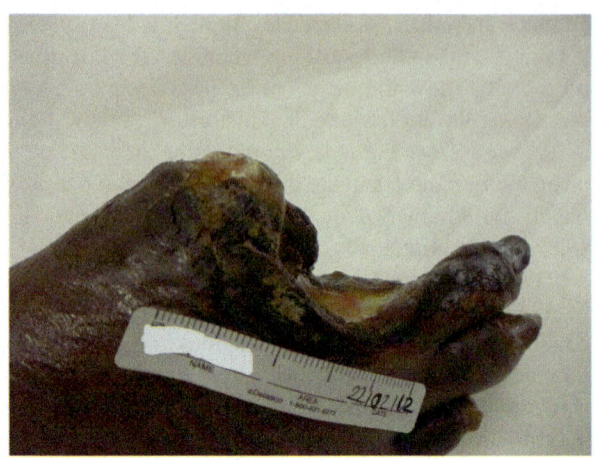

Patient-Centered Concerns

More and more, quality of life and listening to the patient's worries, beliefs, and expectations have become a marker of good healthcare. Especially when treating persons with Diabetes and cutaneous ulcers these aspects of care need to be taken into consideration. Fear of amputation is very common in diabetics who have ulcers. After evaluating the wound, the clinician should discuss the goals of treatment and listen to the patient's understanding of the plan and expectations.

The economic aspects of treatment should also be discussed since advanced wound care modalities, and the healthcare team that needs to be involved in their care, can become costly. Therapies should then be selected based on the ability of the patient or health care system to pay for them. Furthermore, many patients become incapacitated by their wounds, so occupational, and work-related issues should be discussed. Centering care around the patient will identify these as well as other issues related to adherence to treatment, and will aid in establishing a good relationship between physician and patient [32, 33].

Treating the Cause

Once the patient has been properly evaluated, the diagnosis has been established, and goals and expectations of treatment have been discussed with the patient, the single most important measure into achieving wound improvement is treating the cause.

Treatment of the cause will correct, whenever possible, the underlying factors leading to poor healing.

General treatment of the cause in Diabetes focuses directly on optimal glucose control. One must remember that whenever infection or a wound ensues, this may cause glucose levels to vary wildly. Therefore, one must team up with the internist

Table 13.2 Frequent causes of ulcers in the diabetic patient and treatment of the causative factors

Wound	Cause	Treatment
Diabetic foot and hand	Ischemia Infection Pressure	Revascularization Antimicrobial therapy Offloading [34]
Venous leg ulcer	Venous hypertension	Compression therapy [35]
Arterial	Ischemia	Revascularization [36]
Pressure	Pressure	Offloading (pressure shifting) [37, 38] Special surfaces [39]
Other		Treat specific cause

or diabetic care expert to keep glucose under control. Also, Diabetes may co-exist with several comorbidities that affect healing such as lack of circulation, hypertension or hypercholesterolemia. All these should be controlled should also be addressed.

Some of the most common types of ulcers found in diabetics, as well as their cause and specific treatment, are listed in Table 13.2.

Unfortunately, treatment of the cause is not always possible due mainly to either the patient's general condition, or because the cause is still unknown. In these cases, proper wound care preparation will optimize the local conditions to improve the chances of healing.

Principles of Wound Bed Preparation

A concept introduced to the wound care literature first by plastic surgeons, and later adopted by wound care clinicians, wound bed preparation is an organized series of steps or conditions that need to be addressed to optimize wound healing [40]. This approach deals with adequate tissue debridement, diagnosis and treatment of infection, and providing adequate moisture to the wound to allow cell migration and healing. If these aspects have been addressed and the wound is still not healing, the use of advanced wound care modalities may be indicated.

Tissue Debridement

The first step in managing the wound is to remove necrotic tissue from the wound bed, also known as debridement. When dry, necrotic tissue is usually black or brown and easily distinguished from healthy tissues underneath. However, when moist, it becomes a white, stringy, adherent substance known as slough that should not be confused with viable tissue and should be readily removed (Fig. 13.3).

Debridement is vital to preparing the wound for closure. The presence of necrotic tissue in the wound bed causes delays in its repair in several ways. First, it acts as a mechanical barrier that blocks the migration of keratinocytes from the edges of the wound as well wound contraction. Second, it is a constant stimulus for the already chronic inflammatory process that diabetics are especially prone to have. Third, it promotes bacterial infections. Removing necrotic tissue will allow the clinician to properly measure the wound, evaluate for signs of infection and, more importantly, it stimulates the wound to begin the repair process, turning a chronic wound into an acute one [41].

A few conditions must be met before debridement. Patients must be evaluated and treated for conditions that may affect the outcome of the procedure such as hyperglycemia. It is important to remember that diabetics usually have some degree of vascular damage; in order to avoid creating a larger wound that is more prone to infection, the area to be treated should be evaluated for adequate blood supply (see above) [41]. Finally, consider using some kind of analgesic or anesthetic, whether it be topical or systemic. The fact that patients have neuropathy does not mean they may not require pain control during the procedure.

There are several modalities that may be used for tissue debridement. The most common ones are surgical (sharp), mechanical, biosurgical, enzymatic, and autolytic.

Surgical debridement uses sharp instruments such as scalpels, scissors, or curettes to remove necrotic tissue. It is the fastest method and will remove large amounts of necrotic tissue that may involve deeper structures as bone and tendons. Sharp debridement will also reduce bacterial burden effectively so it is indicated whenever a wound is severely infected. The cost may vary greatly depending on whether or not the patient requires the use of an operating room and anesthesia. It also has the advantage of stimulating the wound bed which makes it the method of choice for diabetic wounds [41]. Drawbacks to surgical debridement include a higher risk of bleeding, pain and the fact that it requires the clinician to distinguish devitalized from healthy tissue making it a non-selective method of debridement. Hydrosurgical debridement uses a high-pressure water jet to cut through tissue. It hasn't been shown to be more effective than other options and costs significantly limits its use in daily practice [42].

Mechanical debridement involves the forceful removal of tissue from the wound bed. This can be achieved by several methods and may range from the simple rubbing of gauze on the surface of the wound, to the infamous wet-to-dry. Wet-to-dry debridement consists on applying wet gauze on the wound bed and allowing it to dry. The gauze is then pulled and removed together with necrotic tissue. Wound cleansing debridement involves using a continuous flow of fluid at high pressures to force devitalized tissue out of the wound bed. In whirlpool debridement, the patient is submerged in a whirlpool where water jets help loosens necrotic tissue and bacteria from the wound. These methods are also non-selective and can cause significant pain to the patient which is why they should be avoided if possible [43].

Maggot debridement therapy, also called biosurgery, is the use of medical-grade larvae of the blowfly *Lucilia sericata* to remove necrotic tissue from the wound base. Basically, the larvae are "caged" over the area to be cleaned where they will selectively remove devitalized material while avoiding healthy, viable tissue. Additionally, they have been shown to produce antiseptic substances that may help decrease bacterial load and fight off infection. Advantages of biosurgical debridement include its high selectivity for unviable tissue, low risk, and high effectiveness

(Fig. 13.5a–c). Disadvantages include the need to procure the larvae, which must be bred in a sterile environment, and patient compliance [44].

Wounds can be debrided by applying topical enzymes such as papain, streptokinase and fibrinolysin to devitalized tissue until the wound is completely cleaned; this is known as enzymatic debridement. Since papain may cause cross-sensitivity with latex, the only available enzymatic debridement is through the use of collagenase. Autolytic debridement involves keeping wounds moist with hydrogels, or occlusive dressings to cause naturally occurring enzymes to break down devitalized tissue. These are painless and selective methods; however, if used alone, it can take a long time to clean the wound completely.

The choice between the different types of debridement depends on several factors such as the physician's skill, the conditions of the patient and the wound, availability and costs [45]. Another important factor to consider is the amount of tissue that needs to be removed. Wounds with large amounts of devitalized tissue may take too long to debride with enzymatic or autolytic methods and surgical debridement may represent a better option. Over the course of treatment most patients will require maintenance debriding of small quantities of tissue to maintain the wound bed in optimal conditions; in these cases, less invasive methods such as enzymatic debridement may be considered. Most patients will probably benefit from a combination of methods that maximizes the removal of devitalized tissue and minimized the loss of viable tissue.

Table 13.3 summarizes advantages and disadvantages of different methods of debridement (Table 13.3).

Infection

Host resistance is one of the most important factors in wound infection. Infection occurs whenever the host's ability to counteract bacteria in the wound is surpassed

Table 13.3 Advantages and disadvantages of some of the existing methods for wound debridement

Debridement method	Advantages	Disadvantages
Surgical	– Fast – Allows removal of large quantities of tissue – Reduces bacterial burden – Stimulates wound bed – Variable costs	– Higher risk of bleeding – Pain – Non-selective (depends on clinician's skill)
Mechanical	– Low cost (wet-to-dry and physical) – High cost (pressurized water)	– Non-selective – Pain
Biosurgical	– Selective – May decrease bacterial load – Effective	– Patient compliance – Availability of larvae is limited – May be painful
Enzymatic/ Autolytic	– Selective – Painless	– Slow

[46]. In diabetics, this is particularly important since uncontrolled Diabetes leads to a poor immune response. Furthermore, typical signs of inflammation may not be evident for some time and therefore infections tend to be more severe at the time of diagnosis.

The diagnosis of infection in a wound should always be based on clinical signs. Unfortunately, there is great variability in the available evidence on how to diagnose infection given that complex interactions exist between the host and the bacteria present in the wound.

Whenever a patient develops and ulcer, bacteria will enter deeper tissues and will begin to replicate and invade them. If the host can fight back the bacteria, the bacteria will be eliminated, the wound bed will granulate and eventually the wound edges will advance and heal the wound. Unfortunately, diabetics are prone to infections given the previously discussed alterations caused by chronic abnormal glucose levels. Furthermore, the patient will present for evaluation later, given that most of the time neuropathy will affect the ability to feel pain. Hence, most wounds in diabetics will already have polymicrobial infections.

Signs of local infection or "critical colonization" will include a wound that stalls or wound edges that fail to advance. The wound odor and exudate may increase or even new areas of slough will form. All these signs should warn the clinician that bacterial burden has increased to the point of not allowing the wound to heal [47, 48]. Biofilm formation may ensue and cause increased levels of chronic inflammatory mediators in the wound and repeated acute infections [49].

Deep infection will show the classical signs of inflammation: erythema, increased temperature, edema, loss of function and pain. Increased pain or the appearance of pain in a non-painful wound has been shown to be the best predictor of wound infection [9]. Infection would then need to be classified into mild, moderate or severe according to specific criteria and systemic involvement [50].

Osteomyelitis is a common concern in diabetic patients; in the case of diabetic foot ulcers, research has shown that positive plain x-rays or a positive probe-to-bone test may be enough to diagnose bone involvement [10, 51]. Imaging modalities like MRI or nuclear medicine may be necessary in cases of suspected osteomyelitis associated with other types of ulcers.

Cultures should be obtained whenever infection is suspected to guide proper antimicrobial therapy. Although tissue cultures from the wound bed are ideal, properly obtained swabs have shown to be a good alternative [52]. These swabs should be taken from the deeper part of the wound after debridement of all necrotic tissue. Lately, a new method of molecular bacterial identification, has led to new discoveries on the most common bacteria found in all chronic wounds and may substitute common cultures in the future [53].

Treatment of infection will depend on whether infection is limited to the surface of the wound or bacteria are causing deep infection. As stated above, infection in the diabetic can be lethal and therefore it is important to consider prompt hospitalization and therapy when a severe or even moderate infection is diagnosed. Prompt debridement and adequate antimicrobial therapy should be started immediately after diagnosis and cultures.

Several antimicrobial dressings are now available to treat increased bacterial burden in the wounds. The advantages of these dressings over common materials are that they will deliver the antimicrobial agent continuously in steady concentrations while controlling exudate and minimizing chances of resistance or sensitizations. The most common of these antimicrobials are silver, iodine or polyhexamethylene (PHMB) [54–65]. Briefly, silver may be found in numerous dressings ranging from hydrocolloids to alginates or pure carboxymethylcellulose; ionic silver is slowly released into the wound bed. Cadexomer iodine, a slow-release iodine compound, has been shown to increase wound healing in leg ulcers and diabetic ulcers. Finally, PHMB is a wide-spectrum polymerized biguanide with no reported bacterial resistance. It denatures bacterial proteins causing membrane pores that will destroy bacteria in the wound. This compound may be found in cleansing solutions and dressings as well. It is important to remember that these dressings will only treat the surface of the wound and therefore, if deeper infection is suspected, systemic antibiotics will be necessary. Recently published data indicates that osteomyelitis can be treated with antibiotics alone, challenging the traditional belief that it should always be treated with surgery and antibiotics [66, 67].

Treating increased bacterial burden and infection will lead to better chances of healing and formation of granulation tissue and wound closure. Once granulation tissue begins to appear, one may consider switching to regular advanced wound care dressings that are not impregnated with antimicrobials, but this will depend on the host's ability to fight off infection.

Moisture Balance

For many years, and following Hippocrates' teachings, it was believed that in order for a wound to heal, it should be dried and allowed to form a scab. This concept prevailed for centuries until Winter proved that allowing a wound to dry would slow the healing process [26]. Hinman later corroborated these findings on the arms of healthy volunteers where the use of occlusion with a polyurethane film helped wounds to heal faster and better [27]. The concept of moist healing was then introduced to the medical literature.

Moisture in the wound should be balanced. Uncontrolled exudate usually follows increased inflammation, and may cause maceration of the borders, new ulcer formation and loss of protein and growth factors. Therefore, achieving moisture balance by absorbing excess exudate and providing a moist environment is a goal of therapy.

For this reason, advanced dressings materials were developed to substitute for common cotton gauze that has limited absorbing capabilities and may adhere to the wound, leave residue or allow the wound to dry.

A full list of all the available dressings would be too lengthy for this chapter, but the most commonly used dressings are:

Hydrogels. Previously mentioned in the debridement section, these are gels with high amounts of water that will provide moisture to dry wounds. It may be amorphous or come in wafers.

Polyurethane films. These were the dressings first used by Winter and Hinman. Films will not allow the wound to dry and act mainly by allowing water vapor through without absorbing any fluid. This makes them ideal for wounds with very little exudate, for large amounts of exudate will cause maceration.

Hydrocolloids. Different mixtures of carboxymethyl cellulose, gelatin and pectin create a colloid that may be found in several shapes and sizes. This dressing will form a gel in contact with the exudate (the gel may have a characteristic odor and consistency) that will provide for some exudate absorption while maintaining active autolytic debridement (Fig. 13.11).

Foams. These dressings may range from high-grade polyurethane foams to some hydropolymers that absorb and lock-in exudate. They may hold large quantities of exudate according to their design and may even be used under compression. Foams may also be used as adjuvant therapy to prevent ulcer formation in patients at risk of friction or pressure (Fig. 13.12).

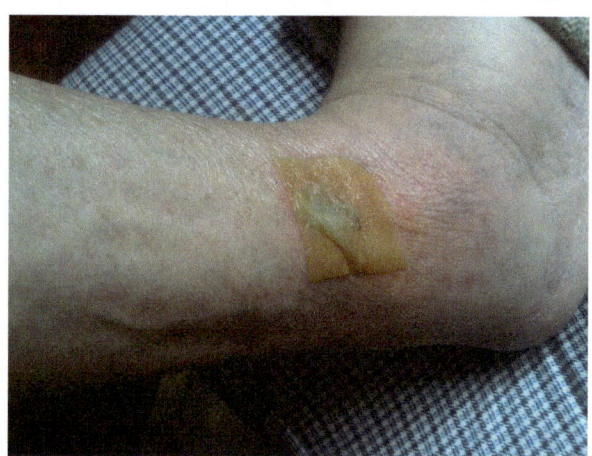

Fig. 13.11 Hydrocolloid dressing after 48 h on a lightly exudative ulcer

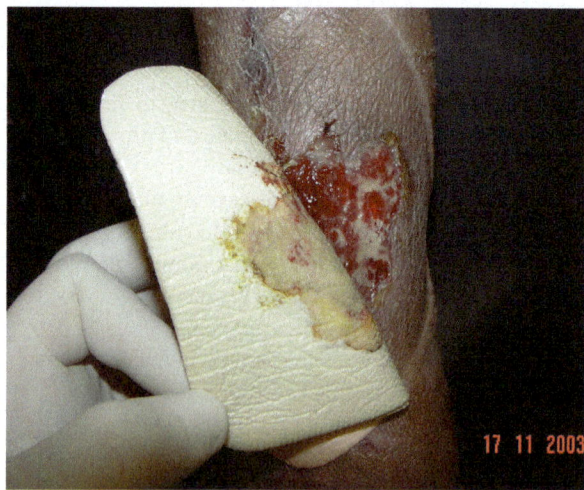

Fig. 13.12 Foam dressing on an ulcer leg

Fig. 13.13 Hydrofiber dressing applied on a wound with moderate to high exudate

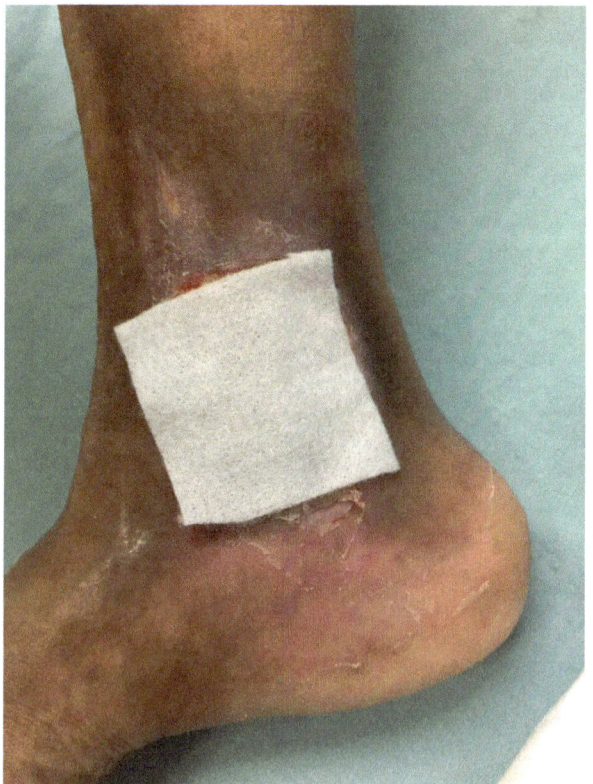

Alginates. Calcium alginate is a highly absorbing soft material that is used in wounds with heavy exudate. This compound is degradable and may be used to pack wounds safely, especially those with large amounts of drainage.

Pure carboxymethyl cellulose fibers. These dressings are also soft and highly absorbent. Their main advantage besides their absorption is that they will not diffuse the exudate beyond the border of the ulcer and are particularly helpful in preventing maceration (Fig. 13.13).

Exudate may also be controlled using devices such as negative pressure wound therapy (see below).

The use of these materials will depend on the amount of exudate, the goals of therapy and the clinician's experience. Once the properties and general principles of these dressings are understood, the clinician may either change the dressings to a less or more absorbing material or increase or decrease the number of days between dressing changes to achieve optimum moisture balance [68, 69].

Advanced Wound Care Modalities

Most wounds will heal after correcting the cause and achieve proper debridement, control of infection and inflammation and providing moist healing. However close to 10% of wounds will take much longer to heal or will require advanced wound

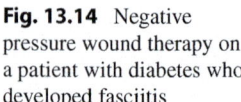

Fig. 13.14 Negative pressure wound therapy on a patient with diabetes who developed fasciitis

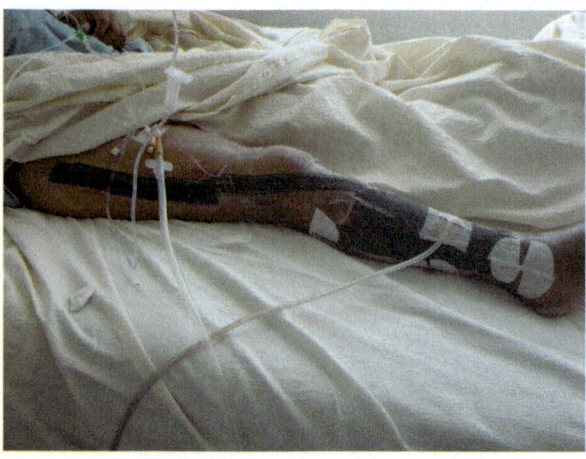

care modalities. Most of these therapies have been developed over the last 20 years and are costly, but some of them have proven to shorten healing times and are backed by strong evidence.

Negative Pressure Wound Therapy

Negative pressure wound therapy (NPWT) is the transmission of vacuum to the surface of the ulcer by means of an interphase (that may be foam or special gauze) and an advanced pump that can graduate the amount of negative pressure to be delivered. NPWT has been shown to provide many advantages on the wound bed. By creating negative pressure, it will help the wound contract towards the center of the ulcer. Granulation tissue is then stimulated through increased cell replication. Since all the exudate is collected in a canister, it will also control moisture by removing excess fluid. This removal of fluid improves local circulation and rids the wound of local lymphatic congestion and edema. Silver interphase foams are available when additional antimicrobial activity is needed [70].

Negative pressure wound therapy has shown to decrease healing times and decrease the number of complications and amputations in diabetic patients [71] (Fig. 13.14).

Hyperbaric Oxygen Therapy

Although initial hypoxia in the wound acts as a potent initiator of healing, oxygen is necessary for the synthesis of collagen and for immune cells to effectively fight back infection. Therefore, wounds that are not properly perfused will not heal, in part, due to lack of oxygenation.

Hyperbaric oxygen therapy (HBOT) is defined as "an intervention in which an individual breathes near 100% oxygen intermittently while inside a hyperbaric chamber that is pressurized to greater than sea level pressure (1 atmosphere absolute, or ATA)" [72]. By increasing the pressure, gases become more soluble and therefore oxygen concentrations in the blood and plasma will increase 1000-fold allowing for underperfused tissues to become oxygenated.

Due to the large variability of the study quality regarding HBOT, and the fact that the therapy is used for unapproved indications, controversy exists regarding its efficacy. However, recent studies have shown that the use of this modality of therapy is well indicated in diabetic foot ulcers and will improve the chances that a wound will heal [73].

Growth Factors

During the healing process, inflammatory cells will produce several growth factors to stimulate collagen synthesis, recruitment and migration of cells necessary to produce new tissue. These growth factors have several effects on the ulcer itself.

With this knowledge, recombinant growth factors have been synthesized to stimulate the wound bed to healing [74, 75]. The first product to be approved for this purpose was becaplermin, a recombinant platelet-derived growth factor. Becaplermin increases healing rate in diabetic foot ulcers and has proven to be cost-effective, however a recent black box warning by the FDA indicates that patients who underwent this therapy may have a higher risk of developing cancer.

Another growth factor that has been used in the treatment of cutaneous ulcers is recombinant epidermal growth factor. In a double-blind comparative trial using this factor, more ulcers healed in the study group than in the control group. Furthermore, recent systematic reviews have shown that this therapy is more efficacious than standard care [76].

Other growth factors have been investigated but their efficacy remains to be proven.

An old therapy that has regained some popularity is platelet-rich plasma where a gel containing activated platelets and growth factors is either injected or applied topically to the wound. Unfortunately, not enough evidence exists to regard it as useful in chronic wounds [77].

Although much more research is needed in these novel therapies, especially in the combined use of several growth factors, some of them have shown promising results.

Cutaneous Substitutes

Cutaneous substitutes are bioengineered dressings that are meant to provide temporary (or permanent) wound coverage while healing takes place. Multiple new dressings have been devised in recent years with this purpose ranging from those without living cells that act as scaffolding in the healing process and inhibit metalloproteases, to skin constructs that look and function as normal skin would [78].

Wound matrices are dressings made of substances commonly found in the dermis such as collagen, fibrin, hyaluronic acid or other components of the granulation tissue. These dressings will act as a temporary dermis allowing for cells to migrate into the matrix and create new tissue and blood vessels. These dressings may range from cadaveric dermis from donors specially prepared to become acellular to complex compounds of these molecules that may even be specifically tailored to a particular wound.

Skin constructs or substitutes consist of bio-dressings containing living cells. These living cells may be of dermal origin, such as fibroblasts, or epidermal

Fig. 13.15 Multi-layer
fibroblast construct on a
patient with a diabetic foot
ulcer

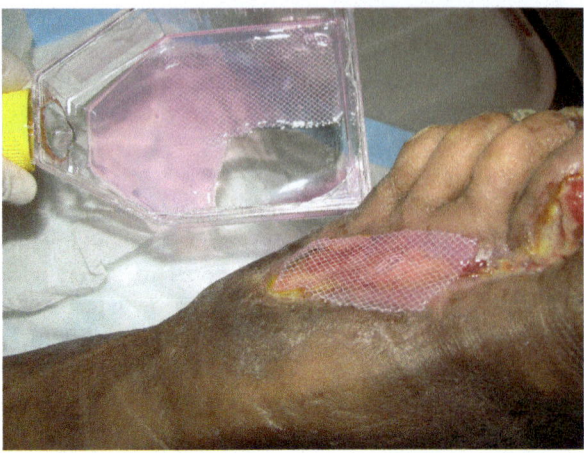

consisting of keratinocytes. The origin of these living cells may be autologous or more commonly from healthy skin donors. Therefore, most of these dressings will not become incorporated, but the living cells within will produce cytokines and growth factors that will stimulate healing while providing a temporary cover for the wound (Fig. 13.15).

Conclusions

Wound healing is a complex process that involves cellular recruitment, matrix synthesis and interactions between the host and the microbiome within the wound. In persons with Diabetes this process may become stalled due to abnormalities caused by increase blood glucose.

Given that amputations in diabetics usually follow a poorly-treated ulcer, it is important to properly assess and readily treat these patients through a multidisciplinary team.

Advanced wound care modalities have allowed to provide the best care to optimize healing, as long as the cause of the ulcer can be treated and the patient and health care team are committed to the treatment.

New technologies are becoming available that will allow for better treatment outcomes for diabetics in the future.

References

1. Schultz GS, Davidson JM, Kirsner RS, Bornstein P, Herman IM. Dynamic reciprocity in the wound microenvironment. Wound Repair Regen. 2011;19:134–48.
2. Greaves NS, Ashcroft KJ, Baguneid M, Bayat A. Current understanding of molecular and cellular mechanisms in fibroplasia and angiogenesis during acute wound healing. J Dermatol Sci. 2013;72:206–17.
3. Baltzis D, Eleftheriadou I, Veves A. Pathogenesis and treatment of impaired wound healing in diabetes mellitus: new insights. Adv Ther. 2014;31:817–36.
4. Young A, McNaught C. The physiology of wound healing. Surgery (Oxford). 2011;29:475–9.
5. Falanga V. Wound healing and its impairment in the diabetic foot. Lancet. 2005;366:1736–43.

6. Lavery LA, Armstrong DG, Wunderlich RP, Mohler MJ, Wendel CS, Lipsky BA. Risk factors for foot infections in individuals with diabetes. Diabetes Care. 2006;29:1288–93.
7. Grigoropoulou P, Eleftheriadou I, Jude EB, Tentolouris N. Diabetic foot infections: an update in diagnosis and management. Curr Diab Rep. 2017;17:3.
8. Lipsky BA, Berendt AR, Cornia PB, et al. 2012 infectious diseases society of america clinical practice guideline for the diagnosis and treatment of diabetic foot infections. J Am Podiatr Med Assoc. 2013;103:2–7.
9. Reddy M, Gill SS, Wu W, Kalkar SR, Rochon PA. Does this patient have an infection of a chronic wound. JAMA. 2012;307:605–11.
10. Aragon-Sanchez J, Lipsky BA, Lazaro-Martinez JL. Diagnosing diabetic foot osteomyelitis: is the combination of probe-to-bone test and plain radiography sufficient for high-risk inpatients. Diabet Med. 2011;28:191–4.
11. Craig AB, Strauss MB, Daniller A, Miller SS. Foot sensation testing in the patient with diabetes: introduction of the quick & easy assessment tool. Wounds. 2014;26:221–31.
12. Slater RA, Koren S, Ramot Y, Buchs A, Rapoport MJ. Interpreting the results of the Semmes-Weinstein monofilament test: accounting for false-positive answers in the international consensus on the diabetic foot protocol by a new model. Diabetes Metab Res Rev. 2014;30:77–80.
13. Sharma S, Kerry C, Atkins H, Rayman G. The Ipswich touch test: a simple and novel method to screen patients with diabetes at home for increased risk of foot ulceration. Diabet Med. 2014;31:1100–3.
14. Margolis DJ, Allen-Taylor L, Hoffstad O, Berlin JA. Diabetic neuropathic foot ulcers: the association of wound size, wound duration, and wound grade on healing. Diabetes Care. 2002;25:1835–9.
15. Jeon BJ, Choi HJ, Kang JS, Tak MS, Park ES. Comparison of five systems of classification of diabetic foot ulcers and predictive factors for amputation. Int Wound J. 2017;14:537–45.
16. Contreras-Ruiz J, Ramos-Hernandez G. Pie diabético. In: Conteras-Ruiz J, editor. Abordaje y Manejo de las Heridas. Ciudad de México: Intersistemas Editores; 2013. p. 297–326.
17. Ince B, Dadaci M, Arslan A, Altuntas Z, Evrenos MK, Fatih KM. Factors determining poor prognostic outcomes following diabetic hand infections. Pak J Med Sci. 2015;31:532–7.
18. Aydin F, Kaya A, Savran A, Incesu M, Karakuzu C, Ozturk AM. Diabetic hand infections and hyperbaric oxygen therapy. Acta Orthop Traumatol Turc. 2014;48:649–54.
19. Gupta V, Gulati N, Bahl J, Bajwa J, Dhawan N. Bullosis diabeticorum: rare presentation in a common disease. Case Rep Endocrinol. 2014;2014:862912.
20. Michael MJ, Mefford JM, Lahham S, Chandwani CE. Bullosis Diabeticorum. West J Emerg Med. 2016;17:188.
21. Wipke-Tevis DD, Rantz MJ, Mehr DR, et al. Prevalence, incidence, management, and predictors of venous ulcers in the long-term-care population using the MDS. Adv Skin Wound Care. 2000;13:218–24.
22. Alavi A, Sibbald RG, Phillips TJ, et al. What's new: management of venous leg ulcers: approach to venous leg ulcers. J Am Acad Dermatol. 2016;74:627–40. quiz 641.
23. Weir GR, Smart H, van Marle J, Cronje FJ. Arterial disease ulcers, part 1: clinical diagnosis and investigation. Adv Skin Wound Care. 2014;27:421–8. quiz 429.
24. Franklin C, Stoffels-Weindorf M, Hillen U, Dissemond J. Ulcerated necrobiosis lipoidica as a rare cause for chronic leg ulcers: case report series of ten patients. Int Wound J. 2015;12:548–54.
25. Ricci JA, Bayer LR, Orgill DP. Evidence-based medicine: the evaluation and treatment of pressure injuries. Plast Reconstr Surg. 2017;139:275e–86e.
26. Winter GD. Formation of the scab and the rate of epithelization of superficial wounds in the skin of the young domestic pig. Nature. 1962;193:293–4.
27. Hinman CD, Maibach H. Effect of air exposure and occlusion on experimental human skin wounds. Nature. 1963;200:377–8.
28. Lozano-Platonoff A, Mejia-Mendoza MD, Ibanez-Doria M, Contreras-Ruiz J. Assessment: cornerstone in wound management. J Am Coll Surg. 2015;221:611–20.
29. Mills JLS, Conte MS, Armstrong DG et al. The Society for Vascular Surgery Lower Extremity Threatened Limb Classification System: risk stratification based on wound, ischemia, and foot infection (WIfI). J Vasc Surg. 2014;59:220–34.e1–2.
30. Rumenapf G, Morbach S. What can I do with a patient with diabetes and critically impaired limb perfusion who cannot be revascularized. Int J Low Extrem Wounds. 2014;13:378–89.

31. Woo KY. Management of non-healable or maintenance wounds with topical povidone iodine. Int Wound J. 2014;11:622–6.
32. Meulepas MA, Braspenning JC, de Grauw WJ, Lucas AE, Wijkel D, Grol RP. Patient-oriented intervention in addition to centrally organised checkups improves diabetic patient outcome in primary care. Qual Saf Health Care. 2008;17:324–8.
33. Ogrin R, Houghton PE, Thompson GW. Effective management of patients with diabetes foot ulcers: outcomes of an Interprofessional Diabetes Foot Ulcer Team. Int Wound J. 2015;12:377–86.
34. Bakker K, Apelqvist J, Lipsky BA, Van Netten JJ, Schaper NC. The 2015 IWGDF guidance on the prevention and management of foot problems in diabetes. Int Wound J. 2016;13(5):1072.
35. Alavi A, Sibbald RG, Phillips TJ, et al. What's new: management of venous leg ulcers: treating venous leg ulcers. J Am Acad Dermatol. 2016;74:643–64. quiz 665.
36. Vouillarmet J, Bourron O, Gaudric J, Lermusiaux P, Millon A, Hartemann A. Lower-extremity arterial revascularization: is there any evidence for diabetic foot ulcer-healing. Diabetes Metab. 2016;42:4–15.
37. Gillespie BM, Chaboyer WP, McInnes E, Kent B, Whitty JA, Thalib L. Repositioning for pressure ulcer prevention in adults. Cochrane Database Syst Rev. 2014;CD009958.
38. Manzano F, Colmenero M, Perez-Perez AM, et al. Comparison of two repositioning schedules for the prevention of pressure ulcers in patients on mechanical ventilation with alternating pressure air mattresses. Intensive Care Med. 2014;40:1679–87.
39. Colin D, Rochet JM, Ribinik P, Barrois B, Passadori Y, Michel JM. What is the best support surface in prevention and treatment, as of 2012, for a patient at risk and/or suffering from pressure ulcer sore? Developing French guidelines for clinical practice. Ann Phys Rehabil Med. 2012;55:466–81.
40. Falanga V. Classifications for wound bed preparation and stimulation of chronic wounds. Wound Repair Regen. 2000;8(5):347.
41. Isei T, Abe M, Nakanishi T, et al. The wound/burn guidelines—3: guidelines for the diagnosis and treatment for diabetic ulcer/gangrene. J Dermatol. 2016;43:591–619.
42. Edwards J, Stapley S. Debridement of diabetic foot ulcers. Cochrane Database Syst Rev. 2010;CD003556.
43. Smith F, Dryburgh N, Donaldson J, Mitchell M. Debridement for surgical wounds. Cochrane Database Syst Rev. 2013;CD006214.
44. Sun X, Jiang K, Chen J, et al. A systematic review of maggot debridement therapy for chronically infected wounds and ulcers. Int J Infect Dis. 2014;25:32–7.
45. Steed DL, Attinger C, Colaizzi T, et al. Guidelines for the treatment of diabetic ulcers. Wound Repair Regen. 2006;14:680–92.
46. Edwards R, Harding KG. Bacteria and wound healing. Curr Opin Infect Dis. 2004;17:91–6.
47. Cutting KF, White RJ. Criteria for identifying wound infection—revisited. Ostomy Wound Manage. 2005;51:28–34.
48. Gardner SE, Frantz RA, Doebbeling BN. The validity of the clinical signs and symptoms used to identify localized chronic wound infection. Wound Repair Regen. 2001;9:178–86.
49. Snyder RJ, Bohn G, Hanft J, et al. Wound biofilm: current perspectives and strategies on biofilm disruption and treatments. Wounds. 2017;29:S1–S17.
50. Lipsky BA, Berendt AR, Deery HG, et al. Diagnosis and treatment of diabetic foot infections. Plast Reconstr Surg. 2006;117:212S–38S.
51. Lam K, van Asten SA, Nguyen T, La Fontaine J, Lavery LA. Diagnostic accuracy of probe to bone to detect osteomyelitis in the diabetic foot: a systematic review. Clin Infect Dis. 2016;63:944–8.
52. Macias Hernandez AE, Alvarez JA, Cabeza de Vaca F, et al. Microbiology of the diabetic foot: is the swab culture useful? Gac Med Mex. 2011;147:117–24.
53. Rhoads DD, Wolcott RD, Sun Y, Dowd SE. Comparison of culture and molecular identification of bacteria in chronic wounds. Int J Mol Sci. 2012;13:2535–50.
54. Health Quality Ontario. Management of chronic pressure ulcers: an evidence-based analysis. Ont Health Technol Assess Ser. 2009;9:1–203.
55. Bianchi J. Cadexomer-iodine in the treatment of venous leg ulcers: what is the evidence. J Wound Care. 2001;10:225–9.

56. Chow I, Lemos EV, Einarson TR. Management and prevention of diabetic foot ulcers and infections: a health economic review. PharmacoEconomics. 2008;26:1019–35.
57. Gethin G, Cowman S, Kolbach DN. Debridement for venous leg ulcers. Cochrane Database Syst Rev. 2015;CD008599.
58. Lipsky BA, Hoey C. Topical antimicrobial therapy for treating chronic wounds. Clin Infect Dis. 2009;49:1541–9.
59. Nelson EA, O'Meara S, Craig D, et al. A series of systematic reviews to inform a decision analysis for sampling and treating infected diabetic foot ulcers. Health Technol Assess. 2006;10. iii-iv, ix.
60. Norman G, Dumville JC, Moore ZE, Tanner J, Christie J, Goto S. Antibiotics and antiseptics for pressure ulcers. Cochrane Database Syst Rev. 2016;4:CD011586.
61. O'Meara S, Al-Kurdi D, Ovington LG. Antibiotics and antiseptics for venous leg ulcers. Cochrane Database Syst Rev. 2008;CD003557.
62. O'Meara S, Al-Kurdi D, Ologun Y, Ovington LG. Antibiotics and antiseptics for venous leg ulcers. Cochrane Database Syst Rev. 2010;CD003557.
63. O'Meara S, Al-Kurdi D, Ologun Y, Ovington LG, Martyn-St James M, Richardson R. Antibiotics and antiseptics for venous leg ulcers. Cochrane Database Syst Rev. 2013;CD003557.
64. O'Meara S, Al-Kurdi D, Ologun Y, Ovington LG, Martyn-St James M, Richardson R. Antibiotics and antiseptics for venous leg ulcers. Cochrane Database Syst Rev. 2014;CD003557.
65. Ubbink DT, Westerbos SJ, Evans D, Land L, Vermeulen H. Topical negative pressure for treating chronic wounds. Cochrane Database Syst Rev. 2008;CD001898.
66. Lazaro-Martinez JL, Aragon-Sanchez J, Garcia-Morales E. Antibiotics versus conservative surgery for treating diabetic foot osteomyelitis: a randomized comparative trial. Diabetes Care. 2014;37:789–95.
67. Tone A, Nguyen S, Devemy F, et al. Six-week versus twelve-week antibiotic therapy for non-surgically treated diabetic foot osteomyelitis: a multicenter open-label controlled randomized study. Diabetes Care. 2015;38:302–7.
68. Broussard KC, Powers JG. Wound dressings: selecting the most appropriate type. Am J Clin Dermatol. 2013;14:449–59.
69. Powers JG, Morton LM, Phillips TJ. Dressings for chronic wounds. Dermatol Ther. 2013;26:197–206.
70. Huang C, Leavitt T, Bayer LR, Orgill DP. Effect of negative pressure wound therapy on wound healing. Curr Probl Surg. 2014;51:301–31.
71. Liu S, He CZ, Cai YT, et al. Evaluation of negative-pressure wound therapy for patients with diabetic foot ulcers: systematic review and meta-analysis. Ther Clin Risk Manag. 2017;13:533–44.
72. Stoekenbroek RM, Santema TB, Legemate DA, Ubbink DT, van den Brink A, Koelemay MJ. Hyperbaric oxygen for the treatment of diabetic foot ulcers: a systematic review. Eur J Vasc Endovasc Surg. 2014;47:647–55.
73. Kranke P, Bennett MH, Martyn-St James M, Schnabel A, Debus SE, Weibel S. Hyperbaric oxygen therapy for chronic wounds. Cochrane Database Syst Rev. 2015;CD004123.
74. Marti-Carvajal AJ, Gluud C, Nicola S et al. Growth factors for treating diabetic foot ulcers. Cochrane Database Syst Rev. 2015;CD008548.
75. Yang S, Geng Z, Ma K, Sun X, Fu X. Efficacy of topical recombinant human epidermal growth factor for treatment of diabetic foot ulcer: a systematic review and meta-analysis. Int J Low Extrem Wounds. 2016;15:120–5.
76. Gomez-Villa R, Aguilar-Rebolledo F, Lozano-Platonoff A, et al. Efficacy of intralesional recombinant human epidermal growth factor in diabetic foot ulcers in Mexican patients: a randomized double-blinded controlled trial. Wound Repair Regen. 2014;22:497–503.
77. Martinez-Zapata MJ, Marti-Carvajal AJ, Sola I, et al. Autologous platelet-rich plasma for treating chronic wounds. Cochrane Database Syst Rev. 2012;10:CD006899.
78. Snyder DL, Sullivan N, Schoelles KM. Skin substitutes for treating chronic wounds. 2012.

Vascular and Neuropathic Foot

14

Adolfo V. Zavala

Diabetic foot is one of the most frequent complications of diabetes, with a high morbimortality, with important health cost, and causing alterations in the quality of life of the patients.

The presence of an ulcer in the feet indicates a high risk of amputation and death. Fifty percent of patients with it die within the next 5 years.

Patients with a history of foot ulcers have a high risk of ulcer recurrence or the involvement of the collateral limb. Therefore, the patient must be considered at a great risk of developing ulcers, and protective and corrective measures must be indicated so that he does not ulcerate.

Diabetic foot is the distal ankle involvement, caused by various causes, mainly due to the interaction of peripheral vasculopathy, neuropathy and alterations in foot biodynamics.

By decreasing the vitality of the foot, and lack of recognition of trauma due to loss of protective sensitivity, pre ulcerative lesions are caused, which, if not detected and treated in time, ulcerate, become infected, causing necrosis leading to amputation, and even the loss of the patient's life.

It is noteworthy that injuries do not occur suddenly, that there is a timeline for the diabetic foot, which must be known to avoid its progression.

We highlight what Bernard Swan said: "I marvel at how much people pay for cutting a leg, and how little they pay to avoid it."

A.V. Zavala
Diabetic Foot and Vasculopathies Clinic at Diabetes Division, Internal Medicine Department,
Hospital de Clínicas José de San Martín, University of Buenos Aires,
Buenos Aires, Argentina
e-mail: info@fuedin.org; fpuchulu@gmail.com

© Springer International Publishing AG 2018   225
E.N. Cohen Sabban et al. (eds.), *Dermatology and Diabetes*,
https://doi.org/10.1007/978-3-319-72475-1_14

Neuropathic Foot

Neuropathy is one of the most frequent complications, being able to be present in more than 50% of diabetics, after 10 years of the disease. The prevalence depends on the diagnostic methods used, increasing when using electromyogram and biopsy.

It can be asymptomatic and is the cause of 80% of foot ulcers (60% pure neuropathic and 20% neuroischemic).

It is noteworthy that it can be present and be asymptomatic, and this is one of the causes of the lesions when the patient does not recognize the presence of pathology and consequently do not take preventive measures, which is why the annual examination of lower limbs is emphasized. By itself, it increases morbidity and mortality, being associated with other complications of diabetes.

The calcification of the middle tunic (Monkerberg's disease) is more frequent in diabetics than in the general population, its pathogenesis is not known with certainty. Edmons et al. argue that it is produced by neuropathy, which we corroborated in a study in diabetics patients with or without calcification. The denervation of arterial walls alters tissue oxygenation, with lack of blood flow regulation, and thus facilitates arterial calcification, with an auto-sympathectomy.

Neuropathy is caused by the individual or associated action of the following processes: sorbitol accumulation, reduction of nerve myo-inositol, reduction in synthesis, quantity and transport of intra-axonal proteins, reduction of ATPase Na/K in the nerve, reduction of the incorporation of glycolipids and amino acids to the myelin, excessive accumulation of glycogen, increased glycosylation of nerve proteins, and nerve hypoxia.

In addition to hyperglycemia, there has been an increased incidence of neuropathy in patients with increased elevated total cholesterol and LDL, increased triglycerides, increased BMI, high levels of von Willebrand factor, microalbuminuria, hypertension and smoking. This highlights the need of a good metabolic control and the reduction of cardiovascular risks factors.

The pathophysiology of neuropathy is not well understood, and is due to metabolic alterations triggered by hyperglycemia. We observe in the figure these alterations: (Fig. 14.1).

To highlight is the elevation of four metabolic pathways:

1. Polyols pathways, with the increase of the sorbitol and decrease of the myo-inositol. This causes increase of the nerve edema and a decrease of the sodium potassium pump.
2. Glycosylation of the nerve proteins (axon and myelin)
3. Oxidative stress, by increasing reactive oxygen species (ROS).
4. Alterations of the δ-6-desaturase, causing prostacyclins decrease and thromboxane increase.

There would be other factors that contribute to nerve damage, such as deficiency of essential fatty acids, immunological and haemorreological alterations.

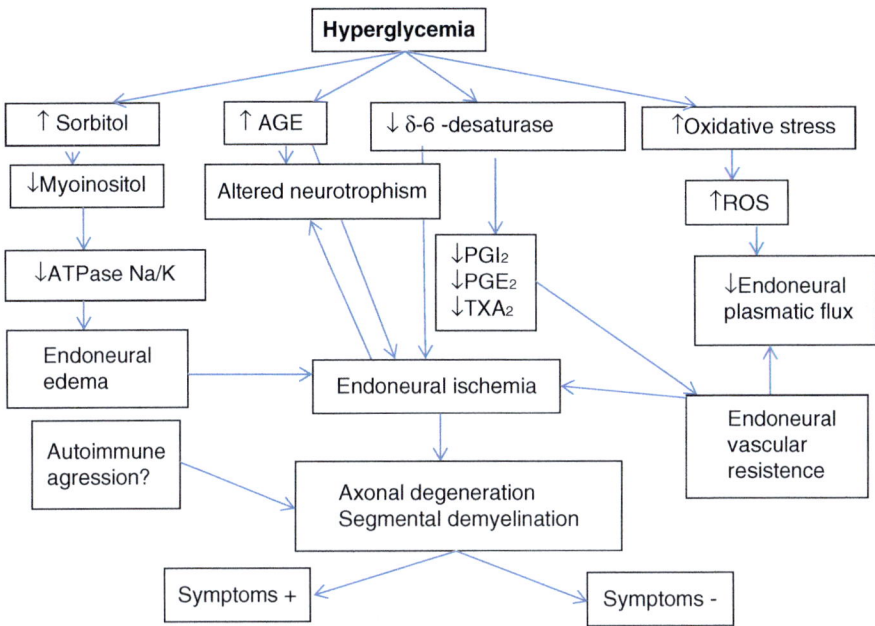

Fig. 14.1 Possible mechanisms by which hyperglycemia determines neuropathy

Table 14.1 Differences between acute and chronic sensitive neuropathy

	Acute sensitive neuropathy	Chronic sensitive motor neuropathy
Start mode	Fast	Insidious, slow
Symptoms	Severe pain and terebrante	Paresthesia, numbness
Severity symptoms	+++	0 to ++

Types of Neuropathy

Neuropathy can affect the foot of the diabetic by individual action or in conjunction with the following categories:

Sensitive Neuropathy

Premature cramps occur specially at night, sensation of walking on cottons, hypoaesthesia and hyperesthesia.

Sensory fibers are affected, losing protection to external and internal aggressions (loss of protective sensitivity).

Sensitivity is altered: tactile, valued with the Semmes-Weinstein filament, vibratory sensitivity (tuning fork or biothesiometer), thermal sensitivity, sensitivity to pain and osteotendinous reflexes.

Acute sensitive neuropathy should be differentiated from chronic, as seen in the Table 14.1.

Motor Neuropathy

The foot muscles (interosseous and lumbrical) are especially affected. This does not permit the toes separation, favoring the action of the extensor tendon, which produces the hammer or claw toes. Foot support points are altered, and chronic hypersupport may result in mallet toes.

Motor neuropathy is potentiated with sarcopenia, which is more frequent in old people, sedentary, with poor diets and with associated chronic pathologies, especially nephropathy.

Autonomic Neuropathy

The skin is dry, with hyperkeratosis, hot with venous dilatation. The temperature is increased and the calcification of the interosseous is favored.

The temperature is elevated and in patches, caused by the increase of flow and the presence of arteriovenous shunt. This causes auto-sypathectomy with calcification of the middle tunic of the vessels.

Osteoarthropathy

With autonomic neuropathy, osteopenia is produced, which facilitates osteoarticular alterations.

The most common involvement is the ankle joint, tarsometatarsal and metatarsophalangeal. It is especially seen in poorly controlled diabetics with peripheral and autonomic neuropathy.

There is hyperkeratosis and edema of the foot, usually without pain. It should be suspected in every patient with long-term Diabetes, with a hot and swollen foot, with peripheral and autonomic neuropathy, with other diabetic complications. Dislocations and fractures occurs which, if not diagnosed early, can produce permanent deformations with metatarsal overloaded and recurrent ulcers.

Neurological Evaluation

For the diagnosis of peripheral neuropathy, a complete clinical and instrumental examination should be performed. It should be done once a year to all diabetic patients despite been asymptomatic, and should be performed more frequently in the presence of symptoms.

Neuropathy should be suspected in long-standing, poorly controlled diabetic patients and with other diabetic complications. In many cases it can be asymptomatic, so it is always necessary to evaluate with instrumental maneuvers.

- Symptoms: pain, especially nocturnal leg cramps, hypoesthesia and hyperesthesia, pallesthesia, tingling, coldness sensation, walking on cotton sensation, etc.
- Evaluation of motor neuropathy: atrophy of the interosseous and lumbrical muscles. Evaluate the magnitude of the muscle strength, the walk and the spreading of the toes. Photo: normal case before separating the toes, and then opening them. In cases of pathological spreading sign, it must be evaluated if there is atrophy of the interosseous spaces (Fig. 14.2).

Before separating fingers   Normal: separate fingers

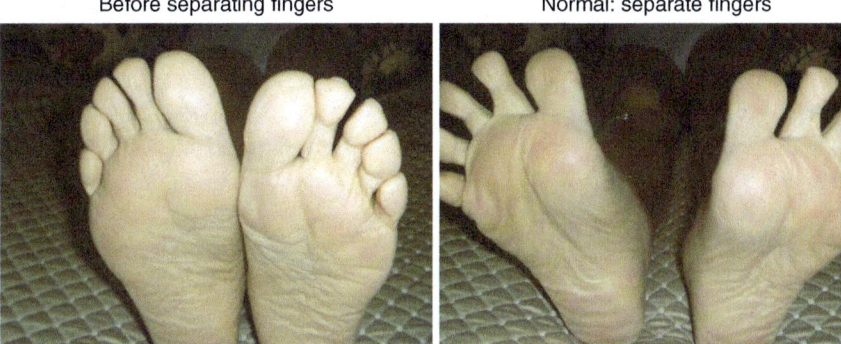

Fig. 14.2 Evaluation of motor neuropathy (**a**) before separating fingers; (**b**) normal: separate fingers

- In the autonomic neuropathy the skin is hot with venous dilatation. At first is hyperhidrosis, but subsequently is dry, it develops an auto-sympathectomy. It is manifested by the decrease or absence of secretion of the sweat and sebaceous glands, causing a decrease in the cutaneous trophism and favoring trophic lesions and/or infections. It is very useful in these cases to measure the temperature by hand and if possible with infrared thermometers, which are more accurate.
- There are other instruments to measure the temperature, including a new podimetric system, which is a mat that marks the temperature, predicting 97% of the recurrence of ulcers.

Score of Sensory Signs

Several scores can be made, we use the University of Texas guidelines, assessing sensitivity to pain, discrimination against cold and heat, vibratory sensitivity, tactile sensitivity with Semmens Weinstein 5.07 monofilament and aquilian reflex.

At least the tactile sensitivity should be measured with the Semmens Weinstein filament (high predictability), vibration sensitivity with the 128 Hz tuning fork or a quantitative meter (Biothesiometer) and the temperature with the infrared thermometer. The latter is highly predictive of the risk of developing ulcers in cases of pre-ulcerative lesions, especially with bone deformations and hyperkeratosis.

Can be seen in the photo, an infrared thermometer, in some countries, patients are indicated to buy it to control their foot temperature. If bone deformities exist, with hyperkeratosis and one or more degree centigrade difference with another zone, it indicates a high risk of ulceration. The patients should rest and consult to the health team. Consensuses mention that it is the most accurate and predictive method of the risk of ulceration.

It is of great value also in the Charcot's foot. In this case, the difference of 2°Centigrades from one zone to another indicates oxidative stress, specific to the acute stage of the disease and when the remission stage begins (Fig. 14.3).

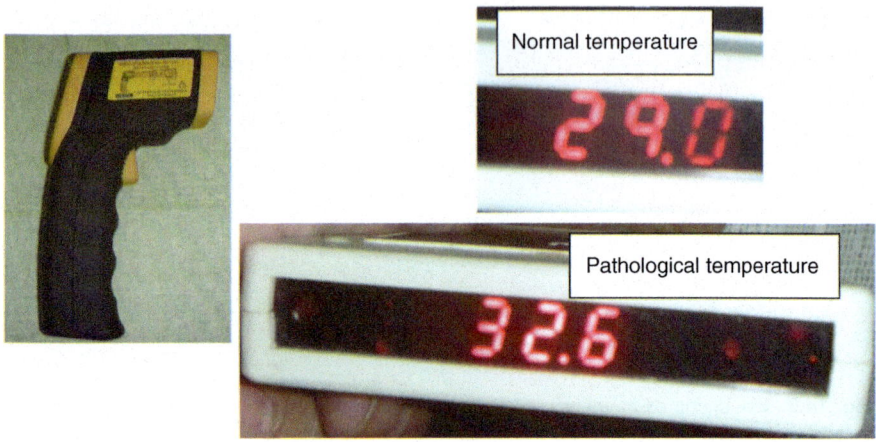

Fig. 14.3 Accessible thermometer. One or more degree centigrade difference with another zone, indicates a high risk of ulceration

Foot Temperature Control

Sensitive Score

There are several schemes; we recommend the evaluation of ten places of the foot (first, third and fifth finger, first, third and fifth metatarsal head, inner edge of foot, external edge foot, heel and back foot. Score and add both feet: 0–3 normal, 3–6 slight alteration, 6–9 moderate alteration and more than 9, lack of protective sensitivity.

This facilitates the production of internal or external traumas, which are warned belatedly by the patient. The diabetic patients can have a bone fracture and continue walking on the affected leg.

- Cold heat sensitivity: Normal 0, pathological 1.
- Pain sensitivity: Normal 0, pathological 1.
- Vibrational sensitivity: Normal 1, pathological 1.
- Tactile sensitivity: Normal 0, altered in some places 1, further altered in most places 2.
- Aquilian reflex: normal 0, decreased 1, absent 2 points.

The Latin American Association of Diabetes states that sensitivity tests can be done in three places (first, third and fifth finger). If there are diagnostic doubts, it is better to do the score in the ten places mentioned.

The autonomics tests and sensory and motor nerve conduction speed with electromyogram are not routine studies in the evaluation of patients, and should be done in case of diagnostic doubts.

Instrumental Studies

- Pallesthesia quantitative measuring devices: the biothesiometer is an objective method of assessment, a threshold lower than 15 mV is normal, and it is pathological when it exceeds 25 mV
- Infrared thermometry. The normal temperature of the skin is between 28 and 31°C. Less than 26° indicates ischemia and there is inflammation when it exceeds 31.5°C. In case of neuropathy, the temperature is not uniform and there may be an elevation of 1–2°C in an area with bone deformation and hyperkeratosis. As mentioned above, this indicates oxidative stress, and a high risk of ulceration.

In Charcot's foot, the temperature is not uniform and there are 2°C more in the affected area. It is an early sign of activity; and the coalescence stage when the temperature decreases.

Electromyogram
It should be done with motor and sensory nerve conduction velocity. Must evaluate the proximal and distal latency, the evoked potentials and the spontaneous activity.

The electromyogram shows fibrillation, loss of motor units, potential for reinnervation and slower conduction velocity. The major compromise is in the distal muscles, with predominance of the lower limbs.

Changes in conduction velocity may reflect underlying pathological structural changes of axons, such as demyelination and atrophy.

These findings suggest a diffuse abnormality of the peripheral nerves function, being able to show subclinical damage in asymptomatic patients.

Neuropathy Classification

According to the findings the patients can be classified:

- **Without clinic neuropathy**: without symptoms, without motor or autonomics signs and a sensitive score lower than 3, being doubtful between 3 and 6. If there are no pathologies, foot must be controlled annually.
- **With clinical neuropathy**: symptoms, other signs and a sensitive score greater than 6. Optimal control of Diabetes, etiological treatment of neuropathy (gamma linoleic or alpha lipoic acid, vitamin E, magnesium), orthosis if indicated and protector shoes should be done. Extreme care of the foot and control of risk factors. Patients should be monitored every 3 months.
- **With severe neuropathy**: With rest pain, ulcers, deformations, Charcot's foot. Treatment must include, local treatment, insoles if necessary, correction of eventual deformations, etc. It is important to consult a team specialized in diabetic foot. Control monthly and after the improvement every 3 months.

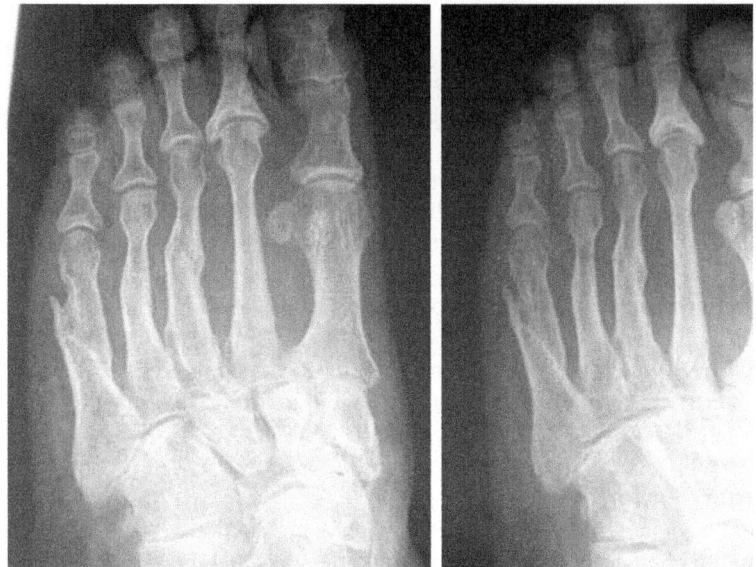

Fig. 14.4 Radiography of a patient with consolidated fractures, in the stage of remission

Charcot's Foot

Is the chronic affection of bones, joints and soft tissues, produced by peripheral and autonomic neuropathy, characterized by an inflammatory process in the initial stages, with the development of bone loss, joint dislocation and fixed deformations.

It is often not diagnosed, with a prevalence of 0.4–13%, increasing to 29%, using radiography, and higher prevalence with nuclear resonance (Fig. 14.4).

Physiopathology

Several factors contribute to its determinism, considering two theories: neuro-traumatic and neuro-vascular due to sympathectomy.

It is currently considered that in susceptible individuals with peripheral neuropathy, an inflammatory process is developed, by activation of the polypeptide receptor activator of nuclear factor kappa B ligand (RANKL), which causes maturation of the osteoclasts. At the same time the nuclear factor kb (NF-kB) stimulates osteoprotegerin production of osteoblasts. The repetitive trauma with lack of pain induces the production of inflammatory cytokines and osteoclasts, causing local osteolysis.

Another possible cause is the decreased secretion of the calcitonin gene, in addition to protein glycosylation, the oxidative stress and the oxidized lipids.

Diagnosis

In the presence of neuropathy, especially autonomic, the clinical presentation with edema, erythema and an increase of 2 °C in the area makes the diagnosis of Charcot's foot.

The radiograph has little sensitivity and its alteration is delayed, being more specific the nuclear magnetic resonance.

Both radiography and nuclear magnetic resonance have different sensitivity according to the stage of development, coalescence or reconstruction.

Treatment

The treatment is conservative, being emphasized the immobilization, the gold standard of the treatment is the total contact cast. Initially it must be changed within 3–7 days, and then every 15 days. Once in the stage of reconstruction, according to the present deformations it must be indicated supportive insoles to correct structural misalignment and orthopedic shoes. In many cases, the patellar dislocation discharge boot is necessary.

Another not so effective possibility is the CROW (Walker).

Bisphosphonates and calcitonin may be indicated to improve osteopenia, and in cases of irreducible deformations, with recurrent ulcers, corrective surgeries must be considered.

Treatment of Neuropathy

The first and fundamental treatment is the improvement of diabetes control, nutrition status and cardiovascular risk factors.

In addition to these measures, normalization of altered metabolic pathways (sorbitol pathway, oxidative stress, proteins glycation, etc.) should be achieved and avoid its consequences. There is evidence of the beneficial effect of lipoic acid.

Haemorheological changes must be improved, avoiding anoxia.

Indication of a healthy diet, with antioxidants, and must be considered the supplementation of taurine, essential fatty acids and myoinositol.

In case of painful neuropathy, the nocturnal pain must be treated to improve quality of life. Can be used antidepressants, mexitilen, pregabalin, opioids, alone or in combination. In specific cases, electrostimulation or nerve blockade are indicated.

Protective and corrective measures are fundamental in order to avoid ulcers.

Early detection is crucial for early immobilization (total contact cast) to avoid deformation.

Must be taken into account that patients who have had a standing ulcer have 50–70% chance of a new ulcer, dying the 50% of the patients in 5 years.

The use of arginine, and nerve growth factors has been postulated.

In case of ulcers, the area must be protected, correct the structural misalignment and the excessive contact, debride all necrotic, hyperkeratotic and devitalized tissues. If there is infection, a tissue sample cultivation must be done with antibiogram, taking the sample with scraping, curettage or biopsy. Gram staining and a colony count should be done, and according to the result, a suitable antibiotic plan, which should be assessed according to the clinical response.

If there is associated osteomyelitis, it is essential to discharge, remove all necrotic bone and establish and adequate antibiotics treatment. According on the depth of the ulcer and the progression, larger debridement, or partial amputations, may arise.

Vascular Foot

Vascular alteration of the lower limbs is less frequent than neuropathy, but is more serious because of the risk of gangrene, with more immediate and long-term mortality, with healing delay, and a higher percentage of amputations.

Approximately 30% of diabetic patients develop peripheral arteriopathy.

In the NHANES study of 1999–2004, was found a prevalence of 5.9% of peripheral vasculopathy (valued with ankle/arm indexes less than 0.9).

Non-diabetics have more affected the aortoiliac or femoral territory. In diabetes is more prevalent the distal affectation or a multiple compromise.

Vasculopathy appears at earlier ages, with several territories affected, and in each area more diseased arteries, with pathology in collaterals, and coronary disease; not being difference between sexes.

20% of people aged over 65 have evidence of peripheral vasculopathy, and only a quarter have symptoms. In the presence of peripheral vascular disease, it is necessary to search the affectation of other territories, especially the heart.

As already mentioned, the international consensus on diabetic foot advises that all diabetics undertake an annually comprehensive foot examination, including vascular evaluation at rest and after exercise. Perform the clinical examination, and the ankle- brachial pressure index. Interrogate on intermittent claudication and resting pain.

Peripheral vasculopathy is more frequent in poorly controlled diabetics with higher cardiovascular risk factors, with greater morbimortality, even if it is asymptomatic. It also has higher mortality than several types of cancer, which highlights its early search and appropriate treatment.

In the BARI 2D study, it was found that every 1% increase in glycosylated hemoglobin it was associated with the 21% increase of peripheral vasculopathy risk at a 5-year follow-up. Diabetic patients have a 50% higher risk of having amputations when they have peripheral vasculopathy.

The prevention of peripheral vasculopathy would be oriented to the intensive treatment of cardiovascular risk factors, and the vascular assessment of the patient should be performed in an integral manner.

Similarly in diabetics as in non-diabetics, the value of vascular risk factors for the development and recurrence of peripheral vasculopathy has been shown; classical risk factors: smoking, dyslipemias, hypertension, obesity, sedentarism, hyperuricemia, microalbuminuria and duration of diabetes; chronic inflammation and oxidative stress, has now been highlighted.

Other factors are associated with hyperglycemia such as: (1) typical diabetic metabolic modifications; (2) variation of insulin levels, (3) microangiopathy and microcirculation disorders; (4) hormonal modifications; and (5) metabolic alterations of the arterial wall, with greater platelet adhesiveness and aggregation, with thrombogenesis increase.

There is a greater susceptibility to complications in certain individuals, relating to family history and various metabolic pathways, especially the decline of antioxidant enzymes.

The natural evolution of 10-year vasculopathy is that of 20 patients, 12 die of vascular events in the heart, brain or aorta, four remain stable, one will need amputation and three vascular surgery.

The early detection of peripheral vasculopathy is essential, to control cardiovascular risk factors and the diabetes, by maximizing the protective and corrective measures of ulcers.

Disease progression, correlates with poor diabetes control, LDL cholesterol elevation, oxidative stress and smoking. This is more atherogenic in diabetics than in the general population, in addition to damage of the endothelium, increases insulin resistance and delays the healing of ulcers.

Classification of Peripheral Vasculopathy

WHO indicates that the peripheral vascular disease presents these stages:

(0) Normal. (1) Asymptomatic foot, but lesion is demonstrated with special studies. (2) Intermittent claudication. (3) Resting pain of ischemic origin. (4) Necrosis or gangrene.

It is common the description of the intermittent claudication pain. It is a pain that appears with the walk and disappears when you suspend it, calming the pain immediately when stopping walking, not needing to lie down or raise the leg.

The most common location is at calf level, but may appear in other areas (buttock, thigh, feet) indicating the area of stenosis. Aortoiliac lesions affect the buttocks or thigh. The femoris in the calf, and those of the tibial peroneal trunk are expressed in the ankle and foot.

Resting pain indicates greater severity of ischemia and a greater need for surgical help. It appears when the patient adopts the horizontal position, relieving himself in the seated position. This is transitory, as it can cause edema, which aggravates ischemia.

Resting pain worsens with cold or walking; being important to differentiate with the resting pain of neuritic origin. For the differential diagnosis, clinical facts must be taken into account, complementing with the doppler flow study. An ankle/arm index greater than 0.50 or an ankle absolute pressure of 90 mmHg is indicative that such pain cannot be due to ischemia.

In any foot lesion, should be determined, if there is critical ischemia with clinical and ankle/arm or finger/arm indices, the patient must be evaluated by a vascular surgery team.

Other Classification

Some authors consider that the WHO classification offers doubts in the clinical management of the patients, so we classify the peripheral vasculopathy in: (a) Normal. (b) Asymptomatic vasculopathy. (c) Clinical vasculopathy (symptoms or signs). (d) Severe ischemia.

It is considered that there is severe ischemia when there is resting pain, ulcers of more than 10 weeks of evolution without improvement with an adequate treatment, necrosis that progresses, ankle/arm index lower than 0.5 and finger/arm index less than 0.3, and transcutaneous oxygen tension less than 30 mmHg.

Valuation of Ischemia

- Symptoms: presence of cold feet and legs, heaviness, intermittent claudication, resting pain mainly at night.
- Skin examination: The skin is cold, shiny, and atrophic, with diminished nail growth, lack of hairs, especially on the fingers (the presence of hairs indicates adequate blood flow). There is also atrophy and loss of subcutaneous fat in the dorsum of the feet.
- The temperature is decreased, less than 26°C with the infrared thermometer, in a room with an adequate temperature.
- Pulse, murmurs, venous filling and capillary refill should be examined at rest and if there are doubts (especially in type 2 diabetic patients, elderly and long-term diabetic patients) the examination must be performed after an exercise or an hyperemia test.
- Take the ankle/arm index, and finger/arm index, with a bidirectional doppler. Pressure controls can also be performed on other areas of the leg and thigh (see below).
- In suspected cases of severe ischemia, pulse waves can be seen, and in more complex equipment, the plethysmographic waves and the evaluation of the transcutaneous oxygen tension.

Ischemia Degrees

According to the findings we classified the patients in:

- **No significant ischemia**: Without signs or symptoms, the ankle /arm index is higher than 0.9, the finger/arm index higher than 0.5 and the transcutaneous oxygen tension over 60 mmHg. Improve diabetes control, foot control (insoles, hyperkeratosis, nails care, fungal infections, etc.) and the correction of cardio-vascular risk factors is indicated; patients should be monitored annually.

- **Clinical ischemia**: There is intermittent claudication or some pathological find-ing (pulses, murmurs, etc.). The ankle/arm index is between 0.9 and 0.5, the finger/arm index between 0.5 and 0.3, and the oxygen tension between 30 and 60 mmHg. In addition to the measures to be taken in the previous category, it is necessary to indicate the vasculopathy treatment (hygienic dietary and vasoac-tive measures), extreme foot care and control it every 3 months.

- **With severe ischemia**: have resting pain, especially nocturnal, necrosis and gan-grene. The ankle/arm and finger/arm indices, and the oxygen tension are lower than the previous category. They must be studied to evaluate whether angioplasty and/or bypass can be performed. If after the procedure there is remaining isch-emia, the intravenous prostaglandins treatment is a possibility, and if there is no improvement, consider amputation. Diabetes care, cardiovascular risk factors and foot care must be extreme to avoid recurrence and the involvement of another member; as well as death due to a vascular episode (cardiac, cerebral or abdominal).

Special Studies

Noninvasive

Doppler Indices
Although there are no symptoms or signs for all diabetics over 35 years of age or with more than 10 years of evolution of the disease, annual determination of ankle and arm pressure must be done with the bidirectional doppler. It is done at rest and if there are doubts, after exercise or the test of hyperemia.

There is autonomic neuropathy in many diabetics, which leads to false positive results due to the opening of the arteriovenous shunt and the calcification of the interosseous arteries. In that case it is more valuable to do the finger/arm index.

Ankle/Arm and Finger/Arm Indices
The pedis and tibial pressure is taken, and the highest value is divided on the arm highest value. A suitable gel should be used, and place the sensor with an adequate pressure and at a 45° angle. The doppler first signal appearance indicates the pres-sure which must be registered and calculate the ratio with the arm values.

The handle of the gauge should be two centimeters above the malleolus in the leg and sensors in the pedis, or the tibial arteries. At the arm 2 cm above the arm bend and the sensor is placed in the radial artery.

The **index values** are:

- Ankle/arm (brachial) index:
  - Normal: 0.91–1.30
  - Clinical ischemia: 0.5–0.9

- Severe ischemia: <0.5
- False positive (autonomic neuropathy, interosseous calcification) over 1.30.
• Finger/arm index:
  - Normal: >0.5
  - Clinical ischemia: 0.3–0.5.
  - Severe ischemia: <0.3.

Sometimes **absolute pressures** must be considered:

• In order to cure an injury to the foot there must be at least an ankle pressure over 50 mmHg.
• In order to cure an injury to the finger, there must be a finger pressure over 30 mmHg.
• An ankle pressure of 90 mmHg discards an ischemic resting pain and suggests a good vascularization for an infrapatellar amputation.
• In case of uncontrolled arterial hypertension, with high arm values, is convenient to consider the absolute pressure at the ankle to evaluate the perfusion.
• Pressure can be taken on the upper and lower thigh and on the calf, determining the segmental pressures, thus suggesting the occlusion site a drop of more than 30 mm of Hg between each sector.
• A thigh index of 1.20 or more indicates the absence of a significant aorto-iliac obstruction. An index of 0.80–1.20 suggests an important but not complete aorto-iliac stenosis and an index of less than 0.80 indicates a probable complete occlusion.
• At the calf level the normal index is from 1 to 1.30; a value from 0.65 to 1 suggests incomplete occlusion of the distal femoral. A complete obstruction at this level is found with an index <0.65.
• At the ankle the normal index is from 1 to 1.30. Incomplete obstruction: 0.5–1, and a complete obstruction of the tibial peroneal trunk or its branches: <0.5.
• As mentioned in pulses and murmurs, the flow study by doppler can show normal values at rest, so it must be done after an exercise or the hyperemia test. The normal result of these test is the increase of the pulse and lower limb pressures. In the case of peripheral arteriopathy, four types of results can be found:
  - Type I: there is a very slight pressure elevation that produces the disappearance of diastolic sound.
  - Type II: the pressure falls, almost 50% of the initial value, but with recovery in 5 min.
  - Type III: there is a more than 50% decrease in pressure values recovering the initial values after 10 min.
  - Type IV: systolic blood pressure drops to almost zero, with a very slow recovery to baseline values (more than 15 min).

Pulse Wave. Plethysmography

The determination of the pulse wave can recognize the arterial stiffness. The normal wave is three phasic, being altered according rigidity and obstruction in biphasic, monophasic and disappearing.

The pneumoplethysmography evaluates the volume changes of the limb according to the systole and diastole; and photoplethysmography studies the change in volume of blood passing through the capillaries.

In each of them are four types of waves: normal, without the dicrotic sign, flattened and lack of wave.

Transcutaneous Oxygen Tension (TCOM)

Is a non-invasive method of measuring the oxygen level of the tissue below the skin. Since oxygen is carried by the blood, TCOM can be used as an indirect measure of blood flow to the tissue. Since blood flow is important for wound healing, TCOM is often used to gauge the ability of tissue to effectively heal.

The transcutaneous oxygen tension may decrease because of the less saturation due to respiratory or cardiac problems, by peripheral vasculopathy, by tissue edema, by microangiopathy, peripheral neuropathy with autonomic alteration with opening of arteriovenous shunts, infections with increased oxygen demand with oxidative stress and local compression (osseous enhancements).

The normal transcutaneous oxygen tension is >60 mmHg, indicating ischemia when it is <30 mmHg. To be healed an amputation there must be a minimum tension in the cutting area of 20 mmHg.

Keep in mind that when an amputation is done, it has to be an adequate flow in the distal area, being useful this study.

In the area to be amputated infection must not exist and we should think about the functionality, the orthosis and avoiding new areas of repeated friction or pressure. The younger the patient's the more the function should be valued.

To amputate it must be extreme the control of Diabetes and the nutritional status, the early rehabilitation of the patient and the prevention of the lesion recurrence and the involvement of the contralateral foot are the clue of a successful treatment.

Contrast Studies

When there is a severe ischemia, in danger of losing the leg and/or life, it must be considered the vascular permeability and the possibility to perform arterial surgery. This requires a contrast arteriography, digital angiography or magnetic resonance angiography.

In order to make an arteriography the contrast substance can be introduced into the artery through the direct injection due to vessel puncture, but it is more convenient introducing a catheter.

The study of the vessels can be done perfectly with this procedure, having very little morbimortality, probably related to the team's experience than the procedure itself.

One advantage of catheterization methods are that allows the study of other vascular territories simultaneously, especially cardiac, carotid arteries, brain and abdomen.

It is essential the visualization of the distal vessels. When there is a chronic arteriopathy it should always be seen contrast substance in the main trunks or collaterals, but the absolute absence of contrast in the leg and/or foot only indicates that insufficient quantity was injected or that the exposure of the radiography was untimely. It should always try to include the foot in the studio, but when it isn't seen permeable vessels useful for the reconstruction in the leg it should be required the presence of contrast in it, either in the collaterals or demonstrating a pedis, posterior tibial or plantar that allows a bypass.

The arterioscopy allows observing the permeability, the vessel diameter and also a stent application.

The magnetic resonance image (MRI), with or without contrast offers a better visualization of the arteries, with less contrast and rays exposure.

Treatment of Vasculopathy

It is also important the adequate control of Diabetes and the cardiovascular risk factors.

Careful must be taken with the use of inhibitors of sodium glucose transport (SGLT2), which may increase the risk of amputations.

It was observed the preventive and curative effect of a diet rich in vegetables and fruits, being detrimental exaggerated red and processed meat consumption.

Very useful is the realization of physical activity. Although patients have intermittent claudication, it must be emphasized walking. It has been observed that tolerance to walk becomes better with simple stretching exercises of the calf. This improves vascular endothelial function, which improves the ability to walk.

Walk works best when exercise lasts a minimum of 30 min, it may be staggered due to pain.

The reduction of the oxygen tension of the muscle or the metabolic alterations on it due to vasculopathy is the angiogenic stimulus.

Training increases flow redistribution from inactive to active muscles; with improvement or reversal of haemorheological disorders.

It is better to include the patients on a controlled exercise program. There is no efficacy data showing the message "go home and walk," which is the most common prescription.

After 4 months of an exercise plan, intermittent claudication (IC) patients require less oxygen at a same physical exigency, improving walking distance with a better quality of life.

To control the walk, pedometers can be used, with a more adherence to treatment. A pedometer that counts steps and measure the whole activity can be used by patients (Fig. 14.5).

Besides health and diet treatment, which should never be missed, it can be indicated an antioxidant and cilostazol treatment in 200 mg per day doses.

In cases of severe ischemia, it should be sent to vascular surgery, to see the possibility of surgery (bypass and/or angioplasty); and if remains residual ischemia or vascular surgery cannot be performed, consider prior to amputation the possibility of treatment with series of intravenous or intra-arterial injections of prostaglandins.

It must be highlighted that the peripheral vascular disease is a marker of systemic atherosclerosis. Therefore, the prevention is oriented to the intensive treatment of the cardiovascular risk factors.

Fig. 14.5 Pedometer

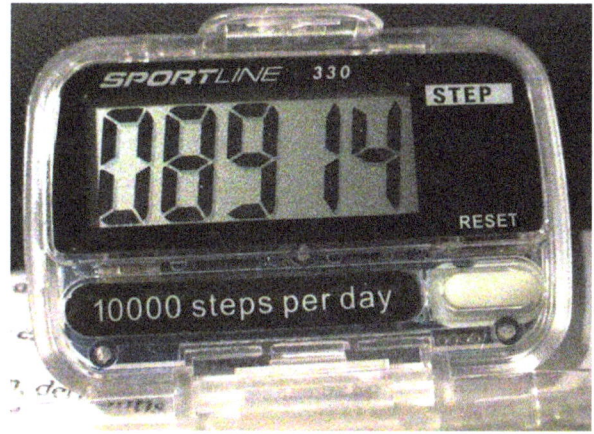

The vascular patient assessment must be comprehensive, ruling out the involvement of coronary and cerebral arteries.

Bibliography

1. Aragon-Sanchez J, et al. Conservative surgery of diabetic for foot osteomyelitis: how can I operate on this patient without amputations. Int J Low Extrem Wounds. 2015;14(2):108–31.
2. Boulton AJM. The pathway to foot ulceration in diabetes. Med Clin N Am. 2013;97:775.
3. Forsythe RO, et al. Peripheral arterial disease and revascularization of the diabetic foot. Diabetes Obes Metab. 2015;17(5):435–44.
4. Javed S, et al. Treatment of painful diabetic neuropathy. Ther Adv Chronic Dis. 2015;6:15.
5. Gmae FE, et al. Effectiveness of interventions to enhance healing of chronic ulcers of the foot in diabetes: a systematic review. Diabetes Metab Res Rev. 2016;32(supl 1):154.
6. Petrova N, et al. Acute charcot neuro/osteoarthropathy. Diabetes Metab Res Rev. 2016;32(suppl 1):281.
7. Ponirakis G, et al. Nerve check for the detection of sensory loss and neuropathic pain in diabetes. Diabetes Technol Ther. 2016;18(12):800–5.
8. Mascarenhas J, et al. Pathogenesis and medical management of diabetic charcot neuroarthropathy. Med Clin N Am. 2013;97:857.
9. Lipsky B. Treating diabetic foot osteomyelitis primarily with surgery or antibiotics: have we answered the questions. Diabetes Care. 2014;37:593.
10. Nicole Lou for PAD, Walking tolerance boosted with simple calf stretching. American Heart Association; May 5, 2017. www.medpagetoday.com/meetingcoverage/additionalmeetings/65055
11. FDA adds boxed warning to canagliflozin for amputation risk. www.fda.gov/mewatch/report.
12. Armstrong D, Lavery LA. Clinical care of the diabetic foot. 3rd ed. Los Angeles: American Diabetes Associations; 2005.
13. Ogilvie R, et al. Dietary intake and peripheral arterial disease incidence in middle aged adults: the Atherosclerosis Risk in Communities (ARIC) Study. Am J Clin Nutr. 2017;105:651–9.
14. Heffron S, et al. Greater frequency of fruit and vegetable consumption is associated with lower prevalence of peripheral artery disease. Arterioscler Thromb Vasc Biol. 2017;37(6):1234–40. https://doi.org/10.1161/ATVBAHA.116.308474.
15. Jeffcotate WJ. Charcot foot syndrome. Diabet Med. 2015;32:760.

Diabetes, Non-Enzymatic Glycation, and Aging

15

Denise Steiner, Carolina Reato Marçon, and Emilia Noemí Cohen Sabban

Introduction

Societal obsession with the process of aging dates back to ancient history, and myths related to the conservation of youth—ranging from a bathing fountain that confers eternal youth to a philosopher's stone that could be used to create an elixir of life—populate both past and contemporary folklore. However, it is only within recent years that aging has been investigated from an empirical approach, as it continues to garner increasing attention from the scientific community. While several hypotheses have been proposed to explain the pathophysiology responsible for senescence, no single theory accounts for the diverse phenomena observed. Rather, aging appears to be a multifactorial process that results from a complex interplay of several factors and mechanisms [1].

Aging is characterized by a decline of anatomical integrity and function across multiple organ systems and a reduced ability to respond to stress. The multisystem decline is associated with increasing pathology, disease, and progressively higher risk of death. Although the true mechanisms that drive the aging process are still a

D. Steiner
Universidade de Mogi das Cruzes, Mogi das Cruzes, São Paulo, Brazil
e-mail: steiner@uol.com.br

C.R. Marçon (✉)
Department of Dermatology, Santa Casa de Misericórdia de São Paulo, São Paulo, São Paulo, Brazil

Universidade de Mogi das Cruzes, Mogi das Cruzes, São Paulo, Brazil
e-mail: carolrmarcon@hotmail.com

E.N. Cohen Sabban, M.D.
Dermatology Department, Instituto de Investigaciones Médicas A. Lanari, University of Buenos Aires (UBA), Buenos Aires, Argentina
e-mail: emicohensabban@gmail.com

© Springer International Publishing AG 2018
E.N. Cohen Sabban et al. (eds.), *Dermatology and Diabetes*,
https://doi.org/10.1007/978-3-319-72475-1_15

mystery, there is evidence that both genetic and environmental factors may affect the rate of appearance of phenotypes characteristic of the aging process. Thus, aging appears in part to be modulated by a genetic–environmental interaction [2]. Studies of gene expression across species and tissues have consistently observed that old age is associated with progressive impairment of mitochondrial function, increased oxidative stress (OS), and immune activation [3]. Interestingly, all these processes can be influenced by modification of nutritional intake. For example, studies of animal species have found that caloric restriction reduces OS and is associated with longer life expectancy. Recent studies have cast doubts on whether humans may be able to maintain a long-term regimen of caloric restriction without unacceptable psychological consequences and whether even caloric restriction may have overall positive health effects in humans [3]. It has been suggested that changes in the quality of the diet could have positive effects on health and longevity and could be more easily implemented compared with caloric restriction.

Nevertheless, stratification of factors and mechanisms contributing to senescence is critical for the development of initial strategies in combating the aging process. The skin is an excellent paradigm for studying aging, in large part due to its easy accessibility. Moreover, in addition to its vulnerability to internal aging processes because of its diverse role in cellular processes, such as metabolism and immunity, the skin is subject to a variety of external stressors as the chief barrier between the body and the environment.

Aging factors can generally be classified as exogenous or endogenous. As ultraviolet (UV) radiation exposure is so strongly associated with a host of age-related skin diseases, endogenous and exogenous factors can theoretically be studied somewhat independently in the skin by differentiating between UVprotected and UV-exposed sites [4]. Endogenously aged skin displays characteristic morphological features with resultant alterations in functionality. These include epidermal, dermal, and extracellular matrix (ECM) atrophy leading to increased fragility, diminished collagen and elastin resulting in fine wrinkle formation, and marked vascular changes disrupting thermoregulation and nutrient supply. Endogenously aged skin also displays decreased mitotic activity, resulting in delayed wound healing, as well as decreased glandular function, resulting in disturbed reepithelialization of deep cutaneous wounds. Also seen is a reduction of melanocytes and Langerhans cells manifesting as hair graying and higher rates of infection, respectively [4–13].

Exogenously aged skin, in which environmental factors such as UV radiation act in concert with endogenous processes, shares many of the characteristics of endogenously aged skin. In addition, exogenously aged skin displays a thickened epidermis and aggregation of abnormal elastic fibers in the dermis (i.e. solar elastosis) [4].

Among the many mechanisms thought to underlie aging, glycation has emerged in recent years as one of the most widely studied processes. Testament to the rapidly growing attention from the scientific community, a cursory literature search will yield thousands of articles related to glycation, the majority of them published in the last decade. *Glycation refers to the non-enzymatic process of proteins, lipids, or nucleic acids covalently bonding to sugar molecules, usually glucose or fructose.* The lack of enzyme mediation is the key differentiator between glycation and glycosylation. Glycosylation occurs at defined sites on the target molecule and is usually critical to the target molecule's function. In contrast, glycation appears to occur at random molecular sites and generally results in the inhibition of the target molecule's ability to function. The products of glycation are called advanced glycation end products.

AGEs were first identified in cooked food as end-products from a non enzymatic reaction between sugars and proteins called the Maillard reaction [14]. The Maillard reaction (non enzymatic glycation (NEG) or browning) in foods has been well studied by the food industry to control food quality. However, it is only 40 years ago that a similar glycation process was recognized in human body by the observation of increased formation of glycosylated haemoglobins in diabetic patients [15] and this would lead to the formation of detrimental AGEs in humans [16].

The body also produces AGEs naturally as it processes sugars. The formation of AGEs is a part of normal metabolism, but if excessively high levels of AGEs are reached in tissues and the circulation they can become pathogenic [17].

The pathologic effects of AGEs are related to their ability to promote OS and inflammation by binding with cell surface receptors or cross-linking with body proteins, altering their structure and function [18]. The formation and accumulation of AGEs is a characteristic feature of tissues in aged people, especially in patients with Diabetes Mellitus (DM), and these products have also been strongly implicated in the pathogenesis of age-related and diabetic complications. Many chronic diseases, including heart diseases, Diabetes and both osteoarthritis (OA) and rheumatoid arthritis are associated with inflammation. It has been reported that AGEs are involved in musculoskeletal diseases such as OA, which is the most common chronic disabling disorder for aged people. Accumulation of AGEs increases stiffness of the collagen network in the bone as well, which may explain some of the age-related increase in skeletal fragility and fracture risk [19]. AGEs can be particularly dangerous for diabetics, as the increased availability of glucose in Diabetes patients accelerates the formation of AGEs.

AGEs are a heterogeneous group of macromolecules that are formed by the NEG of proteins, lipids, and nucleic acids. Humans are exposed to two main sources of AGEs: exogenous AGEs such as tobacco and certain foods [20, 21] and endogenous AGEs that are formed in the body. The Western diet is rich in AGEs. AGEs are formed when food is processed at elevated temperatures, such as during deep-frying, broiling, roasting, grilling; high temperature processing for certain processed foods such as pasteurized dairy products, cheeses, sausages, and processed meats; and commercial breakfast cereals. Endogenous AGEs are generated at higher rates in diabetics due to altered glucose metabolism. AGEs, by increasing OS and through other mechanisms, may accelerate the multisystem decline that occurs with aging and, therefore, reducing intake and circulating levels of AGEs may promote healthy aging and greater longevity [2].

Increased accumulation of AGEs was first directly correlated to the development of diabetic complications. Since then, AGEs have been implicated in a host of other pathologies, including atherosclerosis, end stage renal disease, and chronic obstructive pulmonary disease [22]. (It should be noted that AGE levels have been shown to vary by race and gender, and until larger studies are done to create ethnic- and gender-specific reference values, increased accumulation of AGEs should be defined as levels that are elevated for all demographic groups) [23].

Not coincidentally, many of the pathologies associated with AGEs, including diabetic sequelae, are closely related to senescence.

This extends to aging skin, as methods of AGE detection, such as immunostaining, have demonstrated the prevalence of glycation in aged skin. Glycation results in characteristic structural, morphological, and functional changes in the skin, a process colloquially known as "*sugar sag.*" With glucose and fructose playing such a prominent role in the mechanism, it is not surprising that diet plays a critical role in glycation and thus aging skin [1].

Perhaps more surprising, studies have shown that consumption of AGEs is not only tied to the sugar content of food, but is also affected by the method of cooking. Furthermore, as the connection between diet and aging is more clearly characterized, a host of dietary compounds have surfaced as potential therapeutic candidates in the inhibition of AGE-mediated changes [1].

Until today, more than 300 theories of aging have been proposed, among them the theory of cellular senescence, decreased proliferative capacity and telomere shortening, mitochondrial DNA single mutations, the free radical theory and others, none of which can fully explain all changes observed in aging [24–28]. According to the inflammatory theory of aging, a common characteristic of skin aging factors is their ability to induce or maintain proinflammatory changes and trigger a local inflammatory response which through subsequent immune responses, matrix metalloproteinase (MMP) activation and proinflammatory cytokine production contributes to the structural changes observed in aged skin [29].

In the recent years, the role of AGEs has been increasingly discussed in skin aging, and the potential of anti-AGE strategies has received high interest from pharmaceutical companies for the development of novel anti-aging cosmeceutical compounds [30]. The study of AGE represents one of the most promising areas of research today. Although the initial chemistry behind their formation has been known since the early 1900s, it is only in the last 20 years or so that important work has been done to elaborate on this. The chemical processes and pathways that ultimately lead to AGE formation have, however, yet to be fully clarified [31]. As our knowledge of AGE chemistry increases it is becoming apparent that not all AGE have been isolated, whereas as those that have been characterized are both complex and heterogenous. Thus, the discovery and investigation of AGE inhibitors would offer a potential therapeutic approach for the prevention of diabetic or other pathogenic complications [16].

Biochemistry of AGEs

Glycation is the non-enzymatic reaction between reducing sugars, such as glucose, and proteins, lipids or nucleic acids [32]. Glycation has to be distinguished from glycosylation, which is an enzymatic reaction. Since its first description by Maillard in 1912 and its involvement in food browning during thermal processing by Hodge 50 years later, its presence in living systems and involvement in various pathologies of the human body, including aging and Diabetes, have been an intensive field of research [33, 34].

First described over a century ago, glycation entails a series of simple and complex non-enzymatic reactions. In the key step, known as the Maillard reaction, electrophilic carbonyl groups of the sugar molecule react with free amino groups of amino acids (especially of basic lysine or arginine residues), leading to the formation of a non-stable Schiff base [35]. This non-stable Schiff base contains a carbon-nitrogen double bond, with the nitrogen atom connected to an aryl or alkyl group. The Schiff base rapidly undergoes re-arrangement to form a more stable ketoamine, termed the Amadori product [32, 35]. Schiff bases and Amadori products are reversible reaction products. At this juncture, the Amadori product can: (1) undergo the reverse reaction; (2) react irreversibly with lysine or arginine functional groups to produce stable AGEs in the form of protein adducts or protein cross-links; or (3) undergo further breakdown reactions, such as oxidation, dehydration, and polymerization, to give rise to numerous other AGEs [32, 36]. AGE formation is accelerated by an increased rate of protein turnover, hyperglycemia, temperatures above 120°C (248°F), and the presence of oxygen, reactive oxygen species (ROS), or redox active transition metals [36]. When an oxidative step is involved, the products are called advanced glycoxidation end products [32, 36].

The first, and perhaps most well-known, physiological AGE to be described was glycated hemoglobin (HbA1c), now widely used to measure glycemic control in Diabetes.

Since the discovery of HbA1c in Diabetes, numerous other AGEs have been detected. Some of them have characteristic autofluorescent properties, which simplifies their identification in situ or in vivo [32, 36–47].

However, the most prevalent AGE in the human body, including the skin, is carboxymethyl-lysine (CML), first described by Ahmed which is formed by oxidative degeneration of Amadori products or by direct addition of glyoxal to lysine. It seems to be the major epitope of the commonly used polyclonal anti-AGE antibodies [48].

It is a non-fluorescent protein adduct. In the skin, CML is found in the normal epidermis, aged and diabetic dermis, and photoaging-actinic elastosis [37–39].

Other AGEs detected in skin include pentosidine, glyoxal, methylglyoxal, glucosepane, fructose lysine, carboxyethyl-lysine, glyoxal-lysine dimer, and methylglyoxal-lysine dimer [35, 49].

Pentosidine was first isolated and characterized by Sell and Monnier. It is composed of an arginine and a lysine residue crosslinked to a pentose [50]. Pentosidine is a fluorescent glycoxidation product and forms protein-protein crosslinks [35].

Dicarbonyl compounds like 3-deoxyglucosome, methylglyoxal and glyoxal derive from oxidative degradation or autooxidation of Amadori products and other pathways [32, 51]. These dicarbonyl compounds are very reactive molecules leading to protein crosslinks [32].

Since the discovery of the first glycated protein, glycated hemoglobin in diabetes, numerous other AGEs have been detected. Some of them have characteristic autofluorescent properties, which simplifies their identification in situ or in vivo [32]. To date, numerous AGEs have been identified [36–47].

Environmental factors, such as diet and smoking influence the rate of AGE formation [52, 53]. Moreover, it seems that the level of circulating AGEs levels are genetically determined, as shown in a cohort study of healthy monozygotic and heterozygotic twins [54].

The content of AGEs in the organism is not only defined by the rate of their formation but also by the rate of their removal. Many cells have developed intrinsic detoxifying pathways against accumulation of AGEs [55]. The glutathione-dependent glyoxalase system, comprising of glyoxalase (Glo) I and II, has a key role in the defense against glycation [56]. This system uses reduced glutathione (GSH) to catalyze the conversion of glyoxal, methylglyoxal and other α-oxoaldehydes to the less toxic D-lactate [56]. Other enzymatic systems include fructosyl-amine oxidases (FAOXs) and fructosamine kinases, relatively new classes of enzymes which recognize and break Amadori products [57]. However, FAOXs or "amadoriases" have been found to be expressed only in bacteria, yeast and fungi but not in mammals. They oxidatively break Amadori products but act mostly on low molecular weight compounds [58]. On the contrary, fructosamine kinases are expressed in various genomes including humans [57]. These intracellular enzymes phosphorylate and destabilize Amadori products leading to their spontaneous breakdown [58]. Fructosamine-3-kinase (FN3K), one of the most studied enzymes in this system, is almost ubiquitary expressed in human tissues including the skin. Thus, it plays an important role in the intracellular breakdown of Amadori products [59].

Receptors for AGEs

AGEs not only exert their deleterious actions due to their biological properties per se, but also through their interaction with specific receptors. Receptor for AGEs (RAGE) is a multiligand member of the immunoglobulin superfamily of cell surface receptors, encoded by a gene on chromosome six near the major histocompatibility complex III. It is a pattern recognition receptor binding in addition to AGEs various other molecules such as S-100/calgranulins, high motility group protein B1 (amphoterine), β-amyloid peptides and β-sheet fibrils [52, 60]. The binding of ligands to RAGE stimulates various signaling pathways including the mitogen-activated protein kinases (MAPKs) extracellular signal-regulated kinases (ERK) 1 and 2, phosphatidyl-inositol 3 kinase, p21Ras, stress-activated protein kinase/c-Jun-N-terminal kinase and the janus kinases [52, 60]. Stimulation of RAGE results in activation of the transcription factor nuclear factor kappa-B (NFκB) and subsequent transcription of many proinflammatory genes [60]. Interestingly, RAGE-induced NFκB activation is characterized by a sustained and self-perpetuating action, through induction of positive feedback loops and overwhelming of the autoregulatory negative feedback loops. RAGE activation leads to new synthesis of the transcriptionally active subunit p65, which overwhelms the newly synthesized inhibitor

IκBα. Moreover NFκB increases further expression of RAGE, which itself further stimulates NFκB, forming a vicious cycle of selfrenewing and perpetuating proinflammatory signals [60]. RAGE activation can directly induce oxidative stress by activating nicotinamide adenine dinucleotide phosphate (NADPH)-oxidase (NOX), decreasing activity of superoxide dismutase (SOD), catalase and other pathways, and indirectly by reducing cellular antioxidant defenses, like GSH and ascorbic acid [60–62]. The reduction of GSH leads furthermore to decreased activity of Glo I, the major cellular defense system against methylglyoxal, therefore supporting further production of AGEs [38]. RAGE is almost ubiquitary expressed in the organism, typically at low levels, and its expression is upregulated under various pathologic conditions [60, 63]. In the skin, RAGE expression was observed in both epidermis and dermis, and it was increased in sun-exposed compared with UV irradiation-protected areas. Keratinocytes, fibroblasts, dendritic cells and to a lesser extent endothelial cells and lymphocytes express RAGE [63]. Not only in vivo, but also in vitro, various skin cells types have been shown to express RAGE [61, 63–68].

RAGE is the most studied receptor for advanced glycation end products. Another group of cell surface receptors, AGER1, AGER2 and AGER3 seem to regulate endocytosis and degradation of AGEs, thus counteracting the effects of RAGE [69]. AGER1 has been further shown to counteract AGEs-induced oxidative stress via inhibition of RAGE signaling [70, 71]. Soluble RAGE (sRAGE) is a truncated splice variant of RAGE containing the ligand-binding domain but not the transmembrane domain and has been found in plasma. sRAGE is a soluble extracellular protein without signaling properties and it is considered as a natural decoy receptor of RAGE [72].

Toxicity of Advanced Glycation End-Products (AGEs)

The possible pathophysiological role of AGEs has become a topic of increasing interest over the past few years. With the continued research on the Maillard reaction, it was demonstrated that the Maillard reaction also occurs in vivo and the term *"glycation"* was introduced as a synonym for *"non-enzymatic glycosilation"*, in order to distinguish this from the well known enzymatic glycosilation of proteins [73]. Protein modifications called *"Advanced glycation end-products"* (AGEs), which are formed during aging, Diabetes and in renal failure via comparable chemical pathways as described for heated foods, nowadays are generally accepted to play a pivotal pathophysiological role in several diseases [74]. In vitro studies using human derived endothelial cells exhibited the food-derived AGEs have same protein cross-linking and intracellular oxidant stress actions as their endogenous counterparts. In animal studies like in mice, reduction of dietary AGE intake is accompanied by significant reduction of circulating AGEs levels as well as reduction of diseases related to inflammation and oxidative stress. A low-AGE diet has been associated with a significant increase in mouse lifespan. The human relevance of the in vitro and animal data discussed in a number of studies found independent correlate of the circulating AGEs with the dietary AGEs intake. Moreover, the effect of a low and a high-AGE diet on the inflammatory mediators was also studied by using a group of diabetic subjects. The low-AGE diet significantly reduced serum AGE levels as well as markers of inflammation and endothelial dysfunction. Thus, all these studies demonstrate the associated toxicity of AGEs [16, 75].

AGEs and the Skin

AGEs accumulate in various tissues as a function, as well as a marker, of chronological age [76]. Proteins with slow turnover rates, such as collagen, are especially susceptible to modification by glycation. Collagen in the skin, in fact, has a half-life of approximately 15 years and thus can undergo up to a 50% increase in glycation over an individual's lifetime [77].

Collagen is critical not only to the mechanical framework of the skin but also to several cellular processes, and is impaired by glycation in multiple ways. First, intermolecular cross-linking modifies collagen's biomechanical properties, resulting in increased stiffness and vulnerability to mechanical stimuli [78]. Second, the formation of AGEs on collagen side chains alters the protein's charge and interferes with its active sites, thereby distorting the protein's ability to interact properly with surrounding cells and matrix proteins [79]. Third, the ability to convert L-arginine to nitric oxide, a critical cofactor in the crosslinking of collagen fibers, is impaired [80]. Finally, glycated collagen is highly resistant to degradation by matrix metalloproteinases (MMPs). This further retards the process of collagen turnover and replacement with functional proteins [81].

Other cutaneous extracellular matrix proteins are functionally affected by glycation, including elastin and fibronectin. This further compounds dermal dysfunction [49, 82] as glycation crosslinked collagen, elastin, and fibronectin cannot be repaired like their normal counterparts.

Interestingly, CML-modified elastin is mostly found in sites of solar elastosis and is nearly absent in sun-protected skin. This suggests that UV-radiation can mediate AGE formation in some capacity or, at the least, render cells more sensitive to external stimuli [83]. It is hypothesized that UV-radiation accomplishes this through the formation of ROS (superoxide anion radicals, hydrogen peroxide, and hydroxyl radicals). This induces oxidative stress and accelerates the production of AGEs [84]. AGEs themselves are very reactive molecules and can act as electron donors in the formation of free radicals. Occurring in conjunction with the decline of the enzymatic system that eliminates free radicals during the aging process, these properties lead to a *"vicious cycle"* of AGE formation in the setting of UV exposure.

Formed both intracellularly and extracellularly, AGEs can also have an effect on intracellular molecular function. In the skin, the intermediate filaments of fibroblasts (vimentin) and keratinocytes (cytokeratin 10) have been shown to be susceptible to glycation modification [41]. Analogous to the diverse role of collagen in the skin, intermediate filaments are essential to both the maintenance of cytoskeletal stability and the coordination of numerous cellular functions. Fibroblasts with glycated vimentin demonstrate a reduced contractile capacity, and these modified fibroblasts are found to accumulate in skin biopsies of aged donors [41].

In fact, general cellular function may be compromised in the presence of high concentrations of AGEs. In vitro, human dermal fibroblasts display higher rates of premature senescence and apoptosis, which likely explains the decreased collagen and extracellular matrix protein synthesis observed in both cell culture and aged skin biopsies [65, 85]. Similarly, keratinocytes exposed to AGEs express increased levels of pro-inflammatory mediators, suffer from decreased mobility, and also undergo premature senescence in the presence of AGEs [86].

In addition to intermediate filaments, proteasomal machinery and DNA can undergo glycation. Proteasomal machinery, which functions to remove altered intracellular proteins, decline functionally in vitro when treated with glyoxal [87]. Similar in vitro findings were observed when human epidermal keratinocytes and fibroblasts were treated with glyoxal, leading to accumulation of CML in histones, cleavage of DNA, and, ultimately, arrest of cellular growth [88].

Beyond the modification of host molecular physicochemistry, AGEs also exert detrimental effects through the binding to RAGE. As cited before, RAGE is a multiligand protein that, when activated, can trigger several cellular signaling pathways, that are known to mediate various pathogenic mechanisms through the alteration of cell cycle regulators, gene expression, inflammation, and extracellular protein synthesis [60]. Not surprisingly, RAGE is found to be highly expressed in the skin and is present at even higher levels in both UV-exposed anatomical sites and aged skin [63].

Role of AGEs in the Skin Aging Process

Cutaneous accumulation of AGEs is a feature of skin aging. Accumulation of AGEs has been detected in various tissues during aging and Diabetes, including articular collagen, skeletal and smooth vascular muscles or glomerular basement membranes [89–91]. Accordingly, deposited AGEs in these tissues have been implicated in various Diabetes or age-associated pathologies such as diabetic angiopathy, age and diabetes-associated macular degeneration and osteoarthritis [81, 89–94].

Skin, due to its easy accessibility, offers an excellent opportunity for minimal invasive or even non-invasive investigation of glycation, taking advantage of the characteristic autofluorescent properties of AGEs. Accumulation of AGEs in the skin has been therefore thoroughly studied and is detected not only in Diabetes as expected but also during chronological aging [39, 95, 96]. Glycation associated skin autofluorescence was shown to correlate with chronological aging in a large number of healthy subjects [97].

It is a general perception today that AGE accumulation is dependent on protein turnover rate; therefore long-lived proteins are thought to be mainly modified by glycation [89]. Collagen types I and IV, exhibiting a slow turnover rate of about 10 year, and other dermal long-lived proteins like fibronectin mainly suffer from glycation during intrinsic chronological aging [38, 39]. The appearance of glycated collagen is first observed at the age of 20. It accumulates with a yearly rate of about 3.7% reaching a 30–50% increase at 80 year of age [39, 77]. CML was recently histochemically detected in human epidermis from healthy donors [37]. The upper epidermal layers were mostly involved (stratum spinosum, granulosum and corneum) and the authors identified cytokeratin 10 (CK10) (expressed by differentiated keratinocytes) as a target protein for CML modification. The amount of CML in younger donors seemed to be weak in comparison to the older ones. The latter study had restrictions, as the size of the sample was small and heterogeneous, but indicates a potential involvement of AGEs in epidermal physiology and a possible involvement of more short-lived proteins in glycation chemistry. Moreover, in an in vitro reconstructed organ skin model, both epidermis and dermis, as well as their functions, were modified by glycation [98].

Moreover, smoking, a typical aggravating factor of skin aging, accelerates formation of AGEs and increases their deposition in various tissues including skin [82, 99]. Another important environmental factor for aging is diet. The content of AGEs in food is highly dependent on the method of preparation, like cooking time and temperature. Fried food contains in general far higher amounts of AGEs than boiled or steamed food [100]. Dietary AGEs directly correlate with serum levels of AGEs and inflammatory markers in healthy human subjects, respectively [101].

It has been widely accepted that AGEs, once formed, can be only removed when the modified proteins degrade. However it has now become apparent that in the organism various enzymatic systems seem to be involved in the degradation or removal of AGEs. As mentioned above, Glo I is an enzyme responsible for the removal of reactive α-dicarbonyl compounds. Interestingly, decreased activity of such defense systems against AGEs has been reported during aging [62]. These age-related changes may further increase the extent of deposited AGEs in a living organism over time.

Consequences of AGE deposition in skin. AGEs can be formed intracellularly and extracellularly. Their presence in biological molecules modifies their biomechanical and functional properties. Proteins, lipids and nucleic acids can be targets of advanced glycation, modifying enzyme-substrate interactions, protein-DNA interactions, protein-protein interactions, DNA regulation and epigenetic modulation, thus interfering with numerous physiological functions of the organism. Moreover, AGEs are themselves reactive molecules which through interaction with their receptors activate various molecular pathways in vivo, thus becoming involved in inflammation, immune response, cell proliferation and gene expression.

Extracellular Matrix Proteins

ECM proteins have been regarded as one of the major target structures for glycation. The most abundant collagen type in the skin is type I, whereas collagen IV is being found in the basal membrane. Collagen is one of the strongest proteins. In the skin, it is not only used as a supportive framework for mechanical support for cells and tissues, but represents an active component being able to interact with cells and affect various cellular functions such as migration, differentiation and proliferation.

Collagen glycation impairs its function in various ways. Intermolecular cross-links of adjacent collagen fibers change its biomechanical properties leading to stiffness and decreased flexibility, thus increasing its susceptibility to mechanical stimuli [78]. The change of its charge and the formation of AGEs on side chains of collagen affect its contact sites with cells and other matrix proteins and inhibit its ability to react with them [79]. The precise aggregation of monomers into the triple helix may be affected as well as the association of collagen IV with laminin in the basal membrane [35]. Modified collagen resists degradation by MMPs, thus inhibiting its removal and replacement by newly synthesized and functional one [81]. Accordingly, tissue permeability and turnover is impaired [35, 102].

Other ECM proteins suffering from advanced glycation are elastin and fibronectin, contributing further to dermal dysfunction [38, 39, 42]. Of note, CML-modified elastin has been found almost exclusively in sites of actinic elastosis and not in sun-protected skin, underlining its potential role in photoaging. Indeed, UV irradiation stimulates glycation of elastin in the presence of sugars. Moreover, CML-modified elastin assembled in large and irregular structures, has decreased elasticity and is resistant to proteolytic degradation [83].

It has been shown that in vitro glycated skin samples have impaired biomechanical properties [103]. In vivo, decreased skin elasticity characterizes diabetic subjects in comparison to healthy controls [104].

Intracellular Proteins

Intermediate filaments such as vimentin in fibroblasts and CK10 in keratinocytes have been found to be modified by AGEs [37, 41]. Cytoskeletal proteins are important in providing stability of the cytoskeleton and are crucially involved in numerous cellular functions such as migration and cellular division. Various other intracellular proteins including enzymes and growth factors may be targets of NEG. Glycated basic fibroblast growth factor (bFGF) displays impaired mitogenic activity in endothelial cells [105]. Glycation of enzymes of the ubiquitin-proteasome system and of the lysosomal proteolytic system has been shown to inhibit their action [106]. Antioxidant and other protective enzymes such as Cu-Zn-SOD can be inactivated [107]. Other intracellular components, such as DNA and lipids can be glycated with detrimental effects on their function [32].

Receptors for AGEs: RAGE

AGEs do not only act by altering the physicochemical properties of glycated proteins. As mentioned above, AGEs may bind to their cell surface receptor, RAGE, initiating a cascade of signals influencing cell cycle and proliferation, gene expression, inflammation and extracellular matrix synthesis [60]. Interestingly, RAGE is broadly expressed in human skin and in epidermal keratinocytes, dermal fibroblasts and endo-thelial cells in vitro. It is highly found in sites of solar elastosis, and its expression is induced by AGEs and proinflammatory cytokines like TNFα [63]. In skin cells RAGE has been shown to decrease cell proliferation, induce apoptosis and increase MMPs production. Many of these effects involve NFκB signaling [65].

Effects of AGEs on Resident Skin Cells

AGEs have been shown to affect various functions of skin cells in vitro. They decrease proliferation and enhance apoptosis of human dermal fibroblasts, an effect which is at least partly RAGE dependent and correlates with the activation of NFκB and caspases [85]. In keratinocytes, AGEs decrease cell viability and migration and induce the expression of proinflammatory mediators [86]. Moreover, AGEs are able to induce premature senescence in human dermal fibroblasts and in normal human keratinocytes in vitro [108–110]. Collagen and ECM protein synthesis have been also found to be decreased, while the expression of MMPs is induced [65]. Dicarbonyls such as glyoxal and methylglyoxal impair the signaling of epidermal growth factor receptor (EGFR), a receptor controlling various cellular functions such as proliferation, differentiation, motility and survival, by formation of EGFR crosslinks, blocking of phosphorylation and impaired activation of ERKs and phos-pholipase C [111]. Various other growth factors or proteins significant for cellular functions, like bFGF, may be glycated inhibiting their functions [105]. In the con-text of extrinsic aging, AGEs seem to render cells more sensitive to external stimuli, as UVA irradiated fibroblasts and keratinocytes exhibit decreased viability after exposure to AGEs [112].

The Role of Oxidative Stress

Oxidative stress has been widely accepted to mediate the deleterious effects of solar radiation in the skin during photoaging. Interestingly, in vitro exposure of AGEs to UVA irradiation leads to formation of ROS, such as superoxide anion, hydrogen peroxide and hydroxyl radicals [84]. AGEs can lead to ROS formation in cells by various ways. They can stimulate NOX to induce production of superoxide anion or they can compromise cellular antioxidant defense systems, e.g. inactivation of Cu-Zn-SOD by cross-linking and site-specific fragmentation of this molecule [107]. Moreover, AGEs are themselves very reactive molecules. As early as during their crosslinking reactions they can act as electron donors leading to formation of super-oxide anions [113]. Glycation of proteins creates active enzyme-like centers (cat-ion-radical sites of crosslinked proteins) able to catalyze one-electron oxidation-reduction reactions leading to ROS generation with or without presence of oxygen or transition metals such as iron and copper [113–115]. Finally, autofluo-rescent AGEs, such as pentosidine, can act as endogenous photosensitizers leading to increased ROS formation after UVA irradiation of human skin. UV irradiation of human keratinocytes and fibroblasts in the presence of AGEs led to increased ROS formation and decreased proliferation in vitro [112].

Skin AGEs as Biomarkers of Aging

As AGEs have been etiologically implicated in aging and aging-related pathologies, the idea of using them as biomarkers is appealing. AGEs in the skin have been initially measured by western blots (WB) with polyclonal antibodies or by autofluorescence measurements of skin biopsies, thus restricting the wide use of these measurements. An AGE-Reader (DiagnOptics B.V., Groningen, The Netherlands) has been introduced some years ago as a new, non-invasive method to measure in vivo the skin content of AGEs based on their characteristic autofluorescence [116–118]. Until now it has been shown that skin autofluorescence positively correlates with various diabetes-and age-related complications such as micro and macrovascular complications, renal disease, cardiovascular events, overall mortality, age-related macular degeneration and chronic renal disease [117, 119, 120]. Skin glycation has been proposed as a prognostic factor for the development of diabetic complications [121]. Lately it was shown that skin autofluorescence increases with chronological aging and correlates with skin deposition of AGEs, making this method a potential tool in investigating the effect of various anti-aging products of the cosmetic industry [122].

Dietary Advanced Glycation End-Products (d-AGEs)

A large database of different food items and their AGE contents has been created by measuring CML with ELISA [18, 100]. In general the reported CML contents are correlated with corresponding levels of methyl glyoxal (MG)-derivatives [18]. AGE content of foods as determined by CML and MG levels shows a highly significant linear correlation ($r = 0.8$, $P = 0.0001$) prepared by different cooking techniques. The highly significant internal correlation between two chemically distinct AGEs (CML and MG) in a variety of foods prepared by different methods validates the methodology applied and supports the choice of CML levels as a useful marker of d-AGE content.

As with CML, foods high in protein and fat contained higher amounts of MG than did carbohydrate-rich foods. Recent studies indicate that the meat group contains the highest levels of AGEs because meats are served in larger portions as compared to fats which tend to contain more dAGE per gram of weight. When items in the meat category prepared by similar methods were compared, the highest dAGE levels were observed in beef and cheeses followed by poultry, pork, fish, and eggs. Lamb ranked relatively low in dAGEs compared to other meats.

Higher-fat and aged cheeses, such as full-fat American and Parmesan, contained more dAGEs than lower-fat cheeses, such as reduced-fat mozzarella, 2% milk cheddar, and cottage cheese. Whereas cooking is known to drive the generation of new AGEs in foods, it is interesting to note that even uncooked, animal-derived foods such as cheeses can contain large amounts of dAGEs. This is likely due to pasteurization and/or holding times at ambient room temperatures (e.g., as in curing or aging processes). Glycation-oxidation reactions, although at a slower rate, continue to occur over time even at cool temperatures, resulting in large accumulation of dAGEs in the long term. High-fat spreads, including butter, cream cheese, margarine, and mayonnaise, was also among the foods highest in dAGEs, followed by oils and nuts. As with certain cheeses, butter and different types of oils are AGE-rich, even in their uncooked forms. This may be due to various extraction and purification procedures involving heat, in combination with air and dry conditions, however mild they are. The type of cooking fat used for cooking led to the production of different amounts of dAGEs [16].

In comparison to the meat and fat groups, the carbohydrate group generally contained lower amounts of AGEs due to the higher water content or higher level of antioxidants and vitamins in these foods, which may diminish new AGE formation. The highest dAGE level per gram of food in this category was found in dry-heat processed foods such as crackers, chips, and cookies. This is likely due to the addition of ingredients such as butter, oil, cheese, eggs, and nuts, which during dry-heat processing substantially accelerate dAGE generation. Although AGEs in these snack types of food remain far below those present in meats, they may represent an important health hazard for people who consume multiple snacks during the day or as fast meals [123].

Grains, legumes, breads, vegetables, fruits, and milk were among the lowest items in dAGE, unless prepared with added fats. For instance, biscuits had more than 10 times the amount of dAGEs found in low-fat breads, rolls, or bagels [18].

Nonfat milk had significantly lower dAGEs than whole milk. Whereas heating increased the dAGE content of milk, the values were modest and remained low relative to those of cheeses. Likewise, milk-related products with a high moisture index such as yogurt, pudding, and ice cream were also relatively low in AGEs [18].

Factors Affecting the Rate of Dietary AGEs (d-AGEs) Formation During Cooking

The rate of formation and the diversity of the generated AGEs in food depend on factors such as composition, availability of precursors, presence of transition metals, and availability of pro and antioxidants. Reaction time, processing temperature, concentrations of reactants, availability of water, and pH are particularly well known to have a decisive effect on the rate of the Maillard reaction [124]. As a rule of thumb, the rate of the Maillard reaction at least doubles when the temperature is increased by 10°C. If browning is used to measure the progress of the Maillard reaction, then 4 weeks at 20°C, 3 h at 100°C, and 5 min at 150°C give approximately the same result [125]. Factors like pH [126, 127] and water activity greatly affect the rate of formation of Maillard reaction products (MRPs).

The rate of the Maillard reaction is considered to be low at acidic pH, but increases with increasing pH until a maximum is reached around pH 10 [21]. At higher moisture levels, a decrease in reaction rate is observed due to dilution of the reactants in the aqueous phase. Water is a product of the reaction and it is probable that the law of mass action also leads to a decreased rate of reaction at high moisture levels [128]. Dry heat cooking has been found to promote formation of dietary AGEs as determined by immunological methods. However, AGE formation seems to be reduced by heating in an oven at high humidity, shorter cooking times, lower cooking temperatures, or by the use of acidic ingredients, such as lemon juice or vinegar [16].

Absorption and Bioavailability

Early animal studies reported that MRPs are at least partially absorbed, and those low molecular weights (LMW) MRPs are absorbed to a higher degree than high molecular weight (HMW) MRPs [129]. The absorption of AGEs into the circulation in humans measured by a nonspecific ELISA method was estimated to be about 10% of ingested AGEs [130]. HMWAGEs need to be degraded by gut proteases before the LMW products are liberated. The bioavailability of the partially degraded HMW AGEs will depend on the size of the associated peptide, type of diet, gut environment, and duration of their presence in the gut. Heat-induced changes in proteins can decrease their susceptibility to degradation by gastrointestinal enzymes, and protein and mineral bioavailability have been shown to be influenced negatively by a heat-treated diet [131–133]. Oral bioavailability is thought to be low (10%), secondary to poor absorption from the gastrointestinal tract, as AGE cross link formation is resistant to enzymatic or chemical hydrolysis [130]. The water solubility and amphoteric properties makes LMWAGEs to be absorbed to extracellular and intracellular compartments than HMWAGEs.

The in vivo distribution of CML and CEL after an intravenous injection in rats showed a temporary accumulation in the liver [134], indicating that they may have high affinity to some specific hepatic proteins. In the study of ^{14}C labeled AGEs, it was observed that 60% of the absorbed AGEs were bound in liver and kidney after 72 h, but radioactivity was also observed in lung, heart, and spleen indicating more global distribution and tissue binding [135]. Several animal studies have shown a correspondence between dietary AGE content and serum and tissue AGE levels [136, 137].

Any deterioration in renal function results in AGE accumulation which can lead to endothelial perturbation and hence vascular disease [138]. In vitro studies have proposed that insulin also contributes to AGE elimination from the plasma via the IRS and phosphatidyl-inositol-3-OH kinase (PI3 kinase) pathway [139]. This pathway is thought to be vasculo-protective, leading to a rise in nitric oxide as well as facilitating insulin-mediated glucose transport in adipocytes and skeletal muscle. Recent human studies revealed that about 10% of diet-derived AGEs were absorbed, twothirds of which remained in the body and only one-third of the absorbed AGEs was excreted into the urine within 3 days from ingestion [16, 130, 135].

Dietary Advanced Glycation End-Products (d-AGEs) and Their Health Implications

Nutrient composition, temperature and method of cooking can affect the formation of AGEs in foods. Fats or meat-derived products processed by high heat such as broiling and oven frying contain more AGEs than carbohydrates boiled for longer periods [100, 140]. That is, in the absence of lipids and proteins or heat, sugar content does not necessarily correlate with AGE values in the food. And, the absence of sugars does not necessarily predict low AGE content, as in preparations containing preformed AGElike caramel additives [130].

Food-derived AGEs induce protein cross-linking and intracellular oxidant stress similar to their endogenous counterparts when tested in vitro using human-derived endothelial cells [141]. These pro oxidant and pro inflammatory properties are also found in the circulating AGE fractions derived from these exogenous AGEs. Experiments performed in different animal models have established a significant role for dietary AGEs in inducing T1DM in non-obese diabetic (NOD) [136]. In a group of diabetic subjects, dietary AGE restriction was associated with significant reduction of two markers of inflammation, plasma C reactive protein (CRP) and peripheral mononuclear cell TNF-α, as well as of VCAM-1, a marker of endothelial dysfunction [92]. These observations were later extended to chronic renal failure patients on maintenance peritoneal dialysis, in whom dietary AGE restriction was associated with a parallel reduction of serum AGEs and CRP [142]. The parallel changes of serum AGEs and CRP following dietary AGE modifications are highly suggestive of a role for dietary AGEs in inducing inflammation [16].

Role of Food-Derived AGEs in Vascular Complications in Diabetic Animals

With regards to complications of Diabetes, several different animal models have been used to examine the role of dietary AGEs in the development of kidney disease. In diabetic mouse models, there has been reports of both protective [143] and disparate effects [144] of diets low in AGEs in development of diabetic nephropathy. In remnant kidney models in rats, proteinuria increased during feeding with high AGE diets [145, 146]. Furthermore, high AGE diets were shown to accelerate progression of renal fibrosis [145]. In addition, in a mouse model of obesity, renal impairment developed when high AGEs and a high fat diet were combined. An AGE-poor diet that contained four- to five-fold lower AGE contents for 2 months also decreased serum levels of AGEs and markedly reduced tissue AGEs and RAGE expression, numbers of inflammatory cells, tissue factor, VCAM-1, and MCP-1 levels in diabetic apolipoprotein Edeficient mice [147].

Role of Food-Derived AGEs in Ageing

Aging is associated with increased oxidative stress generation and AGE formation [71]. A life-long restriction of AGE containing diet reduces oxidative stress generation and AGE accumulation which are associated with RAGE and p66 suppression, resulting in extension of lifespan in mice [71]. Oral intake of AGE-containing foods also determines the effects of calorie restriction on oxidant stress, age-related diseases, and lifespan [148]. These observations suggest that restriction of AGE-rich diet may be a novel therapeutic target for prevention of age associated various disorders.

In food analyses, CML has been the most widely used marker for AGEs [149]. The CML content of the same food item can be increased up to 200-fold by increasing the temperature and conditions used in cooking. The CML concentrations of various foods vary widely from about 0.35–0.37 mg CML/kg food for pasteurized skimmed milk and butter to about 11 mg CML/kg food for fried minced beef and 37 mg CML/kg food for white bread crust. Fried meat, sausage, and cookies are high in CML [150]. Other foods that are high in AGEs include many commercial breakfast cereals [151], roasted nuts and seeds [152], ice cream [153], and barbecue sauces [154]. High concentrations of MG, an intermediate product of the Maillard reaction, are found in commercial soft drinks that contain high fructose corn syrup [144]. MG is reactive and readily modifies lysine or arginine residues of proteins to form CEL and hydroimidazolones. Pasteurized milk and sterilized milk contain much higher CML concentrations than raw milk [32]. Evaporated whole milk contains high concentrations of CML, probably due to the high temperatures used in processing the milk. Infant formula contains high concentrations of AGEs [155]. Commercial infant formulas contain a 70-fold higher level of CML than human breast milk, and infants fed infant formula had significantly high plasma CML than breast-fed infants [156]. Foods that are either eaten raw or cooked at lower temperatures are relatively low in AGEs, and such foods include raw fruits and vegetables, raw fish, raw nuts, yoghurt, tofu, pasta, boiled rice, boiled potatoes, and other boiled or simmered foods.

Other processes, besides the formation of AGEs, also take place in food during cooking. It is well-known and described in the literature that heating of food induces degradation and oxidation of heat-sensitive compounds, including vitamins and other bioactive compounds [157–159]. A high versus low AGE diet made by differences in heat treatment will, therefore, have dissimilar content of such compounds and this has also been confirmed when it has been measured in intervention studies [160]. This is a problem, because effects of high AGE diets cannot be directly related only to the AGE content. It cannot be ruled out that a lower content of a range of heat-sensitive nutrients in the diet, e.g., vitamin C, E, and thiamine, could also contribute to these negative effects. Accordingly, AGE levels in body fluids might be markers of the inflammatory and oxidative burden. For example, marginal thiamine deficiency has been shown to increase both markers of oxidative stress and of reactive dicarbonyls [161], and vitamin B6 can also affect AGE formation. Furthermore, extensive heat processing of food can generate Maillard-derived antinutritional and toxic compounds [162, 163]. Such compounds include acrylamide [164, 165], heterocyclic aromatic amines [166] and 5-hydroxymethylfurfural [167], all of which are suspected carcinogens. Thus, simply referring the effects of a less heat-treated diet to effects of AGEs is problematic; the consequences of cooking for the concentrations of AGEs as well as other heat-derived compounds are not tested in the majority of the dietary AGE studies. Only one study has reported the content of acrylamide and 5 hydroxymethylfurfural and they were found to be significantly higher in the high AGE diet [168].

Nevertheless, this shows there is a large range of potentially harmful compounds generated by heat and points to the essential problem with identifying the active compounds. Harmful effects of high AGE diets cannot be directly related to the AGE content. Studies with well-defined compounds outside a complex food matrix (e.g., synthetically produced AGEs) are needed to identify individual effects. Moreover, AGEs are often investigated and discussed as a whole, even though they are a large and heterogeneous group of compounds. The heterogeneity of AGEs makes it difficult to conclude which of these compounds are biologically active and exert which specific effects in vivo. Within the large range of MRPs, not only AGEs have been identified, but also compounds with potential beneficial effects have been described. Melanoidins have been associated with health benefits in some studies and antioxidative properties of MRPs have been observed in a human intervention study [16, 28].

Anti-AGE Strategies: Current Knowledge and Future Perspectives

Since the emergence of AGEs as an important pathogenetic factor in Diabetes and aging the development of strategies against AGEs has been in the center of scientific interest. Substances able to prevent or inhibit formation of AGEs, as well as agents able to break already formed AGEs or those antagonizing their signaling have been identified. Some of them are already being tested in clinical trials [169, 170].

Substances Preventing or Inhibiting AGE Formation

Aminoguanidine was one of the first substances identified limiting the formation of AGEs [171]. Aminoguanidine is a nucleophilic hydrazine and its anti-AGE properties result from trapping of early glycation products such as carbonyl intermediate compounds. It has no effects on more advanced stages of glycation. Despite its potential effects in attenuating various diabetes- and age-related complications in animal models, its use in clinical practice is limited due to adverse effects in clinical trials with diabetic patients [172]. In an in vitro skin aging model it could attenuate collagen glycation, however its effects against AGE induced collagen modification in vivo have been contradictory [173–175]. Studies on topical application of amino-guanidine in the skin are lacking.

Different AGE inhibitors suppress AGE formation at different stages of glycation. For example, aspirin (acetylsalicylic acid) is known to inhibit glycation by acetylating free amino groups of a protein, thereby blocking the attachment of reducing sugars [176, 177] at the early stage of the glycation process. The inhibitory activities against AGE formation of various vitamin B1 and B6 derivatives such as pyridoxamine [178–180] and thiamine pyrophosphate [181] have mainly been attributed to their abilities to scavenge reactive carbonyl compounds [32, 180].

Pyridoxamine, a naturally occurring vitamin B6 isoform, seems to be another tool in the fight against AGEs. Pyridoxamine traps reactive carbonyl intermediates, scavenges ROS and in addition inhibits post-Amadori stages of AGE formation [182]. It has shown promising results in a phase II clinical trial against diabetic nephropathy [183]. Oral intake of pyridoxamine resulted in potent inhibition of skin collagen CML formation in diabetic rats. In addition, penicillamine could reduce the level of AGEs through decreasing the formation of Amadori products [175, 184, 185]. However, its potential against skin aging remains to be shown.

"AGE Breakers"

Chemical substances and enzymes able to recognize and break the Maillard reaction crosslinks have been identified. Such chemical AGE breakers are dimethyl-3-phenayl-thiazolium chloride (ALT-711), N-phenacylthiazolium and N-phenacyl-4,5-dimethylthiazolium [183]. They have been developed to chemically break the prototypical Maillard reaction crosslink via a thiazolium structure [183]. Promising results against cardiovascular complications in Diabetes and aging have been reported, although their actual ability to cleave existing protein crosslinks in tissues has been questioned [184–187].

Interference with intrinsic AGE-detoxifying enzymes like FAOXs, FN3K and the enzymatic system of Glo is another interesting strategy to remove AGEs, as enzymes recognize specific substrates and may be associated with fewer side effects [57, 188, 189]. There are a lot of data supporting the significance of these enzyme systems in aging. As noted above decreased Glo I activity and increased accumulation of AGEs with age have been shown in many tissues and animals [56]. Overexpression of Glo I significantly inhibits hyperglycemia-induced intracellular formation of AGEs in bovine aortic endothelial cells and in mouse mesangial cells by reduction of intra-cellular oxidative stress and apoptosis [190, 191]. A potential in vivo beneficial effect of Glo I against AGEs could be also shown in transgenic rats [192]. Interestingly, it has been recently shown that Glo I is transcriptionally controlled by Nrf2, and that pharmacological Nrf2 activators increase Glo I mRNA and protein levels as well as its activity [56]. The pharmacological induction of such enzymes could represent a novel future strategy against AGEs. Fructosamine phosphokinases are relatively new enzymes and currently under investigation, and until now no inductors or activators of their expression have been found [35]. FAOXs, on the other hand, are not expressed in mammals, and their potential use in humans by enzymatic engineering remains to be discovered [58].

Nutriceuticals

Since oxidation steps are crucially involved in formation of many AGEs, substances with antioxidative or metal chelating properties, may also have antiglycating activities [193]. Thus, a lot of interest has been directed to nutrients and vitamins, so called "nutriceuticals," as natural tools against AGEs [170, 194].

Accordingly, an increasing list of natural antioxidants and chelating agents such as ascorbic acid, α-tocopherol, niacinamide, pyridoxal, sodium selenite, selenium yeast, trolox, rivoflavin, zink and manganese has been shown to inhibit glycation of albumin in vitro [195]. Alpha-lipoic acid was able to reverse tail tendon collagen glycation in fructose-fed rats, an effect which was attributed to its endogenous antioxidant action, its ability to recycle ascorbic acid, α-tocopherol and GSH as well as to its positive influence on glucose uptake and glycaemia [196]. Green tea, vitamins C and E and a combination of N-acetylcystein with taurine and oxerutin could inhibit skin collagen glycation in mice [194, 197]. Another compound, the green tea-derived polyphenol and flavonoid epigallocatechin-3-gallate revealed also promising in vitro effects by antagonizing AGE-induced proinflammatory changes [198]. In healthy human subjects, supplementation of vitamin C significantly decreased serum protein glycation [199].

Many spices and herbs were shown to inhibit glycation of albumin in vitro, among them ginger, cinnamon, cloves, marjoram, rosemary and tarragon [200]. Their protective effects correlated with their phenolic content. Recently, in vivo beneficial effects of some of these compounds were shown in zebrafish [201]. Other promising compounds include blueberry extract and naturally occurring flavonoids, such as luteolin, quercetin and rutin, which can inhibit various stages of AGE formation [202, 203]. Blueberry extract, an AGE-inhibitor and C-xyloside, a glycosaminoglycan synthesis stimulator, were tested for 12 weeks in female diabetic subjects. This treatment resulted in significant improvement of skin firmness, wrinkles and hydration although it failed to show a significant decrease in the cutaneous content of AGEs [202].

In one of the few human studies successfully conducted on anti-AGE therapeutics, L-carnitine supplementation for 6 months in hemodialysis patients significantly decreased levels of AGEs in the skin [204]. L-carnitine, which is naturally abundant in meat, poultry, fish, and dairy products, is an antioxidant. Furthermore, it may function synergistically to neutralize oxidative stress when given with α-lipoic acid [205].

As a well-known nutraceutical product, grape seed extract (GSE) is an abundant source of catechins and proanthocyanidins with a strong antioxidant and free radical scavenging activity [206]. Peng et al. [209] studied the effects of GSE on the formation of Nε—(carboxy-methyl) lysine (CML) in bread. Besides introducing antioxidant activity to bread, GSE also appeared to attenuate CML content in bread crust. In particular, adding 600 and 1000 mg of GSE to bread (500 g) led to over 30% and 50% reduction in bread crust CML content, respectively. Strong antioxidant activities of catechins and proanthocyanidins abundant in GSE may contribute to the reduction of CML in GSE-fortified bread [207]. On the other hand, catechins and proanthocyanidins proved to be able to scavenge the intermediate dicarbonyls (such as MG, glyoxal) [208, 209] in the glycation process, which may also decrease the CML content of GSE-fortified bread.

Caloric Restriction and Dietary Measures

As nutrition is an important factor in skin aging, dietary caloric restriction may be effective in preventing accumulation of AGEs in the human body. In mice restriction of caloric intake increases lifespan and delays many age-related dysfunctions by altering stress response and influencing the expression of various metabolic and biosynthetic genes [210]. Dietary restriction could significantly decrease the levels of AGEs in rat and mice skin collagen [211, 212]. Skin collagen glycation and glycoxidation inversely correlated with lifespan whereas caloric restriction led to decreased accumulation of AGEs and increased lifespan [213]. Dietary restriction may not be a pragmatic option in humans; however a restriction in intake of dietary "glycotoxins" may be more feasible. As outlined above these dietary glycotoxins derive from nutrition. In humans dietary glycotoxins significantly increase concentrations of systemic inflammatory mediators like TNFα, interleukin (IL)-6 and C-reactive protein and are thus considered as diabetogenic, nephrotoxic and proatherogenic [92, 214]. Dietary intake of AGEs correlates with serum AGEs and can induce systemic oxidative stress, increase RAGE expression, decrease antioxidant levels and shorten lifespan in mice [148]. A diet with a low content in AGEs could reduce circulating AGEs and inflammatory biomarkers in patients with Diabetes and renal failure thus seeming to be an important supportive therapy in Diabetes [215, 216]. In mice low dietary AGEs had beneficial effects in wound healing and other DM-associated pathologies [136]. There are no studies investigating the effects of AGE-poor diets on skin aging in humans. However, it has been shown that skin collagen glycation positively correlates with blood glucose levels in Diabetes and that intensive treatment can reduce the levels of skin glycation, implicating that a diet low in AGEs may have a beneficial effect on skin glycation [217, 218].

Targeting RAGE

Another potential strategy against excessive accumulation of AGEs could be the antagonism of RAGE [219]. Possible approaches include gene knock-down of RAGE by siRNA or anti-sense and antagonism of RAGE with putative small molecular inhibitors against RAGE-induced signaling [67, 219]. Promising effects in various systems have been shown in vitro and in vivo with neutralizing anti-RAGE antibodies [60]. Since serum concentrations of sRAGE negatively correlate with AGE-induced pathologies, neutralization of AGEs by these decoy receptors of RAGE may be considered as another anti-AGE strategy. Potential protective effects of sRAGE have been shown in various Diabetes and inflammatory models [60, 62, 63, 220]. Interestingly, sRAGE could also attenuate impaired wound healing in diabetic mice. Therefore, studies will be needed to investigate an analogous effect on skin aging [221].

Others

Molecular chaperones like carnosine have lately shown promise in improving skin appearance in various studies at least in part by reducing the amounts of skin AGEs [222–224].

Combating AGE with Diet

Nearly 70 years ago, Urbach and Lentz reported that the level of sugar both in the blood and in the skin is decreased with a diet low in sugar [225]. Although its significance was not appreciated at the time, this finding demonstrated a quintessential connection between diet and skin health. We now understand that food is a source of both monosaccharides that, in high amounts, catalyze the production of AGEs in the body, and preformed AGEs [226].

Preformed AGEs are absorbed by the gut with approximately 10–0% efficiency. They can then enter the circulation, where they may induce protein cross-linking, inflammation, and intracellular oxidative stress. The end result is the amplification of a similar *"vicious cycle"*, which may be as detrimental as the consumption of excess dietary sugar [227]. Interestingly, preformed AGEs largely result from exogenous synthesis mediated by the food cooking process. Grilling, frying, deep fat frying, and roasting methods are all known to produce higher levels of AGEs in food. In contrast, methods of preparation that are water-based, such as boiling and steaming, produce a logarithmically lower amount of AGEs [21].

A diet low in AGEs correlated with a reduction in inflammatory biomarkers (i.e. TNFα, IL-6 and CRP) in diabetic human patients, as well as an improvement in wound healing and other diabetes-associated sequelae in mice [136, 216]. Other authors have cited the relatively youthful appearance that is often associated with the elderly Asian population as evidence of the long-term impact of employing water-based cooking practices, which are characteristic of Asian cooking [226].

The varying conditions of water and heat play a significant role in the production of dAGE content. As scrambled eggs prepared in an open pan over medium-low heat had about one half the dAGEs of eggs prepared in the same way but over high heat. Similarly, poached or steamed chicken had less than one fourth the dAGEs of roasted or broiled chicken. Moreover, microwaving also did not raise dAGE content to the same extent as other dry heat cooking methods for the relatively short cooking times (6 min or less) that were tested. In nut shell, higher temperature and lower moisture levels coincided with higher dAGE levels [18].

Tight glycemic control over a 4-month period can result in a reduction of glycated collagen formation by 25% [226, 227]. Consumption of a low-sugar diet prepared through waterbased cooking methods would limit both the consumption of preformed exogenous AGES and endogenous production through physiological glycation. Avoiding foods that result in higher levels of AGEs, such as donuts, barbecued meats, and dark-colored soft drinks, can be an effective strategy for slowing *"sugar sag"* [21].

Beans are recommended as suitable foods for diabetic patients in the past mainly for their high fibre and protein contents. Four kinds of beans including mung bean (Vigna radiata) black bean (Phaseolus vulgaris L.), soybean (Glycine max) and cowpea (Vigna unguiculata) were investigated for trapping of MG, a key intermediate compound for the formation of AGEs. The aqueous alcohol extracts of all beans examined have showed significant inhibitory activities at a concentration of 500 ppm with 80.4% inhibition for mung bean, 72.1% for black bean, 70.1% for soybean, and 67.3% for cowpea extract, respectively [208]. Various phenolic antioxidants from plant extracts have been found to inhibit the formation of AGEs, and their inhibition of free radical generation in the glycation process and subsequent inhibition of modification of proteins have been considered as the major mechanisms for mediating their anti-glycation activities. Total phenolics were determined and it was found that mung bean extract had the highest phenolic content and anti-glycation activities of these beans were highly correlated with their total phenolic contents (R2 = 0.95). Two major phenolic compounds from mung bean, vitexin and isovitexin were studied for their activities in direct reapping of MG [208].

Low or acidic pH also arrests the new AGE development. For example, beef that was marinated for 1 h in lemon juice or vinegar formed less than half the amount of AGEs during cooking than the untreated samples [18] Green tea is known well for diabetic people in several ways. It reduces blood glucose level; improves sensitivity to insulin and enhances antioxidant defenses [228, 229]. Furthermore, green tea inhibits the formation of AGEs in an in vitro bovine serum albumin (BSA)/glucose system and in the collagen of aged rats and diabetic rats.

Of interest, several culinary herbs and spices are believed to be capable of inhibiting the endogenous production of AGEs (specifically fructose-induced glycation). These include cinnamon, cloves, oregano, and allspice [195, 196, 200]. Other dietary compounds that have been linked to inhibition of AGE formation based on in vitro data and preliminary animal models include ginger, garlic, α-lipoic acid, carnitine, taurine, carnosine, flavonoids (e.g., green tea catechins), benfotiamine, α-tocopherol,niacinamide, pyridoxal, sodium selenite, selenium yeast, riboflavin, zinc, and manganese [195, 196, 200]. The cosmeceutical industry has taken notice of this data, and several have recently released topical products containing carnosine and α-lipoic acid, with claims related to anti-AGE formation [227]. However, data is lacking as to whether topical administration of these compounds is as effective as dietary delivery in slowing the aging process.

Since glycation is accelerated in the presence of ROS, antioxidants should theo-retically be effective in limiting the production of new AGEs. They may also impact AGE-induced tissue damage. One intriguing study looked at the effects of the anti-oxidant resveratrol. Popularly known for its abundance in red wine, resveratrol is a natural phenol produced by several plants in response to injury and is found in the skin of grapes, blueberries, raspberries, and mulberries. In one study, resveratrol inhibited AGE-induced proliferation and collagen synthesis activity in vascular smooth muscle cells belonging to strokeprone rats [230]. Another study found that it decreased the frequency of DNA breaks in MG treated mouse oocytes. Although resveratrol does not appear to reverse the glycation process itself, these studies sug-gest that it can reduce AGE-induced tissue damage [231]. While these findings are promising, to our knowledge these laboratory results have not yet been demon-strated in human studies.

Numerous traditional herbal infusions, including Luobuma (Apocynum venetum L.), Nagarmotha (Cyperus rotundus), Mate (Ilex paraguariensis) and Guava (Psidium guajava L.) exhibit potent anti-glycation capacities [232–235]. All herbal infusions inhibited the glucose-mediated formation of fluorescent AGEs in a dose-dependent manner at dilutions of 10-fold to 40-fold. At a ten-fold dilution, balm, mint, black tea, green tea and sage almost completely inhibited the formation of fluorescent AGEs. At a 20-fold dilution, only balm retained its capacity to inhibit totally the formation of fluorescent AGEs. Accordingly, comparing the antiglyca-tion capacities of different herbal infusions based on the experimental results obtained from a 40-fold dilution seems logical. At a 40-fold dilution, the anti-glycation capacity of herbal infusions followed the order, balm (89.8%) >mint (47.8%) >black tea (38.0%) >green tea (35.4%), sage (33.4%) and common verbena (30.4%) >rosemary (18.8%) >lemongrass (3.0%) [236].

Based on the current evidence, individuals with Diabetes and/or kidney disease seem to be the population groups deriving most benefit from an AGE-restricted diet and potentially from inhibition of AGE-formation and its associated actions in the body [16, 194, 228, 237].

How to Win the Battle Against AGEs/
Fight Against AGEs in Kitchen

As modern diets are largely heat processed, they are more prone to contain high levels of AGEs [16]. On an average, the intake of dAGE in a cohort of healthy adults from the New York city areas was found to be $14,700 \pm 680$ AGE kU/day [101]. By smart food selection and by changing the way of cooking, the level of AGEs could be lowered in the diet. Overall, moving away from foods high in fat, red meat and processed and fast foods and toward a diet focused more on fruits and vegetables, whole grains and lean meats and fish will not only reduce the AGE intake but help to meet other important nutritional goals as well.

Reducing dAGE may be especially important for people with Diabetes, who generate more endogenous AGEs than those without Diabetes and for those with renal disease, who have impaired AGE clearance from the body [130]. Recently there has been heightened interest in therapeutic diets that are higher in protein and fat and lower in carbohydrate for weight loss, Diabetes and cardiovascular diseases. This type of dietary pattern may substantially raise dAGE intake and thus contribute to health problems over the long term. A safe and optimal dAGE intake for the purposes of disease prevention has yet to be established.

Some tips to win the battle against AGEs in kitchen are as:

- Use of lower cooking temperatures over high cooking temperatures;
- Steming, stewing and poaching are be the cooking methods than frying, grilling and roasting;
- Be wary of browning;
- Higher temperature and lower moisture levels in food during cooking increase dAGE levels;
- Phenolic antioxidants (e.g., in beans) can inhibit the formation of AGEs;
- Addition of acids (e.g., vinegar, lemon juice) lowers AGE levels;
- Green tea inhibits formation of AGEs;
- Cook fresh foods as possible;
- Eat more often at home [16].

Conclusion

Current evidence from many different disciplines lends strong support to the idea that AGEs contribute to the multisystem decline that occurs with aging. AGEs contribute to inflammation and tissue damage through AGE-RAGE binding. AGEs cross-link collagen and other proteins and thus increase the stiffness of tissues such as the major arteries, heart, bone, and muscle.

There is clearly an abundance of in vitro data and a handful of in vivo animal findings that support various options for dietary therapy directed against *"sugar sag."* However, studies in humans are limited by logistical, ethical, and inherent study design issues. Nevertheless, the role of diet in skin aging is undeniable. As our understanding of how accumulation of AGEs affects a rapidly growing number of pathologies, it is inevitable that our research methods will evolve to better address the challenges that currently seem so discouraging.

In the meantime, awareness of the critical impact of AGE formation in both diabetics and non-diabetics must be extended to all patients, regardless of their current health status. That task begins with clinicians. Dietary counseling should be incorporated into our regular interactions with patients, alongside essential discussions about UV-protection and avoidance of tobacco. After all, these are the three most important known exogenous aging factors. Their common grouping is reflective of their interconnected nature and their action in concert to disturb homeostasis.

Finally, there is ample evidence that AGEs play an important role in skin aging. There are also numerous studies investigating potential substances against excessive accumulation of AGEs in tissues. Some of these studies have already shown protective effects against diabetic complications. Modification of intake and circulating levels of AGEs may be a possible strategy to promote health in old age, especially because most Western foods are processed at high temperature and are rich in AGEs. As controlled human studies investigating the effects of these anti-AGE strategies against skin aging are largely missing, this is a hot field for future researches.

References

1. Nguyen HP, Katta R. Sugar sag: glycation and the role of diet in aging skin. Skin Ther Lett. 2015;20(6):1–5.
2. Semba RD, Nicklett EJ, Ferrucci L. Does accumulation of advanced glycation end products contribute to the aging phenotype? J Gerontol A Biol Sci Med Sci. 2010;65(9):963–75.
3. Tosato M, Zamboni V, Ferrini A, Cesari M. The aging process and potential interventions to extend life expectancy. Clin Interv Aging. 2007;2:401–12.
4. Zouboulis CC, Boschnakow A. Chronological ageing and photoageing of the human sebaceous gland. Clin Exp Dermatol. 2001;26(7):600–7.
5. Elias PM, Ghadially R. The aged epidermal permeability barrier: basis for functional abnormalities. Clin Geriatr Med. 2002;18(1):103–20.
6. Ye J, Garg A, Calhoun C, et al. Alterations in cytokine regulation in aged epidermis: implications for permeability barrier homeostasis and inflammation. I. IL-1 gene family. Exp Dermatol. 2002;11(3):209–16.
7. Tsutsumi M, Denda M. Paradoxical effects of beta-estradiol on epidermal permeability barrier homeostasis. Br J Dermatol. 2007;157(4):776–9.
8. Fimmel S, Kurfurst R, Bonte F, et al. Responsiveness to androgens and effectiveness of antisense oligonucleotides against the androgen receptor on human epidermal keratinocytes is dependent on the age of the donor and the location of cell origin. Horm Metab Res. 2007;39(2):157–65.
9. Makrantonaki E, Vogel K, Fimmel S, et al. Interplay of IGF-I and 17betaestradiol at age-specific levels in human sebocytes and fibroblasts in vitro. Exp Gerontol. 2008;43(10):939–46.
10. Ashcroft GS, Horan MA, Ferguson MW. The effects of ageing on wound healing: immunolocalisation of growth factors and their receptors in a murine incisional model. J Anat. 1997;190(Pt 3):351–65.
11. Bhushan M, Cumberbatch M, Dearman RJ, et al. Tumour necrosis factoralpha-induced migration of human Langerhans cells: the influence of ageing. Br J Dermatol. 2002;146(1):32–40.
12. Zouboulis CC, Makrantonaki E. Clinical aspects and molecular diagnostics of skin aging. Clin Dermatol. 2011;29(1):3–14.
13. Chung JH, Yano K, Lee MK, et al. Differential effects of photoaging vs intrinsic aging on the vascularization of human skin. Arch Dermatol. 2002;138(11):1437–42.
14. Cordain L, Eaton SB, Sebastian A, Mann N, Lindeberg S, Watkins BA, O'Keefe JH, Brand-Miller J. Origins and evolution of the western diet: health implications for the 21st century. Am J Clin Nutr. 2005;81:341–54.
15. Rahbar S, Blumenfe O, Ranney HM. Studies of an unusual hemoglobin in patients with diabetes mellitus. Biochem Biophys Res Commun. 1969;36:838–43.
16. Sharma C, Kaur A, Thind SS, Singh B, Raina S. Advanced glycation end-products (AGEs): an emerging concern for processed food industries. J Food Sci Technol. 2015;52(12):7561–76.
17. Ulrich P, Cerami A. Protein glycation, diabetes and aging. Recent Prog Horm Res. 2001;56:21.
18. Uribarri J, Woodruff S, Goodman S, Cai W, Chen X, Pyzik R, Yong A, Striker GE, Vlassara H. Advanced glycation end products in foods and a practical guide to their reduction in the diet. J Am Diet Assoc. 2010;110(6):911–6.

19. Vashishth D, Gibson GJ, Khoury JI, Schaffler MB, Kimura J, Fyhrie DP. Influence of nonenzymatic glycation on biomechanical properties of cortical bone. Bone. 2001;28:195–201.

20. Nicholl ID, Stitt AW, Moore JE, Ritchie AJ, Archer DB, Bucala R. Increased levels of advanced glycation endproducts in the lenses and blood vessels of cigarette smokers. Mol Med. 1998;4:594–601.

21. O'Brien J, Morrissey PA. Nutritional and toxicological aspects of the Maillard browning reaction in foods. Crit Rev Food Sci Nutr. 1989;28(3):211–48.

22. Van Puyvelde K, Mets T, Njemini R, et al. Effect of advanced glycation end product intake on inflammation and aging: a systematic review. Nutr Rev. 2014;72(10):638–50.

23. Mook-Kanamori MJ, Selim MM, Takiddin AH, et al. Ethnic and gender differences in advanced glycation end products measured by skin autofluorescence. Dermatoendocrinol. 2013;5(2):325–30.

24. Medvedev ZA. An attempt at a rational classification of theories of ageing. Biol Rev Camb Philos Soc. 1990;65:375–98.

25. Dimri GP, Lee X, Basile G, Acosta M, Scott G, Roskelley C, et al. A biomarker that identifies senescent human cells in culture and in aging skin in vivo. Proc Natl Acad Sci USA. 1995;92:9363–7.

26. Allsopp RC, Vaziri H, Patterson C, Goldstein S, Younglai EV, Futcher AB, et al. Telomere length predicts replicative capacity of human fibroblasts. Proc Natl Acad Sci USA. 1992;89:10114–8.

27. Michikawa Y, Mazzucchelli F, Bresolin N, Scarlato G, Attardi G. Aging-dependent large accumulation of point mutations in the human mtDNA control region for replication. Science. 1999;286:774–9.

28. Harman D. The free radical theory of aging. Antioxid Redox Signal. 2003;5:557–61.

29. Giacomoni PU, Rein G. Factors of skin ageing share common mechanisms. Biogerontology. 2001;2:219–29.

30. Paraskevi Gkogkolou P, Böhm M. Advanced glycation end products key players in skin aging? Dermato-Endocrinology. 2012;4(3):259–70.

31. John WG, Lamb EJ. Themaillard or browning reaction in diabetes. Eye. 1993;7:230–7.

32. Ahmed N. Advanced glycation end products-role in pathology of diabetic complications. Diabetes Res Clin Pract. 2005;67:3–21.

33. Maillard LC. Action des acides amines sur les sucres: formation des melanoidines par voie methodique. C R Acad Sci (Paris). 1912;154:66–8.

34. Hodge JE. Dehydrated foods, chemistry of browning reactions in model systems. J Agric Food Chem. 1953;1:928–43.

35. Paul RG, Bailey AJ. Glycation of collagen: the basis of its central role in the late complications of ageing and diabetes. Int J Biochem Cell Biol. 1996;28:1297–310.

36. Thorpe SR, Baynes JW. Maillard reaction products in tissue proteins: new products and new perspectives. Amino Acids. 2003;25(3-4):275–81.

37. Kawabata K, Yoshikawa H, Saruwatari K, et al. The presence of N(epsilon)-(carboxymethyl) lysine in the human epidermis. Biochim Biophys Acta. 2011;1814(10):1246–52.

38. Dyer DG, Dunn JA, Thorpe SR, et al. Accumulation of Maillard reaction products in skin collagen in diabetes and aging. J Clin Invest. 1993;91(6):2463–9.

39. Jeanmaire C, Danoux L, Pauly G. Glycation during human dermal intrinsic and actinic ageing: an in vivo and in vitro model study. Br J Dermatol. 2001;145(1):10–8.

40. Fan X, Sell DR, Zhang J, Nemet I, Theves M, Lu J, et al. Anaerobic vs aerobic pathways of carbonyl and oxidant stress in human lens and skin during aging and in diabetes: a comparative analysis. Free Radic Biol Med. 2010;49:847–56.

41. Kueper T, Grune T, Prahl S, Lenz H, Welge V, Biernoth T, et al. Vimentin is the specific target in skin glycation. Structural prerequisites, functional consequences, and role in skin aging. J Biol Chem. 2007;282:23427–36.

42. Mizutari K, Ono T, Ikeda K, Kayashima K, Horiuchi S. Photo enhanced modification of human skin elastin in actinic elastosis by N(epsilon)(carboxymethyl)lysine, one of the glycoxidation products of the Maillard reaction. J Invest Dermatol. 1997;108:797–802.

43. Yu Y, Thorpe SR, Jenkins AJ, Shaw JN, Sochaski MA, McGee D, et al. Advanced glycation end-products and methionine sulphoxide in skin collagen of patients with type 1 diabetes. Diabetologia. 2006;49:2488–98.
44. Taneda S, Monnier VM. ELISA of pentosidine, an advanced glycation end product, in biological specimens. Clin Chem. 1994;40:1766–73.
45. Sell DR, Biemel KM, Reihl O, Lederer MO, Strauch CM, Monnier VM. Glucosepane is a major protein cross-link of the senescent human extracellular matrix. Relationship with diabetes. J Biol Chem. 2005;280:12310–5.
46. Ahmed MU, Brinkmann Frye E, Degenhardt TP, Thorpe SR, Baynes JW. N-epsilon-(carboxyethyl)lysine, a product of the chemical modification of proteins by methylglyoxal, increases with age in human lens proteins. Biochem J. 1997;324:565–70.
47. Frye EB, Degenhardt TP, Thorpe SR, Baynes JW. Role of the Maillard reaction in aging of tissue proteins. Advanced glycation end product-dependent increase in imidazolium crosslinks in human lens proteins. J Biol Chem. 1998;273:18714–9.
48. Reddy S, Bichler J, Wells-Knecht KJ, Thorpe SR, Baynes JW. N epsilon-(carboxymethyl) lysine is a dominant advanced glycation end product (AGE) antigen in tissue proteins. Biochemistry. 1995;34:10872–8.
49. Gkogkolou P, Bohm M. Advanced glycation end products: key players in skin aging? Dermatoendocrinol. 2012;4(3):259–70.
50. Sell DR, Monnier VM. Isolation, purification and partial characterization of novel fluorophores from aging human insoluble collagen-rich tissue. Connect Tissue Res. 1989;19:77–92.
51. Thornalley PJ, Langborg A, Minhas HS. Formation of glyoxal, methylglyoxal and 3-deoxyglucosone in the glycation of proteins by glucose. Biochem J. 1999;344:109–16.
52. Fleming TH, Humpert PM, Nawroth PP, Bierhaus A. Reactive metabolites and AGE/RAGE-mediated cellular dysfunction affect the aging process: a mini-review. Gerontology. 2011;57:435–43.
53. Cerami C, Founds H, Nicholl I, Mitsuhashi T, Giordano D, Vanpatten S, et al. Tobacco smoke is a source of toxic reactive glycation products. Proc Natl Acad Sci USA. 1997;94:13915–20.
54. Leslie RD, Beyan H, Sawtell P, Boehm BO, Spector TD, Snieder H. Level of an advanced glycated end product is genetically determined: a study of normal twins. Diabetes. 2003;52:2441–4.
55. Thornalley PJ. The enzymatic defence against glycation in health, disease and therapeutics: a symposium to examine the concept. Biochem Soc Trans. 2003;31:1341–2.
56. Xue M, Rabbani N, Thornalley PJ. Glyoxalase in ageing. Semin Cell Dev Biol. 2011;22:293–301.
57. Wu X, Monnier VM. Enzymatic deglycation of proteins. Arch Biochem Biophys. 2003;419:16–24.
58. Van Schaftingen E, Collard F, Wiame E, Veiga-da-Cunha M. Enzymatic repair of amadori products. Amino Acids. 2012;42:1143–50.
59. Conner JR, Beisswenger PJ, Szwergold BS. Some clues as to the regulation, expression, function, and distribution of fructosamine-3-kinase and fructosamine-3-kinase-related protein. Ann N Y Acad Sci. 2005;1043:824–36.
60. Bierhaus A, Humpert PM, Morcos M, Wendt T, Chavakis T, Arnold B, et al. Understanding RAGE, the receptor for advanced glycation end products. J Mol Med (Berl). 2005;83:876–86.
61. Loughlin DT, Artlett CM. Precursor of advanced glycation end products mediates ER-stress-induced caspase- 3 activation of human dermal fibroblasts through NAD(P)H oxidase 4. PLoS One. 2010;5:e11093.
62. Ramasamy R, Vannucci SJ, Yan SS, Herold K, Yan SF, Schmidt AM. Advanced glycation end products and RAGE: a common thread in aging, diabetes, neurodegeneration, and inflammation. Glycobiology. 2005;15:16R–28R.
63. Lohwasser C, Neureiter D, Weigle B, Kirchner T, Schuppan D. The receptor for advanced glycation end products is highly expressed in the skin and upregulated by advanced glycation end products and tumor necrosis factor-alpha. J Invest Dermatol. 2006;126:291–9.

64. Fujimoto E, Kobayashi T, Fujimoto N, Akiyama M, Tajima S, Nagai R. AGE modified collagens I and III induce keratinocyte terminal differentiation through AGE receptor CD36: epidermal-dermal interaction in acquired perforating dermatosis. J Invest Dermatol. 2010;130:405–14.

65. Zhu P, Ren M, Yang C, YX H, Ran JM, Yan L. Involvement of RAGE, MAPK and NF-κB pathways in AGEs-induced MMP-9 activation in HaCaT keratinocytes. Exp Dermatol. 2012;21:123–9.

66. Hilmenyuk T, Bellinghausen I, Heydenreich B, Ilchmann A, Toda M, Grabbe S, et al. Effects of glycation of the model food allergen ovalbumin on antigen uptake and presentation by human dendritic cells. Immunology. 2010;129:437–45.

67. Chen Y, Akirav EM, Chen W, Henegariu O, Moser B, Desai D, et al. RAGE ligation affects T cell activation and controls T cell differentiation. J Immunol. 2008;181:4272–8.

68. Tanaka N, Yonekura H, Yamagishi S, Fujimori H, Yamamoto Y, Yamamoto H. The receptor for advanced glycation end products is induced by the glycation products themselves and tumor necrosis factor-alpha through nuclear factor-kappa B, and by 17beta-estradiol through Sp-1 in human vascular endothelial cells. J Biol Chem. 2000;275:25781–90.

69. Vlassara H. The AGE-receptor in the pathogenesis of diabetic complications. Diabetes Metab Res Rev. 2001;17:436–43.

70. Lu C, He JC, Cai W, Liu H, Zhu L, Vlassara H. Advanced glycation endproduct (AGE) receptor 1 is a negative regulator of the inflammatory response to age in mesangial cells. Proc Natl Acad Sci USA. 2004;101:11767–72.

71. Cai W, He JC, Zhu L, Chen X, Wallenstein S, Striker GE, Vlassara H. Reduced oxidant stress and extended lifespan in mice exposed to a low glycotoxin diet: association with increased AGER1 expression. Am J Pathol. 2007;170:1893–902.

72. Ramasamy R, Yan SF, Schmidt AM. RAGE: therapeutic target and biomarker of the inflammatory response-the evidence mounts. J Leukoc Biol. 2009;86:505–12.

73. Brownlee M, Vlassara H, Cerami A. Nonenzymaic glycosylation and the pathogenesis of diabetic complications. Annu Int Med. 1984;101:527–37.

74. Raj DS, Choudhury D, Welbourne TC, Levi M. Age a nephrologist's perspective. Am J Kidney Dis. 2000;35:365–80.

75. Uribarri J. Advanced glycation end products. In: Daugirdas JT, editor. Handbook of chronic kidney disease management. Philadelphia: Lippincott Willliams and Wilkins; 2012. p. 152–8.

76. Hipkiss AR. Accumulation of altered proteins and ageing: causes and effects. Exp Gerontol. 2006;41(5):464–73.

77. Dunn JA, McCance DR, Thorpe SR, et al. Age-dependent accumulation of N epsilon-(carboxymethyl)lysine and N epsilon-(carboxymethyl) hydroxylysine in human skin collagen. Biochemistry. 1991;30(5):1205–10.

78. Avery NC, Bailey AJ. The effects of the Maillard reaction on the physical properties and cell interactions of collagen. Pathol Biol (Paris). 2006;54(7):387–95.

79. Haitoglou CS, Tsilibary EC, Brownlee M, et al. Altered cellular interactions between endothelial cells and nonenzymatically glucosylated laminin/type IV collagen. J Biol Chem. 1992;267(18):12404–7.

80. Goldin A, Beckman JA, Schmidt AM, et al. Advanced glycation end products: sparking the development of diabetic vascular injury. Circulation. 2006;114(6):597–605.

81. DeGroot J, Verzijl N, Wenting-Van Wijk MJ, et al. Age-related decrease in susceptibility of human articular cartilage to matrix metalloproteinasemediated degradation: the role of advanced glycation end products. Arthritis Rheum. 2001;44(11):2562–71.

82. Nowotny K, Grune T. Degradation of oxidized and glycoxidized collagen: role of collagen cross-linking. Arch Biochem Biophys. 2014;542:56–64.

83. Yoshinaga E, Kawada A, Ono K, et al. N(varepsilon)-(carboxymethyl)lysine modification of elastin alters its biological properties: implications for the accumulation of abnormal elastic fibers in actinic elastosis. J Invest Dermatol. 2012;132(2):315–23.

84. Masaki H, Okano Y, Sakurai H. Generation of active oxygen species from advanced glycation end-products (AGEs) during ultraviolet light A (UVA) irradiation and a possible mechanism for cell damaging. Biochim Biophys Acta. 1999;1428(1):45–56.

85. Alikhani Z, Alikhani M, Boyd CM, et al. Advanced glycation end products enhance expression of pro-apoptotic genes and stimulate fibroblast apoptosis through cytoplasmic and mitochondrial pathways. J Biol Chem. 2005;280(13):12087–95.

86. Zhu P, Yang C, Chen LH, et al. Impairment of human keratinocyte mobility and proliferation by advanced glycation end products-modified BSA. Arch Dermatol Res. 2011;303(5):339–50.

87. Bulteau AL, Verbeke P, Petropoulos I, et al. Proteasome inhibition in glyoxal-treated fibroblasts and resistance of glycated glucose-6-phosphate dehydrogenase to 20 S proteasome degradation in vitro. J Biol Chem. 2001;276(49):45662–8.

88. Roberts MJ, Wondrak GT, Laurean DC, et al. DNA damage by carbonyl stress in human skin cells. Mutat Res. 2003;522(1-2):45–56.

89. Verzijl N, DeGroot J, Oldehinkel E, Bank RA, Thorpe SR, Baynes JW, et al. Age-related accumulation of Maillard reaction products in human articular cartilage collagen. Biochem J. 2000;350:381–7.

90. Haus JM, Carrithers JA, Trappe SW, Trappe TA. Collagen, cross-linking, and advanced glycation end products in aging human skeletal muscle. J Appl Physiol. 2007;103:2068–76.

91. Sell DR, Carlson EC, Monnier VM. Differential effects of type 2 (non-insulin-dependent) diabetes mellitus on pentosidine formation in skin and glomerular basement membrane. Diabetologia. 1993;36:936–41.

92. Vlassara H, Cai W, Crandall J, Goldberg T, Oberstein R, Dardaine V, et al. Inflammatory mediators are induced by dietary glycotoxins, a major risk factor for diabetic angiopathy. Proc Natl Acad Sci USA. 2002;99:15596–601.

93. Glenn JV, Beattie JR, Barrett L, Frizzell N, Thorpe SR, Boulton ME, et al. Confocal Raman microscopy can quantify advanced glycation end product (age) modifications in Bruch's membrane leading to accurate, nondestructive prediction of ocular aging. FASEB J. 2007;21:3542–52.

94. Stitt AW. Advanced glycation: an important pathological event in diabetic and age related ocular disease. Br J Ophthalmol. 2001;85:746–53.

95. Sell DR, Lane MA, Johnson WA, Masoro EJ, Mock OB, Reiser KM, et al. Longevity and the genetic determination of collagen glycoxidation kinetics in mammalian senescence. Proc Natl Acad Sci USA. 1996;93:485–90.

96. Schleicher ED, Wagner E, Nerlich AG. Increased accumulation of the glycoxidation product N(epsilon)-(carboxymethyl)lysine in human tissues in diabetes and aging. J Clin Invest. 1997;99:457–68.

97. Corstjens H, Dicanio D, Muizzuddin N, Neven A, Sparacio R, Declercq L, et al. Glycation associated skin autofluorescence and skin elasticity are related to chronological age and body mass index of healthy subjects. Exp Gerontol. 2008;43(7):663.

98. Pageon H. Reaction of glycation and human skin: the effects on the skin and its components, reconstructed skin as a model. Pathol Biol (Paris). 2010;58:226–31.

99. Lutgers HL, Graaff R, Links TP, Ubink-Veltmaat LJ, Bilo HJ, Gans RO, et al. Skin autofluorescence as a noninvasive marker of vascular damage in patients with type 2 diabetes. Diabetes Care. 2006;29:2654–9.

100. Goldberg T, Cai W, Peppa M, Dardaine V, Baliga BS, Uribarri J, et al. Advanced glycoxidation end products in commonly consumed foods. J Am Diet Assoc. 2004;104:1287–91.

101. Uribarri J, Cai W, Peppa M, Goodman S, Ferrucci L, Striker G, et al. Circulating glycotoxins and dietary advanced glycation endproducts: two links to inflammatory response, oxidative stress, and aging. J Gerontol A Biol Sci Med Sci. 2007;62:427–33.

102. DeGroot J. The age of the matrix: chemistry, consequence and cure. Curr Opin Pharmacol. 2004;4:301–5.

103. Reihsner R, Melling M, Pfeiler W, Menzel EJ. Alterations of biochemical and two-dimensional biomechanical properties of human skin in diabetes mellitus as compared to effects of in vitro non-enzymatic glycation. Clin Biomech (Bristol, Avon). 2000;15:379–86.

104. Yoon HS, Baik SH, Oh CH. Quantitative measurement of desquamation and skin elasticity in diabetic patients. Skin Res Technol. 2002;8:250–4.
105. Giardino I, Edelstein D, Brownlee M. Nonenzymatic glycosylation in vitro and in bovine endothelial cells alters basic fibroblast growth factor activity. A model for intracellular glycosylation in diabetes. J Clin Invest. 1994;94:110–7.
106. Uchiki T, Weikel KA, Jiao W, Shang F, Caceres A, Pawlak D, et al. Glycation-altered proteolysis as a pathobiologic mechanism that links dietary glycemic index, aging, and age-related disease (in nondiabetics). Aging Cell. 2012;11:1–13.
107. Ukeda H, Hasegawa Y, Ishi T, Sawamura M. Inactivation of Cu, Zn-superoxide dismutase by intermediates of Maillard reaction and glycolytic pathway and some sugars. Biosci Biotechnol Biochem. 1997;61:2039–42.
108. Berge U, Behrens J, Rattan SI. Sugar-induced premature aging and altered differentiation in human epidermal keratinocytes. Ann NY Acad Sci. 2007;1100:524–9.
109. Ravelojaona V, Robert AM, Robert L. Expression of senescence-associated beta-galactosidase (SA-beta-Gal) by human skin fibroblasts, effect of advanced glycation end-products and fucose or rhamnose-rich polysaccharides. Arch Gerontol Geriatr. 2009;48:151–4.
110. Sejersen H, Rattan SI. Dicarbonyl-induced accelerated aging in vitro in human skin fibroblasts. Biogerontology. 2009;10:203–11.
111. Portero-Otín M, Pamplona R, Bellmunt MJ, Ruiz MC, Prat J, Salvayre R, et al. Advanced glycation end product precursors impair epidermal growth factor receptor signaling. Diabetes. 2002;51:1535–42.
112. Wondrak GT, Roberts MJ, Jacobson MK, Jacobson EL. Photosensitized growth inhibition of cultured human skin cells: mechanism and suppression of oxidative stress from solar irradiation of glycated proteins. J Invest Dermatol. 2002;119:489–98.
113. Yim MB, Yim HS, Lee C, Kang SO, Chock PB. Protein glycation: creation of catalytic sites for free radical generation. Ann NY Acad Sci. 2001;928:48–53.
114. Lee C, Yim MB, Chock PB, Yim HS, Kang SO. Oxidation-reduction properties of methylglyoxal-modified protein in relation to free radical generation. J Biol Chem. 1998;273:25272–8.
115. Qian M, Liu M, Eaton JW. Transition metals bind to glycated proteins forming redox active "glycochelates": implications for the pathogenesis of certain diabetic complications. Biochem Biophys Res Commun. 1998;250:385–9.
116. Meerwaldt R, Links T, Graaff R, Thorpe SR, Baynes JW, Hartog J, et al. Simple noninvasive measurement of skin autofluorescence. Ann NY Acad Sci. 2005;1043:290–8.
117. Mulder DJ, Water TV, Lutgers HL, Graaff R, Gans RO, Zijlstra F, et al. Skin autofluorescence, a novel marker for glycemic and oxidative stress-derived advanced glycation endproducts: an overview of current clinical studies, evidence, and limitations. Diabetes Technol Ther. 2006;8:523–35.
118. Tseng JY, Ghazaryan AA, Lo W, Chen YF, Hovhannisyan V, Chen SJ, et al. Multiphoton spectral microscopy for imaging and quantification of tissue glycation. Biomed Opt Express. 2010;2:218–30.
119. Bos DC, de Ranitz-Greven WL, de Valk HW. Advanced glycation end products, measured as skin autofluorescence and diabetes complications: a systematic review. Diabetes Technol Ther. 2011;13:773–9.
120. Smit AJ, Gerrits EG. Skin autofluorescence as a measure of advanced glycation endproduct deposition: a novel risk marker in chronic kidney disease. Curr Opin Nephrol Hypertens. 2010;19:527–33.
121. Genuth S, Sun W, Cleary P, Sell DR, Dahms W, Malone J, et al. DCCT Skin Collagen Ancillary Study Group. Glycation and carboxymethyllysine levels in skin collagen predict the risk of future 10-year progression of diabetic retinopathy and nephropathy in the diabetes control and complications trial and epidemiology of diabetes interventions and complications participants with type 1 diabetes. Diabetes. 2005;54:3103–11.
122. Beisswenger PJ, Howell S, Mackenzie T, Corstjens H, Muizzuddin N, Matsui MS. Two fluorescent wavelengths, 440(ex)/520(em) nm and 370(ex)/440(em) nm, reflect advanced glyca-

tion and oxidation end products in human skin without diabetes. Diabetes Technol Ther. 2012;14:285–92.

123. Story M, Hayes M, Kalina B. Availability of foods in high schools: is there cause for concern? J Am Diet Assoc. 1996;96:123–6.

124. Vlassara H, Uribarri J. Glycoxidation and diabetic complications: modern lessons and a warning? Rev Endocr Metab Disord. 2004;5:181–8.

125. Ledl F, Schleicher E. New aspects of the maillard reaction in foods and in the human body. Angew Chem Int Ed. 1990;29:565–94.

126. Nursten H. Introduction. In: The Maillard reaction chemistry, biochemistry and implications. Cambridge: The Royal Society of Chemistry; 2005. p. 1–4.

127. Nursten H. Recent advances. In: The Maillard Reaction chemistry, biochemistry and implications. Cambridge: The Royal Society of Chemistry; 2005. p. 31–51.

128. Poulsen MW, Hedegaard RV, Anderson JM, Courten B, Bugel S, Nielsen J, Skibsted LH, Dragsted L. Advanced glycation endproducts in food and their effects on health. Food Chem Toxicol. 2013;60:10–37. https://doi.org/10.1016/j.fct.2013.06.052.

129. Finot PA, Magnenat E. Metabolic transit of early and advanced maillard products. Prog Food Nutr Sci. 1981;5:193–207.

130. Koschinsky T, He CJ, Mitsuhashi T, Bucala R, Liu C, Buenting C, Heitmann K, Vlassara H. Orally absorbed reactive glycation products (glycotoxins): an environmental risk factor in diabetic nephropathy. Proc Natl Acad Sci USA. 1997;94(12):6474–9.

131. Delgado-Andrade C, Seiquer I, Garcia MM, Galdo G, Navarro MP. Increased maillard reaction products intake reduces phosphorus digestibility in male adolescents. Nutr. 2011;27:86–91.

132. Garcia MM, Seiquer I, Delgado-Andrade C, Galdo G, Navarro MP. Intake of Maillard reaction products reduces iron bioavailability in male adolescents. Mol Nutr Food Res. 2009;53:1551–60.

133. Seiquer I, Diaz-Alguacil J, Delgado-Andrade C, Lopez-Frias M, Munoz HA, Galdo G, Navarro MP. Diets rich in maillard reaction products affect protein digestibility in adolescent males aged 11–14 y. Am J Clin Nutr. 2006;83:1082–8.

134. Bergmann R, Helling R, Heichert C, Scheunemann M, Mading P, Wittrisch H, Johannsen B, Henle T. Radio fluorination and positron emission tomography (PET) as a new approach to study the in vivo distribution and elimination of the advanced glycation endproducts N epsilon-carboxymethyllysine (CML) and N epsilon-carboxyethyllysine (CEL). Nahrung. 2001;45:182–8.

135. He C, Sabol J, Mitsuhashi T, Vlassara H. Dietary glycotoxins: inhibition of reactive products by aminoguanidine facilitates renal clearance and reduces tissue sequestration. Diabetes. 1999;48:1308–15.

136. Peppa M, Brem H, Ehrlich P, Zhang JG, Cai W, Li Z, et al. Adverse effects of dietary glycotoxins on wound healing in genetically diabetic mice. Diabetes. 2003;52:2805–13.

137. Hofmann SM, Dong HJ, Li Z, Cai W, Altomonte J, Thung SN, Zeng F, Fisher EA, Vlassara H. Improved insulin sensitivity is associated with restricted intake of dietary glycoxidation products in the db/db mouse. Diabetes. 2002;51:2082–9.

138. Bierhaus A, Ziegler R, Nawroth PP. Molecular mechanisms of diabetic angiopathy clues for innovative therapeutic interventions. Horm Res. 1998;50(Suppl 1):1–5.

139. Sano H, Higashi T, Matsumoto K, et al. Insulin enhances macrophage scavenger receptor mediated endocytic uptake of advanced glycated end products. J Biol Chem. 1998;273:8630–7.

140. Uribarri J, Cai WJ, Sandu O, Peppa M, Goldberg T, Vlassara H. Diet- derived advanced glycation end products are major contributors to the body's AGE pool and induce inflammation in healthy subjects. Ann NYAcad Sci. 2005;1043:461–6.

141. Cai W, Cao QD, Zhu L, et al. Oxidative stress-inducing carbonyl compounds from common foods: novel mediators of cellular dysfunction. Mol Med. 2002;8:337–46.

142. Uribarri J, Peppa M, Cai W, Goldberg T, et al. Restriction of dietary glycotoxins markedly reduces AGE toxins in renal failure patients. J Am Soc Nephrol. 2003;14:728–31.

143. Zheng F, He C, Cai W, Hattori M, Steffes M, Vlassara H. Prevention of diabetic nephropathy in mice by a diet low in glycoxidation products. Diabetes Metab Res Rev. 2002;18:224–37.

144. Tan AL, Sourris KC, Harcourt BE, Thallas-Bonke V, Penfold S, Andrikopoulos S, Thomas MC, O'Brien RC, Bierhaus A, Cooper ME, Forbes JM, Coughlan MT. Disparate effects on renal and oxidative parameters following RAGE deletion, AGE accumulation inhibition, or dietary AGE control in experimental diabetic nephropathy. Am J Physiol Ren Physiol. 2010;298:763–70.
145. Feng JX, Hou FF, Liang M, Wang GB, Zhang X, Li HY, Xie D, Tian JW, Liu ZQ. Restricted intake of dietary advanced glycation end products retards renal progression in the remnant kidney model. Kidney Int. 2007;71:901–11.
146. Sebekova K, Faist V, Hofmann T, Schinzel R, Heidland A. Effects of a diet rich in advanced glycation end products in the rat remnant kidney model. Am J Kidney Dis. 2003;41:48–51.
147. Lin RY, Choudhury RP, Cai W, Lu M, Fallon JT, Fisher EA, Vlassara H. Dietary glycotoxins promote diabetic atherosclerosis in apolipoprotein E-deficient mice. Atherosclerosis. 2003;168:213–20.
148. Cai W, He JC, Zhu L, Chen X, Zheng F, Striker GE, et al. Oral glycotoxins determine the effects of calorie restriction on oxidant stress, age-related diseases, and lifespan. Am J Pathol. 2008;173:327–36.
149. Ames JM. Determination of Ne-(carboxymethyl) lysine in foods and related systems. Ann NY Acad Sci. 2008;1126:20–4.
150. Hartkopf J, Pahlke C, Lüdemann G, Erbersdobler HF. Determination of Ne-carboxymethyllysine by a reserved-phase high-performance liquid chromatography method. J Chromatogr. 1994;672:242–6.
151. Delgado-Andrade C, Rufián-Henares JA, Morales FJ. Study on fluorescence of maillard reaction compounds in breakfast cereals. Mol Nutr Food Res. 2006;50:799–804.
152. Yaacoub R, Saliba R, Nsouli B, Khalaf G, Birlouez-Aragon I. Formation of lipid oxidation and isomerization products during processing of nuts and sesame seeds. J Agric Food Chem. 2008;6:7082–90.
153. Drusch S, Faist V, Erbersdobler HF. Determination of Nepsiloncarboxymethyllysine in milk products by a modified reversed-phase HPLC method. Food Chem. 1999;65:547–53.
154. Chao PC, Hsu CC, Yin MC. Analysis of glycative products in sauces and sauce-treated foods. Food Chem. 2009;113:262–6.
155. Birlouez-Aragon I, Pischetsrieder M, Leclère J, et al. Assessment of protein glycation markers in infant formulas. Food Chem. 2004;87:253–9.
156. Sebekova K, Saavedra G, Zumpe C, Somoza V, Klenovicsova K, Birlouez-Aragon I. Plasma concentration and urinary excretion of Ne-(carboxymethyl)lysine in breast milk- and formula-fed infants. Ann NY Acad Sci. 2008;1126:177–80.
157. Dhuique-Mayer C, Tbatou M, Carail M, Caris-Veyrat C, Dornier M, Amiot MJ. Thermal degradation of antioxidant micronutrients in citrus juice: kinetics and newly formed compounds. J Agric Food Chem. 2007;55:4209–16.
158. Klopotek Y, Otto K, Bohm V. Processing strawberries to different products alters contents of vitamin C, total phenolics, total anthocyanins, and antioxidant capacity. J Agric Food Chem. 2005;53:5640–6.
159. Vikram VB, Ramesh MN, Prapulla SG. Thermal degradation kinetics of nutrients in orange juice heated by electromagnetic and conventional methods. J Food Eng. 2005;69:31–40.
160. Birlouez-Aragon I, Saavedra G, Tessier FJ, Galinier A, Ait-Ameur L, Lacoste F, Niamba CN, Alt N, Somoza V, Lecerf JM. A diet based on high-heat-treated foods promotes risk factors for diabetes mellitus and cardiovascular diseases. Am J Clin Nutr. 2010;91:1220–6.
161. Depeint F, Shangari N, Furrer R, Bruce WR, O'Brien PJ. Marginal thiamine deficiency increases oxidative markers in the plasma and selected tissues in F344 rats. Nutr Res. 2007;27:698–704.
162. Friedman M. Dietary impact of food processing. Annu Rev Nutr. 1992;12:119–37.
163. Perez-Locas C, Yaylayan VA. The Maillard reaction and food quality deterioration. In: Skibsted LH, Risbo J, Andersen ML, editors. Chemical deterioration and physical instability of food and beverages. Cambridge: Woodhead Publishing; 2010. p. 70–94.
164. Gokmen V, Senyuva HZ. Effects of some cations on the formation of acrylamide and furfurals in glucose-asparagine model system. Eur Food Res Technol. 2012;225:815–20.

165. Tareke E, Rydberg P, Karlsson P, Eriksson S, Tornqvist M. Analysis of acrylamide, a carcinogen formed in heated foodstuffs. J Agric Food Chem. 2002;50:4998–5006.
166. Skog KI, Johansson MA, Jagerstad MI. Carcinogenic heterocyclic amines in model systems and cooked foods: a review on formation, occurrence and intake. Food Chem Toxicol. 1998;36:879–96.
167. Janzowski C, Glaab V, Samimi E, Schlatter J, Eisenbrand G. 5-Hydroxymethylfurfural: assessment of mutagenicity, DNAdamaging potential and reactivity towards cellular glutathione. Food Chem Toxicol. 2000;38:801–9.
168. Pouillart P, Mauprivez H, Ait-Ameur L, Cayzeele A, Lecerf JM, Tessier FJ, Birlouez-Aragon I. Strategy for the study of the health impact of dietary maillard products in clinical studies—the example of the ICARE clinical study on healthy adults. Ann NY Acad Sci. 2008;1126:173–6.
169. Farris PK. Innovative cosmeceuticals: sirtuin activators and anti-glycation compounds. Semin Cutan Med Surg. 2011;30:163–6.
170. Elosta A, Ghous T, Ahmed N. Natural products as anti-glycation agents: possible therapeutic potential for diabetic complications. Curr Diabetes Rev. 2012;8:92–108.
171. Edelstein D, Brownlee M. Mechanistic studies of advanced glycosylation end product inhibition by aminoguanidine. Diabetes. 1992;41:26–9.
172. Reddy VP, Beyaz A. Inhibitors of the Maillard reaction and AGE breakers as therapeutics for multiple diseases. Drug Discov Today. 2006;11:646–54.
173. Pageon H, Técher MP, Asselineau D. Reconstructed skin modified by glycation of the dermal equivalent as a model for skin aging and its potential use to evaluate anti-glycation molecules. Exp Gerontol. 2008;43:584–8.
174. Sell DR, Nelson JF, Monnier VM. Effect of chronic aminoguanidine treatment on age-related glycation, glycoxidation, and collagen cross-linking in the Fischer 344 rat. J Gerontol A Biol Sci Med Sci. 2001;56:B405–11.
175. Degenhardt TP, Alderson NL, Arrington DD, Beattie RJ, Basgen JM, Steffes MW, et al. Pyridoxamine inhibits early renal disease and dyslipidemia in the streptozotocin- diabetic rat. Kidney Int. 2002;61:939–50.
176. Caballero F, Gerez E, Batlle A, Vazquez E. Preventive aspirin treatment of streptozotocin induced diabetes: blockage of oxidative status and revertion of heme enzymes inhibition. Chem Biol Interact. 2000;126:215–25.
177. Malik NS, Meek KM. The inhibition of sugar-induced structural alterations in collagen by aspirin and other compounds. Biochem Biophys Res Commun. 1994;99:683–6.
178. Khalifah RG, Baynes JW, Hudson BG. Amadorins: novel postamadori inhibitors of advanced glycation reactions. Biochem Biophys Res Commun. 1999;257:251–8.
179. Metz TO, Alderson NL, Thorpe SR, Baynes JW. Pyridoxamine, an inhibitor of advanced glycation and lipoxidation reactions: a novel therapy for treatment of diabetic complications. Arch Biochem Biophys. 2003;419:41–9.
180. Voziyan PA, Metz TO, Baynes JW, Hudson BG. A post-Amadori inhibitor pyridoxamine also inhibits chemical modification of proteins by scavenging carbonyl intermediates of carbohydrate and lipid degradation. J Biol Chem. 2002;277:3397–403.
181. Booth AA, Khalifah RG, Todd P, Hudson BG. In vitro kinetic studies of formation of antigenic advanced glycation end products (AGEs) Novel inhibition of post-Amadori glycation pathways. J Biol Chem. 1997;272:5430–7.
182. Voziyan PA, Hudson BG. Pyridoxamine: the many virtues of a maillard reaction inhibitor. Ann NY Acad Sci. 2005;1043:807–16.
183. Vasan S, Foiles P, Founds H. Therapeutic potential of breakers of advanced glycation end product-protein crosslinks. Arch Biochem Biophys. 2003;419:89–96.
184. Candido R, Forbes JM, Thomas MC, Thallas V, Dean RG, Burns WC, et al. A breaker of advanced glycation end products attenuates diabetes-induced myocardial structural changes. Circ Res. 2003;92:785–92.

185. Bakris GL, Bank AJ, Kass DA, Neutel JM, Preston RA, Oparil S. Advanced glycation end-product cross-linkbreakers. A novel approach to cardiovascular pathologies related to the aging process. Am J Hypertens. 2004;17:23S–30S.
186. Yang S, Litchfield JE, Baynes JW. AGE-breakers cleave model compounds, but do not break Maillard crosslinks in skin and tail collagen from diabetic rats. Arch Biochem Biophys. 2003;412:42–6.
187. Monnier VM, Sell DR. Prevention and repair of protein damage by the Maillard reaction in vivo. Rejuvenation Res. 2006;9:264–73; 114-117 In the rat ALT-711 showed some promising results on skin hydration
188. Xue M, Rabbani N, Momiji H, Imbasi P, Anwar MM, Kitteringham N, et al. Transcriptional control of glyoxalase 1 by Nrf2 provides a stress-responsive defence against dicarbonyl glycation. Biochem J. 2012;443:213–22.
189. Monnier VM, Wu X. Enzymatic deglycation with amadoriase enzymes from Aspergillus sp. as a potential strategy against the complications of diabetes and aging. Biochem Soc Trans. 2003;31:1349–53.
190. Shinohara M, Thornalley PJ, Giardino I, Beisswenger P, Thorpe SR, Onorato J, et al. Overexpression of glyoxalase-I in bovine endothelial cells inhibits intracellular advanced glycation endproduct formation and prevents hyperglycemia-induced increases in macromolecular endocytosis. J Clin Invest. 1998;101:1142–7.
191. Kim KM, Kim YS, Jung DH, Lee J, Kim JS. Increased glyoxalase I levels inhibit accumulation of oxidative stress and an advanced glycation end product in mouse mesangial cells cultured in high glucose. Exp Cell Res. 2012;318:152–9.
192. Brouwers O, Niessen PM, Ferreira I, Miyata T, Scheffer PG, Teerlink T, et al. Overexpression of glyoxalase-I reduces hyperglycemia-induced levels of advanced glycation end products and oxidative stress in diabetic rats. J Biol Chem. 2011;286:1374–80.
193. Price DL, Rhett PM, Thorpe SR, Baynes JW. Chelatingactivity of advanced glycation end-product inhibitors. J Biol Chem. 2001;276:48967–72.
194. Rutter K, Sell DR, Fraser N, Obrenovich M, Zito M, Starke-Reed P, et al. Green tea extract suppresses theage-related increase in collagen crosslinking and fluorescent products in C57BL/6 mice. Int J Vitam Nutr Res. 2003;73:453–60.
195. Tarwadi KV, Agte VV. Effect of micronutrients on methylglyoxal-mediated in vitro glycation of albumin. Biol Trace Elem Res. 2011;143(2):717–25.
196. Thirunavukkarasu V, Nandhini AT, Anuradha CV. Fructose diet-induced skin collagen abnormalities are prevented by lipoic acid. Exp Diabesity Res. 2004;5(4):237–44.
197. Odetti P, Pesce C, Traverso N, Menini S, Maineri EP, Cosso L, et al. Comparative trial of N-acetylcysteine, taurine, and oxerutin on skin and kidney damage in long-term experimental diabetes. Diabetes. 2003;52:499–505.
198. Rasheed Z, Anbazhagan AN, Akhtar N, Ramamurthy S, Voss FR, Haqqi TM. Green tea polyphenol epigallocatechin- 3-gallate inhibits advanced glycation end product-induced expression of tumor necrosis factor-alpha and matrix metalloproteinase-13 in human chondrocytes. Arthritis Res Ther. 2009;11:R71.
199. Vinson JA, Howard HB. Inhibition of protein glycation and advanced glycation end products by ascorbic acid and other vitamins and nutrients. J Nutr Biochem. 1996;7:659–63.
200. Dearlove RP, Greenspan P, Hartle DK, Swanson RB, Hargrove JL. Inhibition of protein glycation by extracts of culinary herbs and spices. J Med Food. 2008;11:275–81.
201. Jin S, Cho KH. Water extracts of cinnamon and clove exhibits potent inhibition of protein glycation and anti-atherosclerotic activity in vitro and in vivo hypolipidemic activity in zebrafish. Food Chem Toxicol. 2011;49:1521–9.
202. Draelos ZD, Yatskayer M, Raab S, Oresajo C. An evaluation of the effect of a topical product containing C-xyloside and blueberry extract on the appearance of type II diabetic skin. J Cosmet Dermatol. 2009;8:147–51.

203. CH W, Yen GC. Inhibitory effect of naturally occurring flavonoids on the formation of advanced glycation endproducts. J Agric Food Chem. 2005;53:3167–73.
204. Fukami K, Yamagishi S, Sakai K, et al. Potential inhibitory effects of L-carnitine supplementation on tissue advanced glycation end products in patients with hemodialysis. Rejuvenation Res. 2013;16(6):460–6.
205. Hagen TM, Liu J, Lykkesfeldt J, et al. Feeding acetyl-L-carnitine and lipoic acid to old rats significantly improves metabolic function while decreasing oxidative stress. Proc Natl Acad Sci USA. 2002;99(4):1870–5.
206. Liang CP, Wang M, Simon JE, Ho CT. Antioxidant activity of plant extracts on the inhibition of citral off-odor formation. Mol Nutr Food Res. 2004;48:308–17.
207. Peng X, Ma J, Cheng KW, Jiang Y, Chen F, Wang M. The effects of grape seed extract fortification on the antioxidant activity and quality attributes of bread. Food Chem. 2010;119:49–53.
208. Peng X, Cheng KW, Ma J, Chen B, Ho CT, Lo C, et al. Cinnamon bark proanthocyanidins as reactive carbonyl scavengers to prevent the formation of advanced glycation endproducts. J Agric Food Chem. 2008;56:1907–11.
209. Lo CY, Li S, Tan D, Pan MH, Sang S, Ho CT. Trapping reactions of reactive carbonyl species with tea polyphenols in simulated physiological conditions. Mol Nutr Food Res. 2006;50(12):1118–28.
210. Lee CK, Klopp RG, Weindruch R, Prolla TA. Gene expression profile of aging and its retardation by caloric restriction. Science. 1999;285:1390–3.
211. Cefalu WT, Bell-Farrow AD, Wang ZQ, Sonntag WE, MX F, Baynes JW, et al. Caloric restriction decreases age-dependent accumulation of the glycoxidation products, N-epsilon(carboxymethyl)lysine and pentosidine, in rat skin collagen. J Gerontol A Biol Sci Med Sci. 1995;50:B337–41.
212. Reiser KM. Influence of age and long-term dietary restriction on enzymatically mediated crosslinks and nonenzymatic glycation of collagen in mice. J Gerontol. 1994;49:B71–9.
213. Sell DR, Kleinman NR, Monnier VM. Longitudinal determination of skin collagen glycation and glycoxidation rates predicts early death in C57BL/6NNIA mice. FASEB J. 2000;14:145–56.
214. Sebeková K, Somoza V. Dietary advanced glycation endproducts (AGEs) and their health effects-PRO. Mol Nutr Food Res. 2007;51:1079–84.
215. Yamagishi S, Ueda S, Okuda S. Food-derived advanced glycation end products (AGEs): a novel therapeutic target for various disorders. Curr Pharm Des. 2007;13:2832–6.
216. Vlassara H, Striker GE. AGE restriction in diabetes mellitus: a paradigm shift. Nat Rev Endocrinol. 2011;7(9):526–39.
217. Lyons TJ, Bailie KE, Dyer DG, Dunn JA, Baynes JW. Decrease in skin collagen glycation with improved glycemic control in patients with insulin-dependent diabetes mellitus. J Clin Invest. 1991;87:1910–5.
218. Monnier VM, Bautista O, Kenny D, Sell DR, Fogarty J, Dahms W, et al. DCCT Skin Collagen Ancillary Study Group. Skin collagen glycation, glycoxidation, and crosslinking are lower in subjects with long-term intensive versus conventional therapy of type 1 diabetes: relevance of glycated collagen products versus HbA1c as markers of diabetic complications. DCCT Skin Collagen Ancillary Study Group. Diabetes Control and Complications Trial. Diabetes. 1999;48:870–80.
219. Hudson BI, Bucciarelli LG, Wendt T, Sakaguchi T, Lalla E, Qu W, et al. Blockade of receptor for advanced glycation endproducts: a new target for therapeutic intervention in diabetic complications and inflammatory disorders. Arch Biochem Biophys. 2003;419:80–8.
220. Yan SF, Ramasamy R, Schmidt AM. Soluble RAGE: therapy and biomarker in unraveling the RAGE axis in chronic disease and aging. Biochem Pharmacol. 2010;79:1379–86.
221. Goova MT, Li J, Kislinger T, Qu W, Lu Y, Bucciarelli LG, et al. Blockade of receptor for advanced glycation end-products restores effective wound healing in diabetic mice. Am J Pathol. 2001;159:513–25.
222. Babizhayev MA, Deyev AI, Savel'yeva EL, Lankin VZ, Yegorov YE. Skin beautification with oral non-hydrolized versions of carnosine and carcinine: effective therapeutic manage-

ment and cosmetic skincare solutions against oxidative glycation and free-radical production as a causal mechanism of diabetic complications and skin aging. J Dermatolog Treat. 2012;23(5):345–84.

223. Babizhayev MA, Nikolayev GM, Nikolayeva JG, Yegorov YE. Biologic activities of molecular chaperones and pharmacologic chaperone imidazole-containing dipeptide-based compounds: natural skin care help and the ultimate challenge: implication for adaptive responses in the skin. Am J Ther. 2012;19:e69–89.

224. Babizhayev MA, Yegorov YE. Therapeutic uses of drug-carrier systems for imidazole-containing dipeptide compounds that act as pharmacological chaperones and have significant impact on the treatment of chronic diseases associated with increased oxidative stress and the formation of advanced glycation end products. Crit Rev Ther Drug Carrier Syst. 2010;27:85–154.

225. Urbach E, Lentz JW. Carbohydrate metabolism and the skin. Arch Derm Syphilol. 1945;52:301–16.

226. Danby FW. Nutrition and aging skin: sugar and glycation. Clin Dermatol. 2010;28(4):409–11.

227. Draelos ZD. Aging skin: the role of diet: facts and controversies. Clin Dermatol. 2013;31(6):701–6.

228. Wu LY, Juan CC, Ho LT, Hsu YP, Hwang LS. Effect of green tea supplement on insulin sensitivity in Sprague–Dawley rats. J Agric Food Chem. 2004;52:643–8.

229. Babu PVA, Sabitha KE, Shyamaladevi CS. Effect of green tea extract on advanced glycation and cross-linking of tail tendon collagen in streptozotocin induced diabetic rats. Food Chem Toxicol. 2008;46:280–5.

230. Mizutani K, Ikeda K, Yamori Y. Resveratrol inhibits AGEs-induced proliferation and collagen synthesis activity in vascular smooth muscle cells from stroke-prone spontaneously hypertensive rats. Biochem Biophys Res Commun. 2000;274(1):61–7.

231. Liu Y, He XQ, Huang X, et al. Resveratrol protects mouse oocytes from methylglyoxal-induced oxidative damage. PLoS One. 2013;8(10):e77960.

232. Yokozawa T, Nakagawa T. Inhibitory effects of Luobuma tea and its components against glucose-mediated protein damage. Food Chem Toxicol. 2004;42:975–81.

233. Ardestani A, Yazdanparast R. Cyperus rotundus suppresses AGE formation and protein oxidation in a model of fructose-mediated protein glycoxidation. Int J Biol Macromol. 2007;41:572–8.

234. Gugliucci A, Markowicz Bastos DH, Schulze J, Ferreira Souza MF. Caffeic and cholorogenic acids in ilex paraguariensis extracts are the main inhibitors of AGE generation by methylglyoxal in model proteins. Fitoterapia. 2009;80:339–44.

235. Hsieh CL, Lin YC, Ko WS, Peng CH, Huang CN, Peng RY. Inhibitory effect of some selected nutraceutic herbs on LDL glycation induced by glucose and glyoxal. J Ethn. 2005;102:357–63.

236. Ho SC, SP W, Lin SM, Tang YL. Comparison of anti-glycation capacities of several herbal infusions with that of green tea. Food Chem. 2010;122:768–74.

237. Nakagawa T, Yokozawa T, Terasawa K, Shu S, Juneja LR. Protective activity of green tea against free radical- and glucosemediated protein damage. J Agric Food Chem. 2002;50:2418–22.

Nail Disorders in Diabetics

16

Jessica Cervantes, Ana Paula Lamas, Andre Lencastre, Daniel Coelho de Sá, and Antonella Tosti

Anatomy of the Nail

The nail plate is a fully keratinized structure produced by the germinative epithelium of the nail matrix. As it grows, the nail plate emerges from the proximal nail fold and progresses distally lying across and adhering to the nail bed. As the nail plate approaches the tip of the digit, it detaches from the underlying tissues at the level of the hyponychium [1, 2]. The nail is bound proximally by the proximal nail fold, laterally by the lateral nail folds, and distally by the distal nail fold [3]. The main function of the nail apparatus is to act as a protective covering for the dorsal aspect of the distal digits [1–4]. Nails increase sensory perception at the finger pads, facilitate object manipulation and contribute to temperature regulation.

There is a rich arterial blood supply to the nail bed and matrix derived from paired digital arteries, a large palmar and small dorsal digital artery on either side. There is a capillary loop system to the whole of the nail fold, but the loops to the roof and matrix are flatter than those below the exposed nail [1, 5].

Under normal conditions, the mean growth rate of a fingernail is 3 mm/month and that of a toenail is 1 mm/month. Therefore, the fingernails take about 4–6 months

J. Cervantes • A. Tosti (✉)
Department of Dermatology and Cutaneous Surgery, Miller School of Medicine, University of Miami, Miami, FL, USA
e-mail: atosti@med.miami.edu

A.P. Lamas
Private Practice in Dermatology, Aracaju, Brazil

A. Lencastre
Department of Dermatology, Hospital de Santo António dos Capuchos, Centro Hospitalar de Lisboa Central, Lisbon, Portugal

D.C. de Sá
Department of Dermatology, Faculdade de Medicina, Universidade de São Paulo, São Paulo, SP, Brazil

© Springer International Publishing AG 2018
E.N. Cohen Sabban et al. (eds.), *Dermatology and Diabetes*,
https://doi.org/10.1007/978-3-319-72475-1_16

to be completely renewed and the toenails take approximately double the time. Nail growth rate can nonetheless be influenced by several factors, including age, local and/or systemic disease and medications [2].

Pathogenic Mechanisms of Nail Diseases in Diabetes

Diabetes can result in complications affecting all systems of the body. Of particular relevance is peripheral arterial disease. Its presence in diabetics may be compounded by infections, such as onychomycosis and bacterial sepsis, and peripheral neuropathy. Capillary morphological and functional abnormalities occur due to alterations in the function of endothelial cells on local flow regulation, as well as modifications of blood viscosity caused by higher plasma viscosity and increased erythrocytes rigidity and aggregation. Neuropathy and altered autonomous nervous contractile arteriole function and high vascular permeability also play a role [6]. Microvascular walls of arterioles, venules, and capillaries are impaired by biochemical processes, which are based on hyperglycemia, namely non-enzymatic glycation of proteins and altered polyolinositol metabolism. Glycation products also accumulate in structural proteins of the microvasculature. A specific macrophage receptor recognizes proteins to which glycation products are bound and stimulates their removal. Different pathologic processes are then activated, such as increase of endothelial permeability and stimulation of growth factor synthesis by macrophage. As a result, the vessel wall thickens and loses its elasticity. Later, the intensified glycation of hemoglobin leads to hypoxia, which is one of the prerequisites for microangiopathy [7, 8].

Clinical Features

Onychomycosis

Onychomycosis, a fungal infection of the toenails and/or fingernails, is one of the most common diseases of the nail [9]. Several risk factors for onychomycosis have been identified, including ageing, tinea pedis, psoriasis, genetic factors, peripheral arterial disease, peripheral neuropathy, trauma, swimming, smoking, immunodeficiency/immunosuppression, and diabetes [10–12]. Onychomycosis is a well-known complication of diabetes mellitus (DM). Diabetics acquire an increased likelihood of dermatophyte infections, especially on the nails; prevalence studies indicate that approximately one third of diabetics are affected [13]. In a 2016 study of 227 diabetic patients, distal subungual onychomycosis was documented to be the most common fungal infection (34.9%), followed by tinea pedis (26.3%) [14]. Other prevalence studies generally range from 1.2–26% [15].

Development of skin fungal and bacterial infections in diabetic patients is attributed to impaired cellular immunity and diminished phagocytic activity of polymorphonuclear leukocytes due to uncontrolled hyperglycemia [14]. Among diabetics, factors associated with higher rates of infection include increased age, male gender, type 2 diabetes (T2DM), peripheral vascular disease, atherosclerosis, retinopathy, neuropathy, duration of diabetes, poor glycemic control, diabetic foot ulcers, obesity, hypertriglyceridemia, insufficient foot care and improper or absent daily foot washings [16–22].

In diabetic patients with onychomycosis, etiological agents are similar to the general population, with dermatophytes being the most prevalent pathogen. *Trichophyton rubrum* is the most common keratinophilic fungi implicated in onychomycosis and tinea pedis. Other species include *Trichophyton mentagraphytes, Trichophyton tonsurans* and *Epidermophyton floccosum* [23]. The role of Candida in causing onychomychosis is controversial; we believe that in immunocompetent patients, Candida is a contaminant or a colonizer of a dermatophyte infected nail, however others consider yeasts as causative agents of onychomycosis if demonstrated by microscopy and culture of the nail [24, 25]. Yeasts are more commonly isolated from fingernails, particularly from chronic paronychia or onycholysis, where they are only secondary colonizers [26].). Total dystrophic onychomycosis of the fingernail due to Candida is rare and more commonly observed in immunosuppressed patients [10].

The severity of nail disease is significantly associated with the duration of diabetes and infection [13, 15]. The most common clinical pattern is distal-lateral subungual onychomycosis. Affected nails can become markedly thickened, and the keratinous debris under the nail plate imparts a yellow/brown discoloration (Fig. 16.1). Superficial white onychomycosis, as the name implies, involves the surface of the nail. It is characterized by chalky white material that can be scraped off the surface of the nail plate. Proximal subungual onychomycosis is the least common subtype. Infection begins near the lunula, extending distally, and is rare except for immunocompromised patients [10]. Overall, nails with fungal infections become distorted and thick with sharp edges that can abrade or ulcerate the adjacent skin (Fig. 16.1). Abrasions or ulcerations can enlarge, become chronic, and serve as portals for infection resulting in severe complications [23].

Direct microscopy is the most efficient screening technique for onychomycosis. It is important to document infection via culture for a dermatophyte or

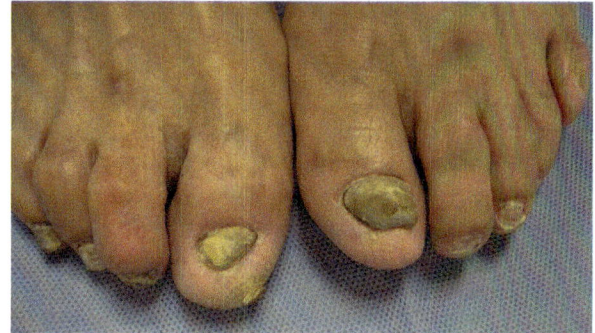

Fig. 16.1 Onychomycosis. Markedly thickened nails with keratinous debris under the nail plate. Nails acquire a yellow/brown discoloration and become distorted and thick with sharp edges that can abrade or ulcerate the adjacent skin

periodic acid-Schiff stain or KOH preparation showing fungal elements prior to the initiation of therapy. The causative microorganisms can be identified by culture or PCR. Considering the vast number of causes of onychodystrophy and its increased frequency among diabetics, despite the absence of fungal infection, documentation will avoid unnecessary medication or delay in the approach to other causes [17, 26, 27]. Proper treatment of onychomycosis is an important aspect of diabetic foot care as it can potentially decrease the risk of foot ulcers, cellulitis, osteomyelitis and amputation [13]. Diabetic patients with onychomycosis have a threefold higher risk of gangrene and/or foot ulcers compared to those without onychomycosis [23]. Dystrophic toenails can damage the surrounding skin and put increased pressure on the underlying toe, compromising its tenuous vascular supply and causing pressure ulcers that can go unnoticed due to coexistent neuropathy. Onychomycosis can become a reservoir for molds and bacteria, which could represent potential invaders of the compromised skin barrier [17, 28, 29]. Patients who belong to susceptible populations, such as diabetics, are more likely to experience recurrence of disease. Patient counseling is an integral part of onychomycosis management. Physicians should educate their patients on the early signs of recurrence and recommend that they contact their physicians at the first signs of disease as likelihood of resolution improves when onychomycosis is detected and treated early [30].

With prompt and adequate treatment, toenails have a greater chance of complete clearance [13]. Appropriate nail hygiene, such as keeping feet cool and dry, discarding or disinfecting old socks and footwear, avoiding going barefoot (especially in public places), trimming nails, and filing down hypertrophic nails, is essential [30]. Topical antifungal prophylaxis and prompt treatment of tinea pedis are other steps that can minimize or prevent disease recurrence as fungal pathogens infecting the skin may serve as reservoirs for reinfection of the nail [30]. Use of proper footwear should likely be emphasized.

Three oral agents are currently prescribed for the treatment of onychomycosis. Terbinafine is a first-line choice in the treatment of onychomycosis in diabetics because of its fungicidal effect [10]. Itraconazole can potentially interact with oral hypoglycemic, such as nateglinide, repaglinide or pioglitazone, putting patients at risk of a hypoglycemic episode when taking itraconazole. However, many of the commonly prescribed hypoglycemic agents (tolbutamide, gliclazide, glibenclamide, glipizide, metformin) are not metabolized by the CYP 3A4 pathway, and data from clinical trials indicate that hypoglycemia in diabetics on itraconazole is infrequent [10, 17, 31]. Fluconazole, also fungistatic, has been shown to be helpful in the treatment of onychomycosis, particularly in cases of suspected Candida nail infection. Like itraconazole, it carries similar risks for drug–drug interactions.

The new topical antifungals efinaconazole 10% solution and tavaborole 10% solution can also be utilized as unique therapy or in conjunction with oral treatments [15]. Laser devices, photodynamic therapy, iontophoresis, and ultrasound are recent device-based therapies that have preliminarily demonstrated fungistatic activity against nail infections. Additional randomized controlled trials are needed to conclude on their efficacy to eradicate fungal infections [32].

Paronychia

Acute Paronychia is often caused by bacterial infection or trauma to the nailfold of one digit. Repetitive trauma, excessive hand immersion in water and contact with chemicals are several contributing mechanisms by which separation of the cuticle from the nail plate may be obtained, facilitating the entrance of environmental particles and micro-organisms beneath the proximal nail fold. The presence of swollen and/or tender lateral or posterior nail folds with purulent fluid collections is diagnostic of acute paronychia.

Chronic paronychia usually arises as a multifactorial inflammatory reaction of the proximal nail fold to irritants and allergens lasting longer than 6 weeks [33]. Prolonged exposure to water, irritating substances, manicures, nail trauma and finger sucking have all been implicated as predisposing factors [34]. Although candida is frequently isolated from the proximal nail fold of patients with paronychia, it is unclear whether Candida infection is responsible for the onset and maintenance of disease. It is more widely accepted that chronic paronychia is a multifactorial eczematous condition [33]. Clinical manifestations of chronic paronychia include nail plate dystrophy, erythema, tenderness, and swelling with retraction of the proximal nail fold and absence of the adjacent cuticle [34]. One or several fingernails are usually affected. The nail plate becomes thickened and discolored, with Beau's lines, and even nail loss. The condition usually has a prolonged course with recurrences [35].

Diabetics often have chronic paronychia and chronic paronychia-like changes addressed above [33, 35]. In a case-control study of 93 children and adolescents with type 1 diabetes mellitus (T1DM) and 100 healthy age-matched controls, Kapellen, Galler and Kiess documented the prevalence of paronychia in T1DM to be 34.4% compared to 23% in controls [32]. Girls were found to have a higher frequency of paronychia than boys. Further, those with longer duration of T1DM were more commonly affected [32]. Vibrational perception was found to be impaired in all regions measured in diabetic patients, compared to non-diabetic peers [32].

First-line treatment of chronic paronychia should include maintenance of strict glycemic control, avoidance of predisposing factors and application of topical steroids [36] and emollients to lubricate the nascent cuticles [34]. In cases of recalcitrant disease, topical or systemic antifungal agents can be used, although oral antifungal therapy is rarely necessary [36]. Antibacterial solutions, acetic acid soaks of 1:1 vinegar to water ratio, and/or oral antibiotics can be used to treat potential secondary bacterial infections. If medical treatment fails, eponychial marsupialization and nail removal is indicated for treatment of chronic paronychia [34, 37].

Ingrown Nails

Ingrown toenail is a frequent foot problem encountered in the general population. In this common condition, the lateral nail fold is penetrated by the edge of the nail plate, resulting in pain, infection and eventually the formation of granulation tissue

[38]. Sometimes, penetrating spicules that have been separated from the nail plate can be found at the edge. The great toes are those most commonly affected. Compression of the toe due to ill-fitting footwear and clipping/cutting the toenails in a half-circle (instead of straight across) are the main contributors to ingrown nails [1, 2, 39]. Ingrown nails is a prevalent dermatologic abnormality seen in diabetic patients. Foot complications occur three to four times more often in diabetics than in non-diabetics controls [38]. There is evidence that people with diabetic neuropathy often wear shoes that are too small in order to increase the sensation of fit [40]. Litzelman demonstrated that diabetic patients with insensate feet tend to buy and wear overly tight shoes, and at least 25% of people with T2DM wear inappropriately sized footwear [41]. Some authors also recognize the importance of prominent lateral nail folds.

Being as ingrown toenail is a risk factor for diabetic foot disease, early recognition and effective treatment is highly recommended to prevent severe complications [42]. Ingrown nails and onychogryphosis (see below) may favor the development of subungual ulcers, which may initially go unnoticed due to the absence of pain or inflammation [43]. Delayed wound healing in diabetics may favor infection, a potentially serious problem.

Treatment may prove difficult and prolonged, especially in patients with diabetes due to delayed wound healing, wound infections, and digital ischemia [44]. It is essential to instruct the patient to cut the nail straight across and wear shoes wide and pliable enough to remove lateral pressure. Abnormalities of foot and toe function should be corrected. Taping is a minimally aggressive method in which the lateral nail fold is taped in an oblique and proximal direction over the pulp of the toe to pull away from the offending lateral nail edge [45]. Use of antiseptics, warm soaks followed by careful drying, powdering, gutter treatment (inserting a small guard between the lateral nail margin and the nail fold), and packing (inserting a pledget of cotton-wool or dental floss between the corner of the nail and the nail fold) may also be helpful [1, 44]. Nail brace application is a simple and inexpensive treatment option that was documented to provide immediate relief of symptoms in diabetic patients by opening the curvature of the nail [38, 45].

If conservative measures fail, operative intervention will be necessary. Surgical removal of the relevant part of the nail plate and chemical matricectomy focusing on the treatment of germinal matrix, to avoid recurrence are the next mainstays. However, uncontrolled tissue destruction, prolonged healing times, and significant postoperative drainage are the limitations of this technique. Postoperative complications should thusly be considered, although this option has been used successfully for the treatment of ingrown toenails in these patients [1, 2, 44, 46, 47].

Pincer Nails

Pincer nail deformity, also referred to as omega nail deformity or trumpet nail deformity, represents a loss in the normal convex shape of the nail with an acquired thickening and transverse overcurvature of the nail plate along its longitudinal axis

[48]. The nail edges press deeply into the lateral nail fold and creates a curvature that increases distally along the nail. This leads to progressive pinching of the nail bed [48–50]. It is usually seen in the toes, with the great toes being most affected.

Pincer nail deformity may be inherited or acquired [1, 2]. Etiology, pathogenesis, and mechanism of inheritance are yet to be fully understood [49]. Acquired pincer nail deformity has been reported most frequently with ill-fitting shoes and in association with medications, but other disorders can be associated such as subungual exostosis, psoriasis, onychomycosis, tumors of the nail apparatus and systemic diseases such as lupus erythematosus, Kawasaki disease, Diabetes, renal disorders, and malignancy [48, 49, 51]. Chronic renal insufficiency in association with Diabetes has been reported to cause endothelial dysfunction and impaired microcirculatory function [52]. However, there is no data showing that a significant change in renal function can affect the nail matrix or its underlying microvasculature [49].

There is no standard therapy for pincer nails. Some conservative treatments, such as nail grinding, placement of a plastic brace, and application of urea paste are available. In cases with severe deformity and high discomfort, surgical therapy should be considered. In vascular high-risk groups, including patients with DM, chronic kidney disease, and/or peripheral vascular disease, a less invasive inverted T-incision method (modified Haneke's technique) is a possible surgical method [53].

Onychodystrophy, Onychauxis and Onychogriphosis

Diabetes is one of the most common diseases presenting with nail dystrophy. Onychodystrophies include Beau's lines, onycholysis, yellowish discoloration, and splinter blood suffusions [54]. Poor peripheral circulation and diabetic neuropathy are responsible for the onychodystrophy present in patients with diabetes [55]. The lesions are possibly more severe in the winter due to functional changes associated with the macro and microangiopathy [54]. The different patterns of diabetic peripheral neuropathy may entail unspecific nail changes on the affected territories, as onychodystrophy is defined simply as malformation of the nail. Diabetic mononeuritis, mononeuritis multiplex or polyneuropathy may be responsible by either symmetrical or asymmetrical pattern of alterations [56], in one or more digits, and thus be a clue to these conditions [57]. Excessive nail thickening and deformity can lead to accumulation of debris and subsequent nail infections. Poor fitting shoes can further aggravate the condition by causing repeated trauma to the injured site [14]. Diabetic foot ulcers may be an unfortunate sequela. To avoid complications, well-fitting shoes, proper nail care, and immediate treatment of nail infections are necessary [55].

Onychauxis refers to enlargement and thickening of the nail plate without deformity, while in onychogryphosis the same kind of changes produce a "ram's horn-like", "oyster-like" or "claw-like" appearance, most likely involving the great toenail. In both cases the nail plate appears uneven, thickened and brown to opaque (Fig. 16.2). Yellow, thickened nails are characteristic of long-standing diabetes [58]. Thickening of the proximal nail folds and skin of the dorsal hands and feet can be

Fig. 16.2 Onychauxis.
Enlargement and
thickening of the nail plate
of the toe nails with
yellowish-brown, uneven
discoloration. Nails
become dystrophic and
opaque

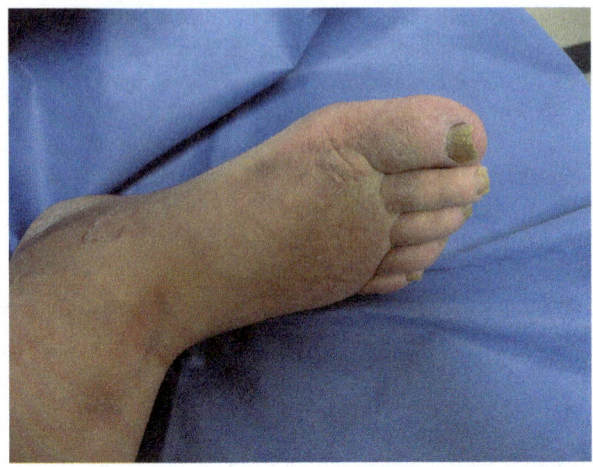

seen in up to 25% of diabetics [58]. Microangiopathic changes of the lower limbs in diabetic patients may be responsible for the toenail thickening and onychogryphosis [58]. Especially in elderly diabetic patients, sudden or minor repetitive trauma, unnoticed due to loss of peripheral sensation and microangiopathy, are major contributors to these conditions.

Diagnosis of these alterations is based on clinical observation and the main differential includes either isolated or superimposed fungal infection. Treatment should address diabetic foot care and optimal shoe fitting: suitable fastening, usage of low heels, personalized footwear if indicated by relevant orthopedic conditions (e.g. Hallux Valgus) [57].

Onycholysis

Diabetes may be associated with distal and/or lateral separation of the nail plate from the nail bed, a clinical sign that is called onycholysis. It is more commonly seen affecting the fingernails than toenails. Fungal infection and blood vessel abnormalities caused by Diabetes favor onycholysis, and age and repetitive involuntary trauma are additional related factors. Nonetheless, onycholysis is essentially an unspecific change that can be idiopathic, associated with numerous dermatologic conditions (e.g. psoriasis, onychomycosis) or systemic diseases (e.g. iron deficiency, hyper or hypothyroidism). If multiple nail units are affected, a systemic cause is more likely the culprit, whereas a single nail unit is more likely caused by a history of trauma or an underlying tumor. Onycholysis itself may be responsible for the subungual space prone to secondary bacterial or fungal colonization. A greenish discoloration of the undersurface of the nail plate is indicative of a secondary infection by *Pseudomonas aeruginosa* [59].

The main causes of toenail onycholysis are onychomycosis and minor trauma. In contrast with toenail onycholysis, pathogenesis at the fingernails may potentially include more frequent exposure to occupational injury, repeated use of cosmetics and lack of efficient protection (when compared to that granted by footwear). The condition may be worsened by overzealous cleaning beneath the nail and thus patients should be instructed keep the nails short, avoid injuring the affected nail, keep the nail bed dry, avoid exposure to contact irritants such as nail enamel, enamel remover or solvents and detergents. As mentioned before, secondary candida colonization is more commonly observed in fingernails. In summary, careful clinical distinction between primary onychomycosis and trauma is essential to guide either drug therapy and/or appropriate trauma-reducing strategies [1, 60].

Vascular Alterations of the Proximal Nail Fold

In DM, capillaroscopic alterations differ significantly from healthy individuals of similar age, gender, and body mass index. The most common alterations include tortuous capillaries, capillary crosslinking, avascular zones, and ectasias [61]. Other common alterations include giant capillaries and ramified capillaries. Compared to control groups, patients with DM present with greater capillary diameter [61]. It is known that hyperglycemia induces intensified metabolism, increased oxygen consumption, causes relative tissue hypoxia, and as a result a dilation of blood vessels [62, 63].

Capillaroscopic alterations are due to progressive endothelial damage. Presence of comorbidities and longer evolution of disease are associated with greater microvascular damage. In a study by Maldonado et al. [61], patients with capillaroscopic alterations had a longer time of disease evolution (12.8 years), compared to those who did not present with capillaroscopic alterations (8.5 years). Reduction in capillary density compared to healthy controls was likewise documented [64].

In Diabetes, diabetic stiff-hand syndrome and sclerodactyly are common complications and need to be distinguished from similar signs in diseases such as scleroderma and early arthritis (See Chap. 7). Capillaroscopic examination may nonetheless be helpful, as it will not show dilated capillaries until the advanced stages of diabetes, while these may be seen earlier in patients with connective tissue disease [43].

Periungual erythema and telangiectasia [65] in the nail folds with or without periungual inflammation are early signs of disease [58]. Periungual telangiectasia are reported in up to 49% of patients with DM [55]. Loss of capillary loops and dilation of remaining capillaries results in formation of telangiectasia in the nail bed [55]. Nail fold erythema, grossly visible dilated blood vessels, fingertip tenderness, and thick cuticles are common presentations [55]. Periungual telangiectasia can be seen with a low-resolution microscope, an ophthalmoscope or a dermatoscope [66, 67].

Treatment is not required [55].

Subungual Hemorrhages

Although common in otherwise healthy individuals, subungual hemorrhages may be observed in a variety of systemic diseases, such as DM. Subungual hemorrhage may serve as an indicator of diabetic microangiopathy severity [68]. Toenail bilateral hemorrhages was described as an early manifestation of previously undiagnosed T2DM in three male patients by Iglesias et al. Hyperglycemia and diabetic retinopathy were present in all three cases suggesting that subungual hemorrhages might be due to microvascular involvement [69]. Impairment of the microcirculation of the nail bed leads to erythrocyte extravasation from capillaries into the dermal ridges resulting in subungual hemorrhages. Poor perfusion of the nail matrix, slow growth of the nail plate, and curvature of the nail with longitudinal ridges are also believed to be provoked by diabetic microangiopathy-induced subungual hemorrhages [68].

Cold Whitlow: Digital Ischemia

Cold whitlow is a pseudoinflammatory nail change where the distal portion of the digit is greatly enlarged and red, simulating paronychia, but the skin temperature is cold or normal. In digital ischemia, the digit is cold and painful. The most common causes include arterial obstruction and peripheral neuropathies causing ischemia (these include carpal tunnel syndrome and Diabetes) [2].

Terry's Nail

Terry's nail describes a physical condition in which finger or toenails appear stark white with a dark band near the ends of the nails (Fig. 16.3). It is a type of apparent leukonychia, in which the white color is due to the pallor of the nail bed not to the nail plate [70]. Apparent leukonychia does not move distally with nail growth and fades with pressure. The nail bed is white, except for its distal 0.5–3.0 mm, before the distal edge of the nail plate that looks red to brownish (Fig. 16.3) [71]. Terry's nails are observed in multiple conditions, including cirrhosis, congestive cardiac failure, chronic renal failure, increased age and adult onset DM [3, 40, 71, 72].

The most important differential diagnosis of Terry's nails is the uremic half-and-half nails (also known as Lindsay's nails) [71]. In Lindsay's nail, the proximal part of the nail is also white, while the distal portion is reddish-brown, occupies 20–60% of the nail bed and does not fade with pressure. Terry's nail, on the other hand, describes a 0.5–3.0 mm brown to pink band with proximal nail bed whiteness on 80% of the nail bed [71]. Although the cause is unclear, the distal reddish-brown band seen in Lindsay's nail is the result of increased concentration of β-melanocyte stimulating hormone and is found in up to 40% of patients with chronic kidney disease [73]. Terry's nails is thought to result from decreased capillary blood flow to the nail bed secondary to an increased growth of connective tissue [1–3]. It is often associated with cirrhosis, chronic congestive heart failure, and adult-onset DM [71, 73].

Fig. 16.3   Terry's nails.
Nail examination of a
patient with Type I Diabetes
mellitus reveals stark white
nails with a dark 0.5–
3.0 mm reddish-brown band
near the ends of the nails, a
characteristic feature of
Terry's nails

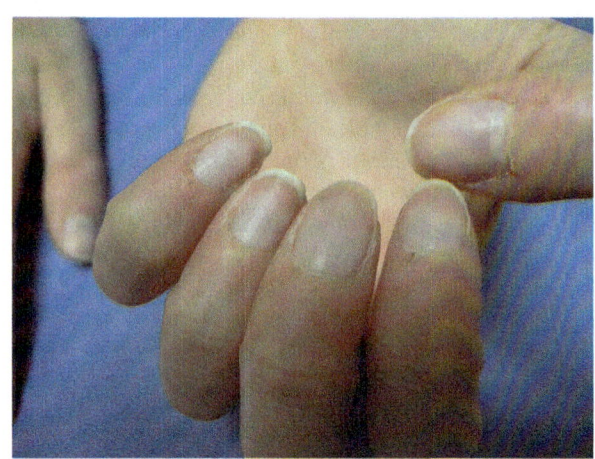

Other

Other nail disorders associated with Diabetes include pitting, pterygium, scleroderma-like changes, trachyonychia, leukonychia, and splinter hemorrhages. Pitting, also known as Rosenau's depressions, are characterized by irregular small pitted craters on the nail plate surface, especially on the middle and ring fingers [17]. They may appear in longitudinal or transverse array or can be scattered at random. Pterygium unguis, both dorsal and ventral, can be seen in diabetics. Arterial spasms, which lead to fusion of the proximal nail fold to the matrix, can result in scarring and dorsal pterygium. Ventral pterygium results in painful obliteration of the hyponychium. Scleroderma-like changes (diabetic cheiroarthropathy) can occur in 20–30% of patients with Diabetes, more commonly in patients with insulin-dependent type. Thickening of the dorsal fingers creates a rough pebbled texture on the skin of the knuckles and nail folds. Trachyonychia, sometimes called sandpapered nails, are also seen in diabetic toenails. Environmental conditions, diabetic microangiopathy and vasomotor dysregulation have been associated with rougher nails in Diabetes. Leukonychia totalis (whitening of the entire nail plate) and leukonychia punctate (white punctate spots on the nails) are suggested to be caused by incorporation of parakeratotic cells into the nail plate due to inadequate blood supply. Splinter hemorrhages have also been documented [59].

Conclusion

Despite the substantial development of imaging and laboratory tools in medicine, a focused physical examination still plays a pivotal role in all medical fields. A wealth of information can be gained from examining the hands. Although early diagnostic clues can be attained from this part of the examination, in particular the examination of the nails, this step is often neglected. In some cases, nail changes are directive for the diagnosis, such as clubbed fingers in pulmonary or cardiovascular disorders. Before other signs of a systemic disease become clinically evident, nail changes may be a presenting feature.

The early recognition of a nail abnormality may lead to earlier diagnosis and treatment, as is the case in DM.

Nailfold capillary microscopy, on the other hand, offers a noninvasive testing method that is simple and quick. It can provide a valuable addition to the present functional testing of peripheral blood vessels. Among the laboratory methods, the most important are mycological and bacteriological investigation. Further, histopathological studies are essential for the diagnosis of tumors [66].

References

1. de Berker DAR, Baran R, Dawber RPR. Disorders of nails. In: Burns T, Breathnach S, Cox N, Griffiths C, editors. Rook's text book of dermatology. 7th ed. Oxford: Blackwell Science; 2004. p. 3139–200.
2. Tosti A, Jorizzo JL, Rapini RP. Dermatology. 1st ed. London: Mosby Elsevier; 2005. p. 1061–78.
3. Fawcett RS, Linford S, et al. Nail abnormalities: clues to systemic disease. Am Fam Physician. 2004;69:1417–24.
4. Grinzi P. Hair and nails. Aust Fam Physician. 2011;40(7):476–84.
5. Bonacci E, Santacroce N, D'Amico N, Mattace R. Nail-fold capillaroscopy in the study of micro-circulation in elderly hypertensive patients. Arch Gerontol Geriatr. 1996;22(Suppl 1):79–83.
6. Halfoun VL, Pires ML, Fernandes TJ, Victer F, Rodrigues KK, Tavares R. Videocapillaroscopy and diabetes mellitus: area of transverse segment in nailfold capillar loops reflects vascular reactivity. Diabetes Res Clin Pract. 2003;61(3):155–60.
7. Bollinger A, Fagrell B. Clinical capillaroscopy—a guide to its use in clinical research and practice. Cambridge: Hogrefe & Huber; 1990. p. 166.
8. Lambova SN, Muller-Ladner U. The specificity of capillaroscopic pattern in connective auto-immune diseases. A comparison with microvascular changes in diseases of social importance: arterial hypertension and diabetes mellitus. Mod Rheumatol. 2009;19(6):600–5.
9. Gupta AK, Konnikov N, MacDonald P, Rich P, Rodger NW, Edmonds MW, et al. Prevalence and epidemiology of toenail onychomycosis in diabetic subjects: a multicentre survey. Br J Dermatol. 1998;139(4):665–71.
10. Finch JJ, Warshaw EM. Toenail onychomycosis: current and future treatment options. Dermatol Ther. 2007;20(1):31–46.
11. Tosti A, Hay R, Arenas-Guzmán R. Patients at risk of onychomycosis--risk factor identification and active prevention. J Eur Acad Dermatol Venereol. 2005;19(1):13–6.
12. Tosti A, Piraccini BM, Mariani R, Stinchi C, Buttasi C. Are local and systemic conditions important for the development of onychomycosis? Eur J Dermatol. 1998;8(1):41–4.
13. Levy L, Zeichner JA. Dermatologic manifestation of diabetes. J Diabetes. 2012;4(1):68–76.
14. Akkus G, Evran M, Gungor D, Karakas M, Sert M, Tetiker T. Tinea pedis and onychomycosis frequency in diabetes mellitus patients and diabetic foot ulcers. A cross sectional—observational study. Pak J Med Sci. 2016;32(4):891–5.
15. Vlahovic TC. Management of onychomycosis in a diabetic population. Podiatry Management Online. 2015.
16. Shahzad M, Al Robaee A, Al Shobaili HA, Alzolibani AA, Al Marshood AA, Al Moteri B. Skin manifestations in diabetic patients attending a diabetic clinic in the Qassim region, Saudi Arabia. Med Princ Pract. 2011;20(2):137–41.
17. Greene RA, Scher RK. Nail changes associated with diabetes mellitus. J Am Acad Dermatol. 1987;16(5 Pt 1):1015–21.
18. Cathcart S, Cantrell W, Elewski B. Onychomycosis and diabetes. J Eur Acad Dermatol Venereol. 2009;23(10):1119–22.

19. Armstrong DG, Holtz K, Wu S. Can the use of a topical antifungal nail lacquer reduce risk for diabetic foot ulceration? Results from a randomised controlled pilot study. Int Wound J. 2005;2(2):166–70.
20. Onalan O, Adar A, Keles H, Ertugrul G, Ozkan N, Aktas H, et al. Onychomycosis is associated with subclinical atherosclerosis in patients with diabetes. Vasa. 2015;44(1):59–64.
21. Gulcan A, Gulcan E, Oksuz S, Sahin I, Kaya D. Prevalence of toenail onychomycosis in patients with type 2 diabetes mellitus and evaluation of risk factors. J Am Podiatr Med Assoc. 2011;101(1):49–54.
22. Takehara K, Oe M, Tsunemi Y, Nagase T, Ohashi Y, Iizaka S, et al. Factors associated with presence and severity of toenail onychomycosis in patients with diabetes: a cross-sectional study. Int J Nurs Stud. 2011;48(9):1101–8.
23. Eba M, Njunda AL, Mouliom RN, Kwenti ET, Fuh AN, Nchanji GT, et al. Onychomycosis in diabetic patients in Fako Division of Cameroon: prevalence, causative agents, associated factors and antifungal sensitivity patterns. BMC Res Notes. 2016;9(1):494.
24. Gupta AK, Drummond-Main C, Cooper EA, Brintnell W, Piraccini BM, Tosti A. Systematic review of nondermatophyte mold onychomycosis: diagnosis, clinical types, epidemiology, and treatment. J Am Acad Dermatol. 2012;66(3):494–502.
25. Saunte DM, Holgersen JB, Haedersdal M, Strauss G, Bitsch M, Svendsen OL, et al. Prevalence of toe nail onychomycosis in diabetic patients. Acta Derm Venereol. 2006;86(5):425–8.
26. Manzano-Gayosso P, Hernández-Hernández F, Méndez-Tovar LJ, et al. Onychomycosis incidence in type 2 diabetes mellitus. Mycopathologia. 2008;166:41–5.
27. Aye M, Masson EA. Dermatological care of the diabetic foot. Am J Clin Dermatol. 2002;3(7):463–74.
28. Pierard GE, Pierard-Franchimont C. The nail under fungal siege in patients with type II diabetes mellitus. Mycoses. 2005;48(5):339–42.
29. Drake LA, Patrick DL, Fleckman P, Andr J, Baran R, Haneke E, et al. The impact of onychomycosis on quality of life: development of an international onychomycosis-specific questionnaire to measure patient quality of life. J Am Acad Dermatol. 1999;41(2 Pt 1):189–96.
30. Tosti A, Elewski BE. Onychomycosis: practical approaches to minimize relapse and recurrence. Skin Appendage Disord. 2016;2(1–2):83–7.
31. Scher RK, Tavakkol A, Sigurgeirsson B, Hay RJ, Joseph WS, Tosti A, et al. Onychomycosis: diagnosis and definition of cure. J Am Acad Dermatol. 2007;56(6):939–44.
32. Ghannoum M, Isham N. Fungal nail infections (onychomycosis): a never-ending story? PLoS Pathog. 2014;10(6):e1004105.
33. Rigopoulos D, Larios G, Gregoriou S, Alevizos A. Acute and chronic paronychia. Am Fam Physician. 2008;77(3):339–46.
34. Rockwell PG. Acute and chronic paronychia. Am Fam Physician. 2001;63(6):1113–6.
35. Daniel CR 3rd, Iorizzo M, Piraccini BM, Tosti A. Grading simple chronic paronychia and onycholysis. Int J Dermatol. 2006;45(12):1447–8.
36. Tosti A, Piraccini BM, Ghetti E, Colombo MD. Topical steroids versus systemic antifungals in the treatment of chronic paronychia: an open, randomized double-blind and double dummy study. J Am Acad Dermatol. 2002;47(1):73–6.
37. Relhan V, Goel K, Bansal S, Garg VK. Management of chronic paronychia. Indian J Dermatol. 2014;59(1):15–20.
38. Erdogan FG, Erdogan G. Long-term results of nail brace application in diabetic patients with ingrown nails. Dermatol Surg. 2008;34(1):84–6. discussion 6–7.
39. Baran R. The nail in the elderly. Clin Dermatol. 2011;29(1):54–60.
40. Parnes A. If the shoe fits...footwear and patients with diabetes. Int J Clin Pract. 2007;61(11):1788–90.
41. Litzelman DK, Marriott DJ, Vinicor F. The role of footwear in the prevention of foot lesions in patients with NIDDM. Conventional wisdom or evidence-based practice? Diabetes Care. 1997;20(2):156–62.
42. Younes NA, Ahmad AT. Diabetic foot disease. Endocr Pract. 2006;12(5):583–92.

43. Bergman R, Sharony L, Schapira D, Nahir MA, Balbir-Gurman A. The handheld dermatoscope as a nail-fold capillaroscopic instrument. Arch Dermatol. 2003;139(8):1027–30.
44. Tatlican S, Eren C, Yamangokturk B, Eskioglu F, Bostanci S. Chemical matricectomy with 10% sodium hydroxide for the treatment of ingrown toenails in people with diabetes. Dermatol Surg. 2010;36(2):219–22.
45. Haneke E. Controversies in the treatment of ingrown nails. Dermatol Res Pract. 2012;2012:783924.
46. Giacalone VF. Phenol matricectomy in patients with diabetes. J Foot Ankle Surg. 1997;36(4):264–7. discussion 328.
47. Felton PM, Weaver TD. Phenol and alcohol chemical matrixectomy in diabetic versus nondiabetic patients. A retrospective study. J Am Podiatr Med Assoc. 1999;89(8):410–2.
48. Hernandez C, Deleon D. Acquired pincer nail deformity associated with renal failure. J Clin Aesthet Dermatol. 2011;4(12):43–5.
49. Kirkland CR, Sheth P. Acquired pincer nail deformity associated with end stage renal disease secondary to diabetes. Dermatol Online J. 2009;15(4):17.
50. Baran R, Haneke E, Richert B. Pincer nails: definition and surgical treatment. Dermatol Surg. 2001;27(3):261–6.
51. Nam HM, Kim UK, Park SD, Kim JH, Park K. Correction of pincer nail deformity using dermal grafting. Ann Dermatol. 2011;23(Suppl 3):S299–302.
52. Stewart J, Kohen A, Brouder D, Rahim F, Adler S, Garrick R, et al. Noninvasive interrogation of microvasculature for signs of endothelial dysfunction in patients with chronic renal failure. Am J Physiol Heart Circ Physiol. 2004;287(6):H2687–96.
53. Jung DJ, Kim JH, Lee HY, Kim DC, Lee SI, Kim TY. Anatomical characteristics and surgical treatments of pincer nail deformity. Arch Plast Surg. 2015;42(2):207–13.
54. Pierard GE, Seite S, Hermanns-Le T, Delvenne P, Scheen A, Pierard-Franchimont C. The skin landscape in diabetes mellitus. Focus on dermocosmetic management. Clin Cosmet Investig Dermatol. 2013;6:127–35.
55. Duff M, Demidova O, Blackburn S, Shubrook J. Cutaneous manifestations of diabetes mellitus. Clin Diabetes. 2015;33(1):40–8.
56. Singh G, Haneef NS, Uday A. Nail changes and disorders among the elderly. Indian J Dermatol Venereol Leprol. 2005;71(6):386–92.
57. Mann RJ, Burton JL. Nail dystrophy due to diabetic neuropathy. Br Med J (Clin Res Ed). 1982;284(6327):1445.
58. Rich P. Nail changes due to diabetes and other endocrinopathies. Dermatol Ther. 2002;15:107–10.
59. Baran R, Dawber RPR. Diseases of the nails and their management. 2nd ed. Oxford; Boston: Blackwell Scientific; 2012. p. 513.
60. Singh G. Nails in systemic disease. Indian J Dermatol Venereol Leprol. 2011;77(6):646–51.
61. Maldonado G, Guerrero R, Paredes C, Rios C. Nailfold capillaroscopy in diabetes mellitus. Microvasc Res. 2017;112:41–6.
62. Shore AC. Capillaroscopy and the measurement of capillary pressure. Br J Clin Pharmacol. 2000;50(6):501–13.
63. Tibirica E, Rodrigues E, Cobas RA, Gomes MB. Endothelial function in patients with type 1 diabetes evaluated by skin capillary recruitment. Microvasc Res. 2007;73(2):107–12.
64. Kuryliszyn–Moskal A, Dubicki A, Zaezycki W, Zonnenberg A, Gorska M. A study on microvascular abnormalities in capillaroscopy in patients with type 1 diabetes mellitus. Diabetol Dosw i Klin. 2006;6(2):98–103.
65. Singal A, Arora R. Nail as a window of systemic diseases. Indian Dermatol Online J. 2015;6(2):67–74.
66. Allevato MA. Diseases mimicking onychomycosis. Clin Dermatol. 2010;28(2):164–77.
67. Baran R, Dawber RPR, Richert B. Physical signs. In: Baran R, Dawber RPR, de Berker DAR, Haneke E, Tosti A, editors. Diseases of the nails and their management. 3rd ed. Oxford: Blackwell Science; 2001. p. 86–103.

68. Chieb S, Baha H, Hali F. Subungual hematoma: clinical appearance of resolution over time. Dermatol Online J. 2015;21(10).
69. Iglesias P, Olmos O, Sastre J, Diez JJ, Fernandez ML, Borbujo J. Subungual hemorrhages. A primary manifestation of diabetes mellitus. Arch Fam Med. 1996;5(3):169–71.
70. Tosti A, Piraccini BM, Starace M. Una. In: Giannetti A, Galimberti RL. Tratado de Dermatología. 1st ed. Padova: Piccin; 2012. p. 245–53.
71. Nia AM, Ederer S, Dahlem KM, Gassanov N, Er F. Terry's nails: a window to systemic diseases. Am J Med. 2011;124(7):602–4.
72. Holzberg M, Walker HK. Terry's nails: revised definition and new correlations. Lancet. 1984;1(8382):896–9.
73. Pitukweerakul S, Pilla S. Terry's nails and Lindsay's nails: two nail abnormalities in chronic systemic diseases. J Gen Intern Med. 2016;31(8):970.

Index

© Springer International Publishing AG 2018
E.N. Cohen Sabban et al. (eds.), *Dermatology and Diabetes*,
https://doi.org/10.1007/978-3-319-72475-1

The manufacturer's authorised representative in the EU is Springer
Nature Customer Service Centre GmbH, Europaplatz 3, 69115 Heidelberg,
Germany. If you have any concerns regarding our products, please
contact ProductSafety@springernature.com

Printed and bound by CPI Group (UK) Ltd, Croydon, CR0 4YY

23/04/2026

02095602-0004